Early Psychosis Intervention

Early Psychosis Intervention

A Culturally Adaptive Clinical Guide

Edited by
Eric Yu-hai Chen, Helen Lee, Gloria Hoi-kei Chan, and
Gloria Hoi-yan Wong

香港大學出版社
HONG KONG UNIVERSITY PRESS

Hong Kong University Press
The University of Hong Kong
Pokfulam Road
Hong Kong
www.hkupress.org

ISBN 978-988-8139-92-7 *(Hardback)*

British Library Cataloguing-in-Publication Data
A catalogue record for this book is available from the British Library.

10 9 8 7 6 5 4 3 2 1

Printed and bound by Liang Yu Printing Factory Ltd. in Hong Kong, China

Contents

List of Illustrations ix
Foreword by Patrick McGorry xi
Foreword by Siow Ann Chong xvii
Preface xix
Acknowledgements xxiii
List of Contributors xxv
List of Abbreviations xxix

Part I Early Psychosis Intervention Developments in Asia

1. Development of Early Intervention Services: Introduction 3
Eric Yu-hai Chen

2. Early Psychosis Services in an Asian Urban Setting: EASY and Other Services in Hong Kong 17
Dicky Wai-sau Chung and Eric Yu-hai Chen

3. Overview of Early Psychosis Service Development in Singapore: The EPIP Story 29
Yee Huei Yong and Swapna Verma

4. Early Psychosis Intervention in an Urban Japanese Setting: Overview of Early Psychosis Services in Japan 37
Masafumi Mizuno, Takahiro Nemoto, and Naohisa Tsujino

5. Overview of the Development of Services for Early Psychosis in Korea 47
Young-chul Chung, Guang-biao Huang, and Keun-Young Oh

Part II Public Awareness and Early Detection in Cultural Context

6. Factors Affecting the Duration of Untreated Psychosis in Hong Kong 67
Eric Yu-hai Chen

7. Public Awareness Approaches in Early Psychosis 75
Gloria Hoi-yan Wong

8. Early Psychosis in the Workplace 87
Eric Yu-hai Chen

9. Enhancing Psychosis Detection through Gatekeepers 93
Chi-wing Law

10. Initial Screening and Assessment: A Phone-Based Two-Stage Screening 101
Sherry Kit-wa Chan, Dana Yuk-yee Chun, and Kin-sheung Wong

11. The Diagnostic Interview in Early Psychosis 111
Wing-chung Chang and Yip-chau Wong

12. Handling At-Risk Mental State 123
May Mei-ling Lam, Chi-chiu Lee, Wing-chung Chang, and Se-fong Hung

Part III Culturally Relevant Psychosocial Case Intervention

13. Implementing Psychological Intervention Programmes in Early Psychosis (PIPE) 137
Suzanne Ho-wai So

14. The PASTE that Binds: Culturally Relevant Psychological Interventions for First-Episode Psychosis Individuals in Singapore 159
Eugene Puay Chong Tay and Lyn Chua

15. Cultural Issues in Early Psychosis Management 175
K. Pushpa

16. Engagement and Outreach in Early Psychosis Management 189
Kai-tai Chan and Gloria Hoi-kei Chan

17. Experience of Stigma in Early Psychosis Patients and Caregivers 199
Desiree Yan Wong, Dicky Wai-sau Chung, and May Mei-ling Lam

18. The Phase-Specific Progress Supervision Model for Case Managers 209
Helen Lee

Part IV Support Programmes in the Community

19. Community Psychosocial Intervention in Early Psychosis 223
Yogeswary d/o Maniam

20. The Peer Support Programme in Early Psychosis Intervention Programme (EPIP) 235
Suying Ang

21. Family Work in Early Psychosis 247
Christopher Loh

22. Working with Non-Governmental Organizations in Early Psychosis 255
Steve Tso and Simon Sai-yu Lui

Part V Medication and Adherence Issues

23. Pharmacological Intervention in Early Psychosis 263
Phyllis Kwok-ling Chan and Edwin Ho-ming Lee

24. Medication Adherence: Specific Issues in Early Psychosis in Asia 273
Christy Lai-ming Hui

Part VI Handling Specific Challenges

25. Relapse Intervention and Related Issues 283
Christy Lai-ming Hui

26. Suicide and Self-Harm Behaviour in Early Psychosis 291
Edwin Pui-fai Pang

27. Comorbid Substance Abuse in Early Psychosis 301
Sherry Kit-wa Chan and Kathy Po-man Chan

28. Handling Patients with Negative Symptoms 311
Wing-chung Chang and Cindy Pui-yu Chiu

Part VII Recovering from Early Psychosis

29. Recovery from Psychosis 323
Chi-wing Law

30. Concepts of Recovery in Early Psychosis: A Cognitive Linguistic Approach 335
Eric Yu-hai Chen

31. Experiential Aspects of Recovery in Early Psychosis: Focus Group Findings 345
May Mei-ling Lam

Part VIII Evaluation and Research

32. Database Design and Management 359
Kin-sheung Wong

33. Research and Outcome Evaluation in Early Psychosis 367
Eric Yu-hai Chen

Index 375

Illustrations

Figures

Figure 2.1	Duration of untreated psychosis (DUP) in Hong Kong prior to the introduction of early psychosis services	18
Figure 7.1	Public misconception about psychosis in Hong Kong	77
Figure 7.2	Stigmatizing attitudes and behaviours towards psychotic patients in Hong Kong	77
Figure 10.1	Workflow of the EASY referral system	102
Figure 10.2	Referring system of EASY	104
Figure 13.1	Psychosocial intervention for first-episode psychosis	139
Figure 15.1	Religious distribution in Singapore	175
Figure 18.1	Supervision model for EPIP case managers	212
Figure 30.1	Container image schema	339
Figure 30.2	Path image schema	340
Figure 32.1	ER diagram of the EASY system	362
Figure 32.2	Implementation of EASY system in site office	364

Tables

Table 4.1	Characteristics of "Il Bosco"	41
Table 4.2	Leading research and clinical centres in Japan	43
Table 5.1	Summary of results from self-administered questionnaires used for mass screenings to identify individuals at high risk for psychosis	51
Table 5.2	Pros and cons of proposed candidate names	57
Table 7.1	JCEP's key public awareness messages	84
Table 13.1	Engagement with psychotic patients	144

Table 14.1	Components of PASTE	161
Table 17.1	Caregivers' reactions towards the diagnosis of psychotic disorder	205
Table 18.1	Case manager's role across different phases of recovery	211
Table 18.2	Case manager characteristics in the beginner phase	214
Table 18.3	Case manager characteristics in Level 1	216
Table 18.4	Case manager characteristics in Level 2	217
Table 18.5	Case manager characteristics in Level 3	218
Table 20.1	Discussion topics of peer support groups	238
Table 20.2	Job description of peer support specialist	240
Table 21.1	Results of pre- and post-tests of the caregivers' workshop in 2009	252
Table 24.1	Ratings on Medication Adherence Rating Scale	278
Table 24.2	Sensitivity and specificity of clinicians' detection of non-adherent behaviours	278
Table 26.1	Static, dynamic and future risk factors for suicide	296
Table 30.1	The journey metaphor of life events	341
Table 31.1	Eight principles of recovery described by Anthony (1993)	347

Foreword

Patrick McGorry

It is now just over a decade since the first early psychosis programmes were established in Asia, representing a critical frontier in global early psychosis reform. In the intervening years an increasing number of clinical and research programmes have been developed and flourished in various Asian cities. It is inspiring to see that so many pioneering Asian psychiatrists, psychologists and academic leaders have recognized that prevention and early intervention are key potential strategies in the struggle to reduce the burden of mental illness in our rapidly changing societies and have taken effective action. Quite apart from the human cost, the economic impact of untreated or poorly treated mental disorders is a major threat to happiness and prosperity world-wide. In its 2011 report on the impact of non-communicable diseases, the World Economic Forum has shown that mental illness will equal cardiovascular disease as the major threat to GDP in both the developed and the developing economies over the next two decades (Bloom et al., 2011). This is because mental disorders are the "chronic diseases of the young", with 75% of onsets occurring before the age of 25 years, and most between puberty and the mid-twenties (Kessler et al., 2005). Obviously, this is especially relevant in the developing countries with their young populations and rapidly changing societies.

In both the western and eastern hemispheres, despite compelling logic, a substantial emerging evidence base which almost uniformly indicates that the early intervention paradigm is as valid in mental health as it is in physical health, and a great many islands of real world progress, timely and appropriate early intervention remains aspirational for the average patient experiencing the onset of a mental illness. This is in part a reflection of the inequity in terms of access to and quality of care that people living with mental ill health around the world still suffer, but it is also a reflection of a certain degree of lack of confidence and maturity within our own mental health community to invest in “best buys”. Despite two decades of indicative evidence, and the early intervention field having been led by an international array of academic clinicians deeply committed to evidence-based medicine, there has been not only excessive conservatism, but also an attempt by a small group of academics to use the evidence-based paradigm selectively to introduce doubt and undermine reform (McGorry, 2012). Scepticism is central to science and necessary, but a double standard is at work here, since similar doubts have not been fuelled, nor has there been a level playing field in terms of judgements on the evidence, in relation to relevant aspects of the status quo of traditional mental health care, nor even in relation to more modest yet competing reform ideas linked to the provision of care to established illnesses.

Fortunately the dichotomy between early intervention and decent long-term care is demonstrably false, since investment in early intervention has been shown to be cost-effective, especially in relation to psychosis, where at least five studies all point to substantial savings, which can actually be channelled into enhancing care programmes for the substantial and cumulative minority whose recovery is prolonged or elusive (Cullberg, 2006; Goldberg, 2006; McCrone, 2012; Mihalopoulos, 2009; Valmaggia; 2009). Many, though admittedly not all, of those who come to need such programmes do so precisely because they have received late, desultory or poor quality intervention from pessimistic and poorly resourced cultures of care, despite the best efforts of dedicated clinicians desperately propping up the latter.

We need to redouble our efforts to reconceptualize mental ill health in a more holistic way that accommodates both the reality of human distress and the need for psychosocial care, as well as the role for new therapies flowing from progress in neuroscience. An urgent priority is the reform, refinancing and re-engineering of our systems of care so that people receive holistic care. Otherwise people with mental illness and their families will continue to suffer what Dr Thomas Insel, Director of the National Institute of Mental Health, calls “the soft bigotry of low expectations”. In Australia, things are becoming more optimistic, with the Australian government constructing 90 new youth mental health platforms, known as *headspace* centres, and 16 early psychosis or EPPIC services to be in place by 2015, among other significant investments in more holistic mental health care. These youth-oriented reforms are slowly being mirrored in Ireland and in some other parts of the world.

In this context the publication of this comprehensive and high quality volume is extremely timely and impressive, and the editors and authors of

Early Psychosis Intervention: A Culturally Adaptive Clinical Guide deserve our full admiration and support. It is only a few years ago that *Time* magazine highlighted the fact that the care of the mentally ill in Asia was lagging way behind the region's economic growth and development (Beech, 2003). This book showcases Asian innovation and leadership in mental health and provides a detailed account of how to detect, engage, treat and maximize recovery in people with early psychosis, particularly in the context of Asian cultures. Pioneering endeavours in early intervention for psychosis are described in Hong Kong, Korea, Japan and Singapore that are not only laying the foundations for new knowledge in this burgeoning field, but also creating impetus for a transformation of the system of mental health care in these countries.

The Hong Kong group, led by Professor Eric Chen, has just celebrated the 10th anniversary of its establishment, and has developed an impressive early psychosis service, encompassing several key platforms, for the whole population of Hong Kong. They have shown on an unprecedented scale that outcomes can be improved, suicide rates reduced and cost-effectiveness demonstrated. Similarly, from 2001, under the leadership of Professor Siow Ann Chong and Dr Swapna Verma in Singapore, a large-scale early psychosis programme is producing much better symptomatic and vocational outcomes for people with previously disabling and stigmatizing illnesses. Things are perhaps a little more challenging in Japan and Korea, where the mental health systems face broader challenges, yet here too we have gifted and determined leaders in Professor Masafumi Mizuno and Dr Young Chul Chung and their respective colleagues, who are focusing on early intervention as a key solution.

Early Psychosis Intervention does not merely showcase systemic reform but provides a truly comprehensive and culturally adapted collection of strategies and skills to achieve the goal of maximum recovery from potentially serious psychotic illness especially in young people. The book covers system development, public awareness, recognition and engagement including the challenges of subthreshold illness and need for care, and all the key biopsychosocial dimensions of treatment, recovery and relapse prevention. Community care, family and vocational interventions and specific guidelines on the sophisticated use of medications are also covered. Comorbidity including physical illness and substance use disorders are included as critical issues for the next decade. Finally, in including a chapter on research and evaluation, the authors recognize that notwithstanding wonderful progress over the past decade, early psychosis is still a young field and new knowledge and skills are still urgently required. A commitment to evidence-based medicine has served the field well as it challenges the conventional model of care, and will sustain progress well into the future. Ultimately all people especially teenagers and emerging adults, who bear the main burden, along with their parents and families, of these potentially threatening and sometimes devastating illnesses, deserve timely access to the best quality of stage-linked care from the beginning and for as long as they need it. Early intervention has been a missing pillar of modern mental health care; this scholarly yet practical resource book adds another solid foundation to the construction of 21st century mental health knowledge and care, not only in Asia, but all around the world.

Patrick McGorry
Professor of Youth Mental Health, the University of Melbourne
Director of Orygen Youth Health and Orygen Youth Health Research Centre, Victoria, Australia

References

Beech H. (2003). Hidden away. *Time Magazine*, Monday, 10 November.

Bloom D. E., Cafiero E. T., Jane-Lopis E., Abrahams-Gessel S., Bloom L. R., Fathima S. et al. (2011). *The Global Economic Burden of Non-Communicable Disease*. Geneva, World Economic Forum.

Cullberg J., Mattsson M., Levander S., Tomsmark L., Elingfors C., Wieselgren I. M. (2006). Treatment costs and clinical outcome for first episode schizophrenia patients: A 3-year follow-up of the Swedish "Parachute Project" and two comparison groups. *Acta Psychiatr Scand*, *114*, 274–281.

Goldberg K., Norman R., Hoch J. S., Schmitz N., Windell D., Brown N., Malla A. (2006). Impact of a specialised early intervention service for psychotic disorders on patient characteristics, service use, and hospital costs in a defined catchment area. *Can J Psychiatry*, *51*, 895–903.

Kessler R. C., Berglund P., Demler O., Jin R., Merikangas K. R., Walters E. E. (2005). Lifetime prevalence and age-of-onset distributions of DSM-IV disorders in the National Comorbidity Survey Replication. *Arch Gen Psychiatry*, *62*, 593–602.

McCrone P., Craig T. K., Power P., Garety P. A. (2012). Cost-effectiveness of an early intervention service for people with psychosis. *Br J Psychiatry*, *196*, 377–382.

McGorry P. (2012). At Issue: Cochrane, early intervention, and mental health reform: Analysis, paralysis, or evidence-informed progress? *Schizophr Bull*, *38*, 221–224.

Mihalopoulos C., Harris M., Henry L., Harrigan S., McGorry P. (2009). Is early intervention in psychosis cost-effective over the long term? *Schizophr Bull*, *35*(5), 909–918.

Valmaggia L. R., McCrone P., Knapp M., Woolley J. B., Broome M. R., Tabraham P., et al. (2009). Economic impact of early intervention in people at high risk of psychosis. *Psychol Med*, *39*, 1617–1626.

Foreword

Siow Ann Chong

An adage of modern medicine states that early detection and treatment of a disorder is the key to achieving better outcomes. However, this concept has arrived rather belatedly in mental health.

The understanding that psychoses afflict much suffering on both individuals and their families, and exact an enormous toll in social and economic costs from lost productivity also needs little emphasis. The possibility that these losses could be ameliorated by knowledge which we already have makes the situation even more tragic.

Fortunately, in the past two decades, much hard work has been done and much gain has been achieved in the fight to alleviate distress and impairments in those experiencing psychosis. Notably, there are now many early detection and intervention programmes in UK, Europe, North America, and Asia.

The earliest of such programmes in Asia started in Hong Kong and Singapore almost simultaneously. Both have in successive years grown in strength, emerged as leading centres in the region, and contributed significantly to the field. There are now programmes in South Korea and Japan too. But much still remains to be done in the world's largest and most populous continents, such as China and Africa, where there are still many countries and regions that do not even have the rudiments of such infrastructures.

The development and implementation of such programmes are similar world-wide, and yet dissimilar; each country having unique challenges and different variables including the amount of resources available, the level of priority allocated to mental health by local policy-makers, and the cultural values and attitudes of the general population towards mental disorders.

Despite these differences, much can be learnt from the experiences of these programmes. What is implicitly evident from the chapters contained within this volume is that the leaders of these programmes have adopted a "leap-frogging" approach that delivers best outcomes. They have done this by learning and adapting best practices from each other and from around the world, and through integration and innovation. This would be one of the valuable lessons for those who read this book.

The chapters represent a distillation of knowledge of thoughtful practitioners and researchers whose collective experiences have been forged from many years of frontline work, and undoubtedly from lessons learnt through mistakes made. The dialogue offers perspectives on how to make services accessible to patients and their families, how to establish links in the community, how to engage the public, how to deliver culturally sensitive interventions, and how to set up a database for evaluation and research. The latter contribution is important as there is "no such thing as a free lunch". These wise, pragmatic practitioners know they need to show a return for policy-makers' investments in these programmes, as well as counter critics and detractors.

This book will be a useful resource for mental health professionals and for policy-makers involved in mental health, as well as residents in psychiatry and trainees in other mental health professions. As information and ideas covered in this book are not generally available, this volume will stimulate readers and will be a springboard for greater proactivity in this on-going fight for people suffering from psychosis.

Siow Ann Chong
Institute of Mental Health, Singapore

Preface

This book discusses the practice of early psychosis intervention in various sociocultural contexts. Grounded in more than a decade of clinical and research experience in locations across Asia, outside the conventional "Western" system, the essays address a comprehensive range of topics pertinent to the central question of how to improve patient care in the early stages of psychosis. The discussion enriches and complements existing accounts of early intervention for psychosis (EI) by highlighting the interaction between cultural factors and efforts to improve care for early psychosis patients.

Psychotic disorders affect 1–3 per cent of the population, and are one of the most disabling conditions confronting humankind. The causes for psychosis are complex and not yet fully understood. This illness affects a person's core experiences: how they engage and respond to the "realities" around them. Underlying the condition are complex interactions between genetic, developmental, brain structural, neurochemical, cognitive, and psychosocial factors. The disorders manifest as distortions in the perception and interpretation of social situations, but also affect other cognitive and motivational systems in the brain. Symptoms are primarily situated in the subjective experience of the patient and cannot be directly observed from outside. Typically, patients are unaware of the illness. Treatment by antipsychotic medications can reduce psychotic experiences, but relapses are frequent. Other cognitive, motivational, and functional problems cannot be directly addressed by medication. Moreover, psychotic disorders are still heavily stigmatized in society, which adds to the suffering of patients and caregivers.

Patients present to mental health services only after a long period of delay during which adverse experiences and risks can multiply. The illness pathway in the initial years can be turbulent and may influence long-term outcomes in various ways. Conventional mental health care systems are poor at providing timely care for patients with early psychosis. Optimal treatment requires specialized adaptation of care systems, as well as skilful integration of biomedical and psychosocial interventions by well-trained professionals.

This book has two main objectives; the first is to provide a pragmatic summary of the valuable experiences and clinical wisdom for frontline practitioners and clinical leaders working in settings that call for cultural sensitivity. The rich and detailed material, clinical examples, and guidelines offered will be useful in suggesting approaches for clinicians, case managers, administrators, policy-makers, psychologists, social workers, and other mental health professionals in the field of early psychosis, whether they are working in a primarily non-Western setting, a multicultural setting, or even, with the benefit of reflections offered, a conventional Western setting.

The second objective is to increase awareness of the roles culture plays in the evolving developments during early intervention for psychosis.

EI approaches initially developed out of centres in Australia, Europe, and North America (collectively described here as "Western"). Although cultural and societal diversity must already have confronted practitioners in these locations, the diversities are relatively small compared with that countered when EI approaches take the leap out of the "Western" system to land amongst a much wider diversity of cultural and service environments.

In this process, the core principles of EI confront and interact with a wide range of cultural and societal environments; some of these facilitate aspects of EI work, while others are unaccommodating. EI services in such diverse cultural ecologies have to respond with more explorations, more innovations, and more adaptations, and a heightened expectation that some initiatives will survive and thrive, but others will not. Optimal EI systems that evolve for each distinct cultural and societal ecology are expected to be different from the ancestral (Western) prototypes, and also from one another. As such, the ongoing development of EI systems in non-Western settings offers a unique opportunity to reflect on how mental health service systems take shape, and the factors that might have critical influence over their eventual forms and structures.

In the midst of this remarkable ongoing evolution, this book is but a small interim, even initial, reflection. The discussion will have served its purpose if it facilitates the sharing of hard-won experiences and increases the awareness of the need for innovations, adaptations and evaluations, thereby inspiring the developments of new initiatives, so that more patients are served in better ways in some hitherto unreached niches.

The EI teams whose work this book describes consist of exceptionally dedicated individuals, who took on the arduous task of exploring and constructing the best approaches to improving outcome in one of the most challenging and complex clinical conditions, often amidst improvised systems with few resources and high levels of stigma. They are, however, supported by a collegiate network of EI leaders internationally, as well as by a large number of government and non-governmental agencies in their respective localities. Most importantly, their work, such as those described in this volume, has been sustained by patients and caregivers whose encouragement and participation has been vital.

Eric Yu-hai Chen, Helen Lee, Gloria Hoi-kei Chan, and Gloria Hoi-yan Wong
Hong Kong
April 2013

Acknowledgements

This book is the fruit of years of hard work of many dedicated people in early psychosis services.

We are extremely fortunate to have received enormous help from our colleagues in various early intervention programmes in Hong Kong, Japan, Korea, and Singapore. In particular, we would like to thank the very dedicated and enthusiastic team of clinicians, case managers, and researchers in the EASY (Early Assessment Services for Young People with Psychosis) project and PSI (Psychosis Studies and Intervention) programme in Hong Kong, EPIP (Early Psychosis Intervention Programme) in Singapore, and various governmental and non-governmental organizations, hospitals, and universities in Asia. Without their unreserved support in sharing their invaluable experience and knowledge, this book would not have been possible.

In the process of editing and producing this book, we have been privileged to have the guidance and assistance from Christy Leung of Hong Kong University Press. Our gratitude goes to all our dear friends who have reviewed the manuscript, and have given time and provided very useful critiques and important advice to help improve this volume. Special thanks are due to Professor Siow Ann Chong from Institute of Mental Health, Singapore, and Professor Patrick McGorry from ORYGEN Youth Health, Australia, and International Early Psychosis Association for their feedback and encouragement.

Finally, and most importantly, this book and early intervention services would have no place without the support from our patients and their family members. They have given us their trust in the journey of fighting a difficult illness, and have inspired us to advance our services.

Contributors

Editors

Eric Yu-hai Chen, Professor, Psychosis Studies and Intervention Programme, Department of Psychiatry, Li Ka Shing Faculty of Medicine, The University of Hong Kong; Convenor, Early Psychosis Group, Hospital Authority, Hong Kong.

Helen Lee, Principal Case Manager and Team Leader, Early Psychosis Intervention Programme, Institute of Mental Health, Singapore.

Gloria Hoi-kei Chan, Case Intervention Officer, Psychosis Studies and Intervention Programme, Department of Psychiatry, Li Ka Shing Faculty of Medicine, The University of Hong Kong.

Gloria Hoi-yan Wong, Post-doctoral Fellow, Psychosis Studies and Intervention Programme, Department of Psychiatry, Li Ka Shing Faculty of Medicine, The University of Hong Kong.

Contributors

Suying Ang, Senior Case Manager, Early Psychosis Intervention Programme, Institute of Mental Health, Singapore.

Kai-tai Chan, Associate Consultant, Department of General Adult Psychiatry, Castle Peak Hospital, Hong Kong.

Phyllis Kwok-ling Chan, Consultant Psychiatrist and Team Head, Child and Adolescent Psychiatry, Department of Psychiatry, Queen Mary Hospital, Hong Kong.

Sherry Kit-wa Chan, Clinical Assistant Professor, Psychosis Studies and Intervention Programme, Department of Psychiatry, Li Ka Shing Faculty of Medicine, The University of Hong Kong.

Kathy Po-man Chan, Psychiatrist, Hong Kong.

Wing-chung Chang, Clinical Assistant Professor, Psychosis Studies and Intervention Programme, Department of Psychiatry, Li Ka Shing Faculty of Medicine, The University of Hong Kong.

Cindy Pui-yu Chiu, Honorary Clinical Assistant Professor, Department of Psychiatry, Li Ka Shing Faculty of Medicine, The University of Hong Kong.

Lyn Chua, Adjunct Associate Professor, Department of Psychological Medicine, Yong Loo Lin School of Medicine, National University Hospital System and Mount Elizabeth Medical Centre, Singapore.

Dana Yuk-yee Chun, Case Manager, Early Assessment Service for Young People with Psychosis, Hong Kong.

Dicky Wai-sau Chung, Chief of Service, Department of Psychiatry, New Territories East, Hong Kong.

Young-chul Chung, Professor, Department of Psychiatry, Chonbuk National University Medical School, Jeonju, Korea.

Guang-biao Huang, Researcher, Department of Psychiatry, Chonbuk National University Medical School, Jeonju, Korea.

Se-fong Hung, Honorary Clinical Professor, Department of Psychiatry, Chinese University of Hong Kong.

Christy Lai-ming Hui, Research Officer, Psychosis Studies and Intervention Programme, Department of Psychiatry, Li Ka Shing Faculty of Medicine, The University of Hong Kong.

May Mei-ling Lam, Honorary Clinical Assistant Professor, Department of Psychiatry, Li Ka Shing Faculty of Medicine, The University of Hong Kong.

Chi-wing Law, Honorary Clinical Assistant Professor, Department of Psychiatry, Li Ka Shing Faculty of Medicine, The University of Hong Kong.

Chi-chiu Lee, Consultant Psychiatrist, Kwai Chung Hospital, Hong Kong.

Edwin Ho-ming Lee, Clinical Assistant Professor, Psychosis Studies and Intervention Programme, Department of Psychiatry, Li Ka Shing Faculty of Medicine, The University of Hong Kong.

Christopher Loh, Case Manager and Family Therapist, Early Psychosis Intervention Programme, Institute of Mental Health, Singapore.

Simon Sai-yu Lui, Associate Consultant, Department of Psychiatry, Castle Peak Hospital, Hong Kong.

Yogeswary d/o Maniam, Senior Occupational Therapist, Early Psychosis Intervention Programme, Institute of Mental Health, Singapore.

Masafumi Mizuno, Professor and Chair, Department of Neuropsychiatry, Toho University Faculty of Medicine, Japan.

Takahiro Nemoto, Associate Professor, Department of Neuropsychiatry, Toho University Faculty of Medicine, Japan.

Keun-Young Oh, Psychiatrist, Heemang Hospital, Gimje, Jeonbuk, Korea.

Edwin Pui-fai Pang, Associate Consultant, Department of Psychiatry, United Christian Hospital, Hong Kong.

K. Pushpa, Senior Case Manager and Deputy Team Leader, Early Psychosis Intervention Programme, Institute of Mental Health, Singapore.

Suzanne Ho-wai So, Assistant Professor, Department of Psychology, Chinese University of Hong Kong.

Eugene Puay Chong Tay, Senior Counsellor, Early Psychosis Intervention Programme, Institute of Mental Health, Singapore.

Steve Tso, Consultant, Siu Lam Hospital, Hong Kong.

Naohisa Tsujino, Assistant Professor, Department of Neuropsychiatry, Toho University Faculty of Medicine, Japan.

Swapna Verma, Associate Professor, Chief of Early Psychosis Intervention Programme, Senior Consultant of Institute of Mental Health, Associate Professor of DUKE-NUS, Singapore.

Kin-sheung Wong, Community Psychiatric Nurse, Shatin Hospital, Hong Kong.

Desiree Yan Wong, Research Coordinator, Psychosis Studies and Intervention Programme, Department of Psychiatry, Li Ka Shing Faculty of Medicine, The University of Hong Kong.

Yip-chau Wong, Associate Consultant, Department of Psychiatry, Tai Po Hospital, Hong Kong.

Yee Huei Yong, Case Manager, Early Psychosis Intervention Programme, Institute of Mental Health, Singapore.

Abbreviations

AED	accident and emergency department
AMPQ	Adolescent Mental Health and Problem-Behaviour Questionnaire
ARMS	at-risk mental state
AWWA	Asian Women's Welfare Association
BDI	Beck Depression Inventory
BPRS	Brief Psychiatric Rating Score
BSABS	Bonn Scale for the Assessment of Basic Symptoms
CAARMS	Comprehensive Assessment of At-Risk Mental States
CAMI	Caregivers' Association of the Mentally Ill
CAPE	Community Assessment of Psychic Experiences
CAST	Consultation and Support Service in Toyama
CBCL	Child Behaviour Checklist
CBT	cognitive-behavioural therapy
CDC	Community Development Council in Singapore
CHAT	Community Health Assessment Team
CMS	Clinical Management System in Hong Kong
CPSQ	Child Problems Screening Questionnaire
DEEP	Detection of Early Psychosis Project
DSM	*Diagnostic and Statistical Manual of Mental Disorder*
DUI	duration of untreated illness
DUP	duration of untreated psychosis

EASY	Early Assessment Service for Young People with Psychosis
EPIP	Early Psychosis Intervention Programme in Singapore
EPISO	Early Psychosis Intervention Society in Hong Kong
EPPIC	Early Psychosis Prevention and Intervention Centre in Australia
EPS	extrapyramidal side-effects
ERIroas	Early Recognition Inventory Retrospective Assessment of the onset and course of schizophrenia and other psychoses
ESI	Eppendorf Schizophrenia Inventory
FCSs	family service centres in Singapore
FES	first-episode schizophrenia
FGAs	first-generation antipsychotics
GAF	Global Assessment Functioning Scale
GP	general practitioner
GRAPE	Green Programme for Recognition and Prevention of Early Psychosis
HSREDS	Hillside Study of Risk and Detection of Schizophrenia
ICCMW	Integrated Community Centre for Mental Wellness
ICD	*International Classification of Diseases*
IMH	Institute of Mental Health in Singapore
IROAS	Interview for the Retrospective Assessment of the Onset of Schizophrenia
IQ	intelligence quotient
JCEP	Jockey Club Early Psychosis Project
JSEIP	Japanese Society for Prevention and Early Intervention in Psychiatry
JSPN	Japanese Society of Psychiatry and Neurology
K-NEP	Korean Network of Early Psychosis
MARS	Medication Adherence Rating Scale
MCT	Mobile Crisis Team in Singapore
MEMS	Medication Event Monitoring System

MEST	Ministry of Education, Science and Technology in Korea
MHWL	Japanese Ministry of Health, Welfare, and Labour
MSDN	Microsoft Developer Network
MSW	Medical Social Work Department in Singapore
MW	Ministry for Health and Welfare in Korea
NGO	non-governmental organization
NICE	National Institute for Health and Clinical Excellence
NNT	number needed to treat
OPD	outpatient department
OTP	optimal treatment project
PACE	Personal Assistance and Crisis Evaluation in Melbourne, Australia
PANSS	Positive and Negative Syndrome Scale
PASTE	Personal and Strategic Coping Therapy for Early Psychosis
PDI	Peters Delusions Inventory
PET	positron emission topography
PIPE	Psychological Intervention Programme in Early Psychosis
PQ	Prodromal Questionnaire
PRIME	Prevention through Risk Identification, Management, and Education Study
RDBMS	relational database management system
RPS	relapse prevention study in Hong Kong
SAF	Singapore Armed Forces
SAFE	Sendai At-Risk Mental State and First Episode Service
SAMH	Singapore Association for Mental Health
SCC	Simei Care Centre in Singapore
SCS	Strauss and Carpenter Prognostic Scale
SGAs	second-generation antipsychotics
SIPS	Structured Interview for Prodromal Syndromes

SOPS	Scale of Prodromal Syndromes
SRS	Silver Ribbon Singapore
STEP	Social Treatment for Early Psychosis
SWAP	Support for Wellness Achievement Programme
TOPP	Early Treatment of Psychosis Project in Norway
UHR	ultra-high risk
WAKABA	Youth Mental Support Center in Matsuzawa
WEE	Wee Education Emotion Centre
WHO	World Health Organization
YMSC MIE	Youth Mental Support Centre Mie
Y-PARQ	Youth Psychosis At-Risk Questionnaire
YSR	Youth Self-Report

Part I

Early Psychosis Intervention Developments in Asia

1
Development of Early Intervention Services: Introduction

Eric Yu-hai Chen

The Idea of Early Intervention

The concept of "early intervention" is not foreign to medical practice. The idea is rooted in the recognition that many illnesses evolve as a progression over time involving the accruement of irreversible adverse processes. Consequently, the timing of intervention becomes a prime factor affecting outcomes.

The challenge confronting the field of early psychosis is that many of these pathological processes and their interactions are not yet clearly understood. In the meantime, clinicians and patients must nevertheless manage with the best possible judgements they choose.

One uncontroversial fact in psychosis is that the condition nearly always has negative impacts on the quality of life of sufferers and carers (Chan et al., 2007; Law et al., 2005); the longer psychosis stays untreated, the longer the patients and their carers have to suffer. Thus, the devastating nature of the illness calls for the earliest healthcare intervention possible. In fact, the notion of early intervention is recognized by the East and the West alike. In English, the idiom "a stitch in time saves nine" spells out the wisdom that anything that needs doing is better to be done sooner rather than later. In Chinese, an equivalent concept is found in the saying *bing xiang qian zhong yi* (病向淺中醫), which literally means it is better to get treatment before an illness takes root. The undesirability of delay is taken for granted in many areas of medicine such as treatment of cancer, heart disease, and hypertension.

The Concept of Schizophrenia and Early Detection

In view of the obvious desirability of early intervention, it is intriguing that in the management of mental illnesses, particularly psychotic disorders such as schizophrenia, the concept of early intervention was never integrated from the beginning. This was perhaps partly due to heavy stigmatization associated with the condition, and partly to pessimism towards treatment outcomes. Such pessimistic attitudes towards the illness can be traced back to at least 1899 when Emil Kraepelin coined the term "dementia praecox" (where "praecox" refers to the adolescent onset and "dementia" denotes a downhill course of the disease) to describe the condition of progressive decline in patients with psychotic symptoms. At that time, Kraepelin and others viewed the condition as a brain disease comparable to dementia, with both conditions destined for progressive deterioration. Later, Bleuler in his 1908, *Dementia Praecox* or the *Group of Schizophrenias*, replaced the term "dementia praecox" by "schizophrenia", emphasizing the heterogeneity of the illness and suggesting variability in outcomes (Fusar-Poli & Politi, 2008). Nevertheless, Kraepelin's concept of schizophrenia as brain deterioration prevailed.

The perception of psychosis (particularly schizophrenia) as a serious condition has been commonly shared by patients and their families, doctors, social workers, and the general public, rendering it difficult to accept such a diagnosis. Such negative attitudes towards the condition was further reinforced by clinics and hospitals' sample bias, namely, clinicians and patients alike had an inaccurate impression that psychosis was a more serious condition than it actually is. This view may have come about because the patients whom clinicians frequently review probably have a need to remain in more regular contact with the care system, possibly reflecting the presence of more complex and resistant symptoms. In fact, the subset of patients appearing more regularly in a hospital setting, and more likely over-represented in research studies, are those with the most severe form of the illness along the phenotypic continuum and do not represent the underlying population (Bak et al., 2005). Even though clinicians are aware of such bias, pessimism towards the illness is not easily dismissed.

These perspectives foster a perception that the schizophrenia diagnosis involves irreversible damage to the brain or mind, leading to permanent changes that affect the core of a person's individuality and personality. The treatment outcomes of schizophrenia have also been viewed as generally hopeless. In some Asian languages, the official translation of the term "schizophrenia" (精神分裂症) pose some language-specific problems. Rendering an explicit reference to a "broken mind" has led to further aggravation of the negative connotation (see Chapter 5, "Overview of the Development of Services for Early Psychosis in Korea"). Introduction of a novel term for "schizophrenia" and for "psychosis" has been the response for some locations (see Chapter 2, "Early Psychosis Services in an Asian Urban Setting: EASY and Other Services in Hong Kong", Chapter 5, "Overview of the Development of Services for Early Psychosis in Korea", and Chapter 7, "Public Awareness Approaches in Early Psychosis).

In the *perceived* absence of effective intervention, early diagnosis may be viewed as a process that only brings earlier suffering and helplessness. Haunted by these biased and negative views towards mental illness, it is not surprising that mainstream psychiatry in the early days did not invest much effort on early diagnosis and outcome improvement for psychotic disorders. This has led to an unfortunate scenario where pathways to care were relatively neglected and research and intervention were severely inadequate (Lincoln & McGorry, 1995).

In recent decades, a number of studies have revisited the long-term outcomes of schizophrenia and provided data that suggest recovery is possible in many patients (Harding et al., 1987; Harding, Zubin, & Strauss, 1987; McGlashan, 1984). There has also been increasing evidence suggesting that delay in treatment is associated with poorer outcomes. These developments have coincided with the focusing of research effort in first-episode illness, providing a rich knowledge base about the early course of the disorder, as well as providing an opportunity for studying the prospective longitudinal outcomes for these samples, thus avoiding excessive negative bias in outcome data (see Chapter 33, "Research and Outcome Evaluation in Early Psychosis"). These data provide fresh impetus for early psychosis work.

The Duration of Untreated Psychosis (DUP)

With the development of standardized instruments for measuring the duration of untreated psychosis (DUP) (e.g. Hafner et al., 1992), more robust data supporting the association between DUP and clinical outcomes have also been emerging (e.g. Amminger et al., 2002; International Early Psychosis Association Writing, 2005; Johannessen, Larsen, & McGlashan, 1999; Malla et al., 2002; Marshall et al., 2005; Oosthuizen et al., 2005). Such efforts have revealed the unfortunate phenomenon that the DUP in many countries is unacceptably long (averaging one to two years or longer). This delay in treatment is not confined to developing regions of the world, but also appears in many Western countries with well-resourced mental health services. This universal trend of delays in treatment of psychosis can be ascribed to a number of factors. Apart from stigmatization and a negative outlook for the illness, psychosis is commonly associated with social withdrawal and lack of insight. Social withdrawal results in reduced communication between the patient and his/her social network, resulting in less likelihood that psychotic symptoms are detected. Patients' lack of ability to recognize their experiences as a possible consequence of an illness also leads to less active help-seeking behaviours. In this volume, a detailed study of DUP and the factors associated with long DUP, which leads to a strategy on public awareness work for the Hong Kong population, is discussed (see Chapter 6, "Factors Affecting the Duration of Untreated Psychosis in Hong Kong").

Early Intervention Services as Counter-Measures

Given these unique challenges, conventional healthcare delivery systems (which rely on more active help-seeking) are ill-designed to handle psychosis. Care systems specifically designed for psychosis patients are called for. Investigations by researchers such as Falloon (1992) have suggested the need for early intervention (EI) service for psychotic disorders. Following this, pioneering efforts were made in Melbourne (Australia) and Norway to pilot services that target the needs for early identification and treatment (McGlashan & Johannessen, 1996; McGorry et al., 1996). The success of these initial programmes has provided impetus for the development of service and research programmes in an increasing number of locations (Chen et al., 2011; Craig et al., 2004; Hegelstad et al., 2012; Henry et al., 2010; Petersen et al., 2005). The International Early Psychosis Association (IEPA) was formed in 1998, with the aims of fostering scientific research and service development. In the last two decades, increasing development of early psychosis intervention teams took place in Europe, Australia, New Zealand, and North America.

Early Psychosis Work in Asia

Meanwhile in Asia, EI programmes have started to be developed in a few centres. Prior to this, however, EI services were set up primarily in the above-mentioned populations with a "Western" culture, despite local variations in service delivery systems. The need for adaptation to cultural diversity in these

Western services is relatively small. As EI work continues to expand outside these societies, the role of cultural factors becomes more prominent and significant. The interplay between culture and psychosis presentation and management could significantly modulate the effectiveness and success of intervention. It is no longer possible to simply graft existing programmes from one location to another. In addition, there is a much greater diversity in societal attitudes to psychosis and in mental health service delivery systems across Asia. How to take these factors into consideration in designing optimal care is one of the main themes of this volume.

Development of comprehensive early psychosis programmes in Hong Kong and Singapore started in 2001 (see Chapter 2, "Early Psychosis Services in an Asian Urban Setting: EASY and Other Services in Hong Kong" and Chapter 3, "Overview of Early Psychosis Service Development in Singapore: The EPIP Story"). Both locations have had established links with "Western" systems for specialist training, service model and research collaborations. Hong Kong has a predominantly Chinese culture while Singapore is more multi-ethnic. Both are metropolitan cities with high economic standards but relatively deprived mental health services.

At present, EI developments are also underway in many Asian locations including Mainland China, India, Indonesia, Japan (see Chapter 4, "Early Psychosis Intervention in an Urban Japanese Setting: Overview of Early Psychosis Services in Japan"), Korea (see Chapter 5, "Overview of the Development of Services for Early Psychosis in Korea"), Malaysia and Taiwan. Clinicians, intervention professionals, and researchers working in EI programmes in these regions have established the Asian Network of Early Psychosis (ANEP) to foster communication and sharing of experiences. Recently, the ANEP published an Early Psychosis Declaration for Asia, emphasizing the unique challenges and agenda for EI services in Asia (Asian Network of Early Psychosis, 2012). On the other hand, as each site develops according to local resources and opportunities, there are both similarities and differences between programmes. While all EI programmes in Asia started with a similar general framework, the final form of a particular programme is essentially the result of an interaction between the disorder, local culture, and societal factors.

General Framework and Cultural Relevance of Early Psychosis Work

Goals of early intervention

Early psychosis intervention encompasses several distinct but interacting basic components. The ultimate goal of early intervention is to improve the long-term outcome for psychotic disorders. In order to attain favourable long-term outcomes, early intervention advocates propose that optimal management of the initial few years following onset of psychosis (the critical period) is of utmost importance (Birchwood, Todd, & Jackson, 1998). This strategy is argued primarily from the observation that early outcome after the initial few years often account for much of the overall variations in long-term outcome (e.g., see Harrison et al., 1996; Harrison et al., 2001). The critical period hypothesis leads to the suggestion that where there are resource limitations, there is a significant advantage gained by giving priority to management of the early course of the illness by providing a specialized early psychosis team and case managers for patients during the first few years of illness.

To achieve optimal critical period outcome, three distinctive strategies have been widely adopted, namely (1) early detection; (2) at-risk mental state detection and intervention; and (3) critical period interventions. The latter includes casework, community care, medications, specific programmes for clinical scenarios such as relapses and self-harm, and recovery in psychosis.

Early detection

Early detection aims to reduce the delay of initiating effective treatment (i.e. the duration of untreated psychosis, see Chapter 6, "Factors Affecting the Duration of Untreated Psychosis in Hong Kong"), given that DUP is often unacceptably lengthy (see Chapter 2, "Early Psychosis Services in an Asian Urban Setting: EASY and Other Services in Hong Kong"; Chapter 3, "Overview of Early Psychosis Service Development in Singapore: The EPIP Story"; Chapter 4, "Early Psychosis Intervention in an Urban Japanese Setting: Overview of Early Psychosis Services in Japan"; and Chapter 6, "Factors Affecting the Duration of Untreated Psychosis in Hong Kong"). During the DUP, patients' functioning and quality of life are compromised, with concomitant breakdown of social networks and occupational opportunities. DUP is likely to be determined by a number of factors, which include the abruptness of symptom onset, the recognition of the symptoms by patients or caregivers, and the process of seeking help. Chapter 6 provides an example of studying how some of the factors contributed to a long DUP in Hong Kong. As shortening of DUP is a goal for many EI programmes, an EI programme has to change what happens *before* the patient is engaged with the service. Commonly adopted strategies include enhancing public awareness for psychosis in the general population (see Chapter 7, "Public Awareness Approaches in Early Psychosis") and training gatekeepers (those who are more likely to be in contact with patients) to identify and refer potential patients (see Chapter 8, "Early Psychosis in the Workplace" and Chapter 9, "Enhancing Psychosis Detection through Gatekeepers"). Removing barriers to help-seeking is a major issue in heavily stigmatizing societies. Chapter 10 ("Initial Screening and Assessment: A Phone-Based Two-Stage Screening") describes a telephone-based screening designed to address this. In Chapter 11 ("The Diagnostic Interview in Early Psychosis"), issues related to the initial diagnosis are discussed, including the importance of the assessment setting and engagement techniques.

At-risk mental state detection and intervention

Based on the observation that in a proportion of patients, first-episode psychosis is preceded by a prodromal phase or at-risk mental state (Hafner & Maurer, 2006), it may be possible to identify vulnerable individuals and intervene earlier to prevent onset of a full-blown psychosis. Services using this approach have been started in several locations including Japan, Korea, and Singapore (Chapters 3–5). Chapter 12 ("Handling At-Risk Mental State") introduces comprehensively the issues related to screening and intervention for at-risk mental states, using empirical data from Hong Kong to illustrate many key issues.

Models of critical period intervention

The main part of this volume explores working with patients diagnosed with a first-episode psychotic disorder. In line with the critical period hypothesis, as soon as a patient is identified, optimal intervention should be offered for the initial few years to attain the best possible outcome.

Early psychosis case work

Current approaches in most EI programmes provide a case manager, who will tailor-make a set of psychosocial interventions for the patient according to a case formulation and care plan, bearing in mind that these psychosocial interventions require integration of local cultural factors to be effective. In Part III "Culturally Relevant Psychosocial Case Intervention", the core approaches are described in detail by experienced clinicians, psychologists, and case managers who have been working within these cultural settings. Extensive use of clinically oriented discussion and informative case examples underline the pragmatic issues encountered in real-life practice. Chapter 13 ("Implementing Psychological Intervention Programmes in Early Psychosis [PIPE]") introduces the conceptual framework of a three-tier psychological intervention system adopted by the Hong Kong EI programme. This is followed by a description of a culturally relevant psychosocial intervention programme in Singapore (see Chapter 14, "The PASTE that Binds: Culturally Relevant Psychological Interventions for First-Episode Psychosis Individuals in Singapore"). To further highlight the significance of cultural considerations, Chapter 15 ("Cultural Issues in Early Psychosis Management") focuses on some cultural themes in managing patients with psychosis. Chapter 16 ("Engagement and Outreach in Early Psychosis Management") discusses EI in the cultural context of Asian societies. Importantly, Chapter 17 ("Experience of Stigma in Early Psychosis Patients and Caregivers") explores the central issue of stigma as experienced by patients and caregivers. Arguably, stigma has a heightened role in Asian societies and may exert inordinate influence on patients and caregivers' behaviours. Understanding the role of stigma is thus crucial to any culturally relevant psychosocial intervention approach.

Chapter 18 ("The Phase-Specific Progress Supervision Model for Case Managers") deals with a vital but often neglected topic: the supervision and development of case managers specializing in early psychosis. Given the important understanding that case managers are core personnel who may have a decisive effect on patients' outcome, early psychosis casework becomes a highly specialized profession with high demand on knowledge and skills. Building up a capable and committed workforce is key to the success of any EI team.

Community care programmes

In many service settings, core early psychosis casework is backed up by a variety of community-based programmes. Chapter 19 ("Community Psychosocial Intervention in Early Psychosis") describes a Singaporean community day-care service focusing on functional outcomes. Chapter 20 ("The Peer Support Programme in Early Psychosis Intervention Programme [EPIP]") introduces the setting up of peer worker programmes, which is followed by a discussion about support programmes for families and caregivers (see Chapter 21, "Family Work in Early Psychosis"). The closing account looks at how health services could collaborate with non-governmental organizations in Hong Kong (see Chapter 22, "Working with Non-Governmental Organizations in Early Psychosis").

Medication treatment

Antipsychotic medication remains the core of treatment and control of early psychosis. Frequently encountered questions about antipsychotic treatment are presented in Chapter 23 ("Pharmacological Intervention in Early Psychosis"). This essay is followed by in-depth discussion of an evidence-based approach to the complexity of adherence behaviour in psychotic patients that includes many pragmatic tips to improve adherence in Chapter 24 ("Medication Adherence: Specific Issues in Early Psychosis in Asia").

Modulating the course of illness

In the critical period, the patient's illness may unfold along several possible trajectories. Awareness of adverse complications is important for timely responses. A number of commonly encountered situations are described together with suggestions for their identification and management. Chapter 25 ("Relapse Intervention and Related Issues") continues to discuss all-important issues in relapse prevention, a common problem that could have a decisive influence over outcomes. Suicide and self-harm behaviour is considered in Chapter 26 ("Suicide and Self-Harm Behaviour in Early Psychosis"), with specific consideration to detection and management of self-harm in early psychosis. This is particularly significant as the critical period is also the period when suicide risk is the highest along the lifetime course of psychotic disorders. Even though the patterns of substance abuse in the sampled Asian populations differ from those encountered in the West, comorbid substance abuse is particularly important as it is invariably associated with poor outcomes in psychosis (see Chapter 27, "Comorbid Substance Abuse in Early Psychosis"). Chapter 28 ("Handling Patients with Negative Symptoms") addresses the problems of prominent negative symptoms, with practical tips for assessment and management in the Asian context.

Recovery

The concept of recovery is a complex notion in psychosis in view of its highly complicated causes, course, and outcomes. Often after a single episode of illness, patients lack sufficiently helpful mental models with which to understand their experiences of the illness. This gap may have important implications for the patient's outlook, functional outcomes, as well as treatment engagement behaviours. Chapter 29 ("Recovery from Psychosis") starts with description of the conventional clinical understanding of recovery, leading to an in-depth exploration of the concept of recovery using a cognitive linguistic approach in Chapter 30 ("Concepts of Recovery in Early Psychosis: A Cognitive Linguistic Approach"). This is complemented by an experiential study of the patients' own views and expressions about their subjective concepts of recovery (see Chapter 31, "Experiential Aspects of Recovery in Early Psychosis: Focus Group Findings"). Understanding these perspectives is critical to effective early psychosis care.

Evaluating EI Services in Asia

The adaptation of EI service in Asia has come a long way, and models continue to emerge that fit cultural and societal factors unique to this region. Research data from these programmes are of particular importance to map how close outcomes are to being optimal. Chapter 32 ("Database Design and Management") gives a detailed description of the practicalities of building an information system useful for evaluating EI programmes. Chapter 33 ("Research and Outcome Evaluation in Early Psychosis") gives a comprehensive overview of research approaches, highlighting the importance of a constant feedback loop between research data and clinical practice.

Conclusion

This book showcases pearls of wisdom from real-world early interventions in Asia during the decade 2000–2010. Looking ahead, early intervention efforts already underway are predicted to sustain full impetus. In Asia, the specific challenges to the development of EI work, including heavy stigmatization, limitation in manpower, training, and physical space, as well as extremely diverse systems of mental health care service delivery may persist but reflecting upon these challenges and sharing ways to overcome them remain central to the purpose of this publication. Foreseeably, the burgeoning interest in early intervention approaches for psychosis will not slacken despite these hardened challenges and difficulties.

References

Amminger, G. P., Edwards, J., Brewer, W. J., Harrigan, S., & McGorry, P. D. (2002). Duration of untreated psychosis and cognitive deterioration in first-episode schizophrenia. *Schizophrenia Research, 54*(3), 223–230. doi: S092099640100278X [pii]

Asian Network of Early Psychosis. (2012). The early psychosis declaration for Asia. *East Asian Archives of Psychiatry, 22*(3), 90–93.

Bak, M., Drukker, M., van Os, J., & Delespaul, P. (2005). Hospital comorbidity bias and the concept of schizophrenia. *Social Psychiatry Psychiatric Epidemiology, 40*(10), 817–821. doi: 10.1007/s00127-005-0971-0

Birchwood, M., Todd, P., & Jackson, C. (1998). Early intervention in psychosis: The critical period hypothesis. [Review]. *The British Journal of Psychiatry. Supplement, 172*(33), 53–59.

Chan, S. W., Hsiung, P. C., Thompson, D. R., Chen, S. C., & Hwu, H. G. (2007). Health-related quality of life of Chinese people with schizophrenia in Hong Kong and Taipei: A cross-sectional analysis. *Research in Nursing and Health, 30*(3), 261–269. doi: 10.1002/nur.20189

Chen, E. Y., Tang, J. Y., Hui, C. L., Chiu, C. P., Lam, M. M., Law, C. W., et al. (2011). Three-year outcome of phase-specific early intervention for first-episode psychosis: A cohort study in Hong Kong. *Early Intervention in Psychiatry.* doi: 10.1111/j.1751-7893.2011.00279.x

Craig, T. K., Garety, P., Power, P., Rahaman, N., Colbert, S., Fornells-Ambrojo, M., et al. (2004). The Lambeth Early Onset (LEO) Team: Randomised controlled trial of the effectiveness of specialised care for early psychosis. [Clinical Trial Comparative Study Randomized Controlled Trial Research Support, Non-U.S. Government]. *British Medical Journal, 329*(7474), 1067. doi: 10.1136/bmj.38246.594873.7C

Falloon, I. R. (1992). Early intervention for first episodes of schizophrenia: A preliminary exploration. *Psychiatry, 55*(1), 4–15.

Fusar-Poli, P., & Politi, P. (2008). Paul Eugen Bleuler and the birth of schizophrenia (1908). *American Journal of Psychiatry, 165*(11), 1407. doi: 165/11/1407 [pii]10.1176/appi.ajp.2008.08050714

Hafner, H., & Maurer, K. (2006). Early detection of schizophrenia: Current evidence and future perspectives. *World Psychiatry, 5*(3), 130–138.

Hafner, H., Riecher-Rossler, A., Hambrecht, M., Maurer, K., Meissner, S., Schmidtke, A., et al. (1992). IRAOS: An instrument for the assessment of onset and early course of schizophrenia. *Schizophrenia Research, 6*(3), 209–223.

Harding, C. M., Brooks, G. W., Ashikaga, T., Strauss, J. S., & Breier, A. (1987). The Vermont longitudinal study of persons with severe mental illness, II: Long-term outcome of subjects who retrospectively met DSM-III criteria for schizophrenia. *American Journal of Psychiatry, 144*(6), 727–735.

Harding, C. M., Zubin, J., & Strauss, J. S. (1987). Chronicity in schizophrenia: Fact, partial fact, or artifact? *Hospital Community Psychiatry, 38*(5), 477–486.

Harrison, G., Croudace, T., Mason, P., Glazebrook, C., & Medley, I. (1996). Predicting the long-term outcome of schizophrenia. [Research Support, Non-U.S. Government]. *Psychological Medicine, 26*(4), 697–705.

Harrison, G., Hopper, K., Craig, T., Laska, E., Siegel, C., Wanderling, J., et al. (2001). Recovery from psychotic illness: A 15- and 25-year international follow-up study. [Multicenter Study Research Support, Non-U.S. Government]. *British Journal of Psychiatry, 178*, 506–517.

Hegelstad, W. T., Larsen, T. K., Auestad, B., Evensen, J., Haahr, U., Joa, I., et al. (2012). Long-term follow-up of the TIPS early detection in psychosis study: Effects on 10-year outcome. *American Journal of Psychiatry, 169*(4), 374–380. doi: 10.1176/appi.ajp.2011.11030459

Henry, L. P., Amminger, G. P., Harris, M. G., Yuen, H. P., Harrigan, S. M., Prosser, A. L., et al. (2010). The EPPIC follow-up study of first-episode psychosis: Longer-term clinical and functional outcome 7 years after index admission. *Journal of Clinical Psychiatry, 71*(6), 716–728. doi: 10.4088/JCP.08m04846yel

International Early Psychosis Association Writing, G. (2005). International clinical practice guidelines for early psychosis. *British Journal of Psychiatry. Supplement, 48*, s120–124. doi: 187/48/s120 [pii]10.1192/bjp.187.48.s120

Johannessen, J. O., Larsen, T. K., & McGlashan, T. (1999). Duration of untreated psychosis: An important target for intervention in schizophrenia? *Nordic Journal of Psychiatry, 53*(4), 275–283. doi: 10.1080/080394899427089

Law, C. W., Chen, E. Y., Cheung, E. F., Chan, R. C., Wong, J. G., Lam, C. L., et al. (2005). Impact of untreated psychosis on quality of life in patients with first-episode schizophrenia. *Quality of Life Research, 14*(8), 1803–1811. doi: 10.1007/s11136-005-3236–6

Lincoln, C. V., & McGorry, P. (1995). Who cares? Pathways to psychiatric care for young people experiencing a first episode of psychosis. *Psychiatric Services, 46*(11), 1166–1171.

Malla, A. K., Norman, R. M., Manchanda, R., Ahmed, M. R., Scholten, D., Harricharan, R., et al. (2002). One-year outcome in first episode psychosis: Influence of DUP and other predictors. *Schizophrenia Research, 54*(3), 231–242. doi: S0920996401002547 [pii]

Marshall, M., Lewis, S., Lockwood, A., Drake, R., Jones, P., & Croudace, T. (2005). Association between duration of untreated psychosis and outcome in cohorts of first-episode patients: A systematic review. *Archives of General Psychiatry, 62*(9), 975–983. doi: 62/9/975 [pii]10.1001/archpsyc.62.9.975

McGlashan, T. H. (1984). The Chestnut Lodge follow-up study. II. Long-term outcome of schizophrenia and the affective disorders. *Archives of General Psychiatry, 41*(6), 586–601.

McGlashan, T. H., & Johannessen, J. O. (1996). Early detection and intervention with schizophrenia: Rationale. *Schizophrenia Bulletin, 22*(2), 201–222.

McGorry, P. D., Edwards, J., Mihalopoulos, C., Harrigan, S. M., & Jackson, H. J. (1996). EPPIC: An evolving system of early detection and optimal management. *Schizophrenia Bulletin, 22*(2), 305–326.

Oosthuizen, P., Emsley, R. A., Keyter, N., Niehaus, D. J., & Koen, L. (2005). Duration of untreated psychosis and outcome in first-episode psychosis. Perspective from a developing country. *Acta Psychiatrica Scandinavica, 111*(3), 214–219. doi: ACP448 [pii]10.1111/j.1600-0447.2004.00448.x

Petersen, L., Jeppesen, P., Thorup, A., Abel, M. B., Ohlenschlaeger, J., Christensen, T. O., et al. (2005). A randomised multicentre trial of integrated versus standard treatment for patients with a first episode of psychotic illness. *British Medical Journal, 331*(7517), 602. doi: bmj.38565.415000.E01 [pii]10.1136/bmj.38565.415000.E01

2

Early Psychosis Services in an Asian Urban Setting: EASY and Other Services in Hong Kong

Dicky Wai-sau Chung and Eric Yu-hai Chen

The first specialized early psychosis service in Hong Kong, the Early Assessment Service for Young People with Psychosis (EASY), was launched in 2001. EASY is a Hospital Authority initiative in Hong Kong. The programme consists of specialized early intervention teams providing services for young adults aged 15 to 25 years with first-episode psychosis. In 2009, an adult early psychosis service became available with the support of the Hong Kong Jockey Club Charities Trust. The Jockey Club Early Psychosis (JCEP) Project provides case management service to 1000 patients aged between 26 and 55 years under the care of the Hospital Authority. Subsequently, the Hong Kong Hospital Authority adopted this service direction and also extended the EASY programme to include adult-onset patients. This chapter gives an overview of early psychosis service development in Hong Kong with a focus on the design and implementation of the EASY programme.

The Situation before Early Intervention Services

Prior to the establishment of early intervention services, psychosis patients in Hong Kong were managed under general psychiatric services, with no special provision for the initial phase of the disorder. Stigmatization was heavy, and this often resulted in a long delay of help-seeking until a crisis arose, after which the patient was often admitted through accident and emergency departments (AEDs) to psychiatric inpatient units, sometimes involving compulsory admissions. After hospitalization, the patient would be followed up in the outpatient clinic where there were a large number of patients per session (more than 30 patients per 3 hour session). Psychiatrists in an outpatient clinic session saw a mixture of various psychiatric conditions, such as substance abuse, personality disorders, mood disorders, and so on. As can be seen in many other parts of Asia, outpatient services were characterized by limited clinician contact (less than 10 minutes of consultation time per patient, focusing mainly on medication and side-effects) and lack of other supportive interventions. This kind of standard care was inadequate to deal with the complex needs associated with young people with an early onset of psychosis (Hui et al., 2008).

In the period before the introduction of early intervention services, long delays in help-seeking were common. Only about one-third of the psychotic patients received treatment within a month of illness onset, about half within 6 months, and about another one-third later than 1 year after onset. The mean delay was about 1.5 years with a median of 5 months (Chen et al., 2005). Figure 2.1 shows the distribution of DUP in a local sample of first-episode psychosis patients before early intervention services were available (unpublished data).

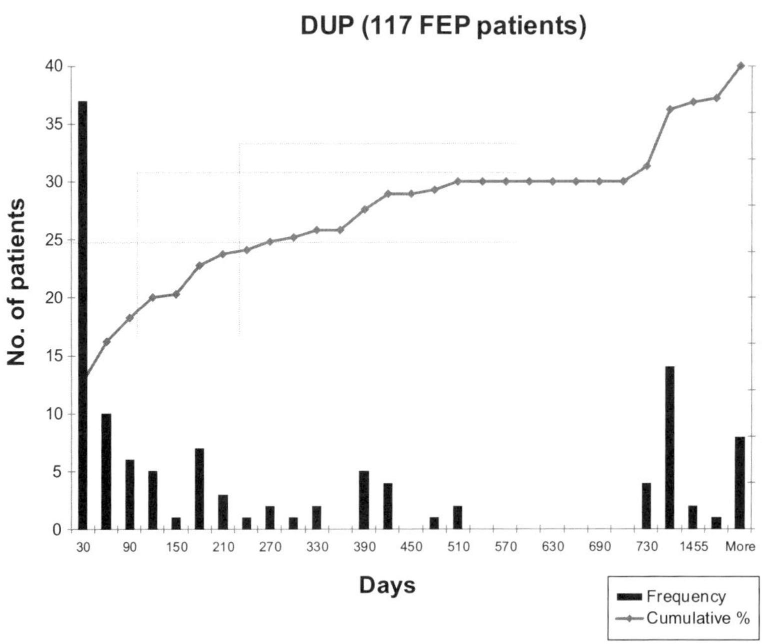

Figure 2.1

Duration of untreated psychosis (DUP) in Hong Kong prior to the introduction of early psychosis services

Patients in their untreated psychotic episodes often had very poor quality of life, with severe impairment in a wide range of life domains (Law et al., 2005).

Data also show that the mode of onset (acute, subacute, or insidious presentation) of the illness had a significant effect on the delay. In particular, patients with acute onset tended to have a shorter delay. Another important observation was that the family's previous experience with psychosis had an effect on the delay. Specifically, if the family has previous experience of another family member falling ill, the delay was significantly shorter than that in families who were experiencing the illness for the first time (Chen et al., 2005). This trend suggested that delays may be a result of the patients' families and the general public in Hong Kong not being well informed about the signs and symptoms of psychotic illnesses, as well as treatment pathways. Thus, providing basic information about psychotic symptoms and making that information available to the general public through media was considered to be an important strategy to reduce delay.

Distinctive Processes in the EASY Service

In view of the unmet needs in early psychosis intervention services, the EASY programme was designed with three main components.

Public awareness and education about psychosis

In Hong Kong, the goal of recognizing people with hallucinations and delusions as displaying a psychotic illness and bringing them to assessment is challenging. Studies conducted prior to the programme revealed that, although the general public had some ideas about mental states and stress, they were not able to differentiate various types of conditions, or between conditions that need medical treatment and those due to general stress. For example, when individuals were presented a case vignette of a patient with distinctive, first-rank symptoms of schizophrenia and asked what they thought the individual might need, a typical answer would be that the person needed some help, but in the form of rest or relaxation rather than medical assessments (Lam, Chan, & Chen, 1996). An intensive informational and educational campaign was therefore set up to inform the public about psychotic symptoms. Through community education programmes, the EASY team reached the public in places such as local housing estates and exhibitions in shopping centres, passing on information about psychosis in the form of games and fun activities (see Chapter 7, "Public Awareness Approaches in Early Psychosis").

Addressing stigmatization and naming of psychosis

At the beginning of the EASY programme, a taskforce was set up to deliberate on a new Chinese term for "psychosis", as a strategy to ameliorate any social stigma attached to the condition. The existing Chinese translations for the terms "psychosis" and "schizophrenia" found in dictionaries were *zhongxing jingshenbing* (重性精神病) and *jingshen fenliezheng* (精神分裂症), respectively. *Zhongxing* means "severe" while *jingshenbing* means mental illness. *Jingshen fenliezheng* in Chinese characters concretely and pictorially portrays a splitting (*fen*) and fracturing (*lie*) of the mind (*jingshen*), which easily misleads people to think of some irreversible damage of the mind or personality.

The taskforce invited suggestions from professionals for a novel translation of the term "psychosis", and finally selected the Chinese term *sijue shitiao* (思覺失調) for psychosis. To the public, the new term still connotes that this condition is an abnormal mental state, depicting a "syndrome" or "symptom cluster". In fact, the term "psychosis" is diagnostically "plastic" without differentiating the condition into any individual formal diagnoses, unlike schizophrenia, bipolar disorder, or delusional disorder. Such a strategic move avoids premature stereotypes and subsequent stigmatization. Also, in practice, the stability of the diagnostic categories at this stage of the illness has been questioned (Chang et al., 2009). The term *sijue* (思覺), meaning thinking and perception, describes the main symptoms in psychosis and *shitiao* (失調), imbalance or dysregulation, convey two messages about early psychosis: first, that psychosis is biological in nature, and second, brings functional impairment, not a permanent damage, and thus is potentially reversible.

At about the same time, a new term for "schizophrenia" was introduced in Japan, referring to an integrative dysregulation (Sugiura et al., 2001). The deliberate choice of *sijue shitiao* (思覺失調) for "psychosis" instead of "schizophrenia" expresses the belief that for the purpose of facilitating early detection and help-seeking, it is more important to communicate with the public about the syndrome of psychosis rather than the diagnosis of schizophrenia (Chiu et al., 2010).

The National Alliance of Mentally Ill in the US endorses the strategy of highlighting the "brain disease" model to explain the nature of schizophrenia to the public. This Chinese name of psychosis is aligned with this notion, aiming to reduce any public misperception that mental patients are personally responsible for bringing about the illness, and that they can choose to control their behaviours. This selection can be compared to the use of *shenjing shuairuo* (神經衰弱), or neurasthenia, a medical term commonly used by Chinese people, which is more publicly acceptable as a minor psychiatric disorder, involving anxiety, depression, and somatization. This term also carries a biological connotation, hinting at fatigue and weakness as a result of problems with the central nervous system.

Easily accessible referral channel

The design of a readily accessible and user-friendly care system also ensures that patients do not need to go through any barriers before receiving medical treatment and assessment, such as seeing a primary care physician, getting a referral, and queuing up in an outpatient clinic, which can sometimes take months.

A flexible assessment system, composed of open referral channels (e.g., a telephone-based assessment system), was designed for EASY. After an initial telephone-based screening assessment, a face-to-face diagnostic assessment was arranged for at-risk cases within one week (median five days). Individuals diagnosed as having a psychotic disorder proceeded to the intervention programme whereas those who fulfilled criteria for at-risk mental states (e.g., in a prodromal stage) were simply monitored. Cases with disorders other than psychosis were referred to other appropriate services if necessary (for details see Chapter 10, "Initial Screening and Assessment: A Phone-Based Two-Stage Screening").

Intensive phase-specific intervention

In order to improve patients' treatment outcomes, the third step, a phase-specific intervention programme was offered to patients for the first two years following the diagnosis of a psychotic disorder.

Protocol-based case management approach

The EASY service is characterized by a case management approach. Each patient and his/her family are assigned a case manager (who may have a nursing, social service, or occupational therapy background). The case manager, who delivers a protocol-based psychoeducational programme (So, Wong, & Chong, 2002) and provides supportive intervention, is available to the family for consultation as required. The case manager makes contact through community visits or interviews in the respective outpatient clinic.

Phase-specific service

The intervention service of EASY aims at addressing specific issues in a particular illness stage to enhance patients' psychosocial functioning. For example, maintenance medication and recovery issues among stabilized first-episode patients who have not relapsed are very different from those of chronic patients. Individuals going through their first episode also hold different ideas about recovery compared with those who have been ill for many years. With phase-specific services, such issues can be addressed in a focused way.

Broad supportive management

With the EASY service, management no longer focuses only on medication control of psychotic symptoms; rather, case managers and clinicians aim at broader goals such as functional recovery as well as psychological adaptation and maintenance of well-being. This differs from services in general psychiatric clinics, in which clinicians usually do not have the time to handle issues other than symptoms and medications.

The caseloads of EASY case managers (around 1 to 100) are much heavier than that in early intervention teams in the West (around 1 to 20/30). Thus, instead of providing intensive intervention such as cognitive-behavioural therapy or family therapy, intervention focuses on basic supportive care and psychoeducation. Case managers provide patients and their caregivers with the information they need for appraising and managing the disorder. Caregivers are particularly important in Hong Kong, as most patients live with their families. In general, family carers are well motivated to provide care and collaborate with clinical teams during the early phase of the illness.

Proactive timely intervention

Time is an important dimension in early psychosis service delivery, both for patients and clinicians. Every EASY clinician and case manager is aware of the

2-year time frame available for working with a particular patient, during which defined tasks have to be completed to try to achieve satisfactory outcomes. This protocol differs from that in general outpatient clinics, where clinical sessions are often brief and appointments are spaced over a long period of time. In the EASY programme, focused interventions with proactive and prospective planning are provided for each patient; clinicians follow a management guideline for early psychosis, which takes references from international guidelines with some local adaptations (Chee, Ng, & Kua, 2005).

Service Planning and Development

The planning and implementation of the EASY programme was carried out under a steering committee consisting of representative psychiatrists and other mental health professionals from each local service cluster. The steering committee coordinates the overall development of service, training, audit, and educational programmes. These include defining the structure and processes of the EASY teams, and negotiating external collaboration with media, non-government organizations (NGOs), and other relevant agencies. The steering committee also coordinates staff training and development.

Based on international and census data of Hong Kong's population structure, the EASY caseload was estimated to be about 700 new cases per year. In order to detect cases early, a screening system was required and, taking into account that some of the cases screened may be false-positives, a larger number of assessments were catered for. As the early intervention team looked after patients during the first two years of their illness after assessment, planners estimated that there would be around 1,200–1,400 cases receiving EASY service at any one time. More recently the service has been extended to provide for an additional estimated 600 new cases aged above 25 years.

There were five district-based EASY teams covering different geographical catchment areas in Hong Kong, and they shared central development so that work was not duplicated. Two additional teams were established after extension and all remain responsible for frontline day-to-day operations and assessment, as well as networking with the respective local community. Each team has two psychiatrists (one associate consultant and one medical officer) and three psychiatric nurses (most of whom are community nurses) who look after about 500 cases and assess approximately 180 cases each year. There is one clinical psychologist who is primarily responsible for conducting direct psycho-education sessions, educational programmes, and training of case managers.

Staff development and training is an important element of EASY. Given the resource limitations, prioritization of available manpower is essential in order to deliver the best possible care to patients. To achieve this, in-house training programmes and monthly meetings cover different practical topics (e.g., engagement, relapse prevention) in handling needs of patients and their caregivers. There is also an annual retreat during which all EASY teams spend a day together for brainstorming sessions. During these retreats, the aims and practices of the EASY programme are discussed and reflected upon.

Service Evaluation and Research

Evidence-based evaluation is an important aspect of the early intervention services in Hong Kong as in other parts of the world. Much emphasis has been put on real-life data in the EASY programme, with an aim to obtain useful insights through clinical practice, which can then be tested and translated back to practice (see Chapter 33, "Research and Outcome Evaluation in Early Psychosis"). EASY's basic research model optimizes the opportunity to work with homogeneous patient groups (i.e., in the same clinical stage of the same disorder) to increase the chances of identifying the different risk factors, and exploring ways of modifying the risk factors through intervention.

Outcomes of EASY Services

Outcome evaluation of the EASY service is also the subject of research. As the programme is territory-wide, there is no concurrent control group to compare outcome with. Thus, outcomes in a group of patients before implementation of the EASY service (historical control) were investigated (Chen et al., 2011).

Clinical and functional outcomes

Patients who have received the EASY service show better occupational functioning outcomes over three years compared with historical controls under standard care. Clinically, the EASY service is associated with milder positive and negative symptoms, as well as fewer and shorter hospitalizations. While cumulative relapse rate remains unchanged with the early intervention service, there are fewer EASY patients with multiple relapses. Patients who have received early intervention service also have a lower risk of suicide and death of any causes (1.2% compared with previously over 3% in the first three years, Chen et al., 2011).

DUP

In areas where DUP has been recorded before and after the introduction of an early intervention programme, such as Norway (Larsen et al., 2001), Melbourne (Krstev et al., 2004), and Australia (McGorry & Yung, 2003), a significant reduction in DUP has been reported. However, a significant reduction in DUP has not yet been demonstrated after the implementation of EASY in Hong Kong. This is possibly due to the fact that with the EASY service, some cases with lengthy DUP who were previously unknown to healthcare services are engaged by the more accessible service (Chen et al., 2011).

Destigmatization

The term *sijue shitiao* has been well accepted since the launch of early psychosis services in Hong Kong and has become a short form of an abnormal mental condition with hallucinations, delusions, and thought disorders. However, the mass media's use of this new translation of early psychosis in Hong Kong is only the first step in ameliorating stigma. Continuous efforts to improve public attitudes towards psychosis are necessary to avoid *sijue shitiao* becoming yet another name for people to mock others with odd behaviour. Much public awareness work has been conducted by the charitable organization, the Hong Kong Early Psychosis Intervention Society (EPISO), to further this aim.

Cost-benefit analysis

A brief cost-benefit analysis of the EASY programme compared the direct spending in the first two years of illness and revealed that the extra staff and medication cost of EASY was offset by a significant reduction in hospitalization, relapse, and treatment of the first episode (Wong et al., 2011). In other words, EASY is cost-neutral with improved clinical outcomes. This was true before indirect costs such as quality of life and suicide rate were taken into consideration, which may suggest larger cost-benefit advantages of EASY compared with standard care.

Conclusion

In summary, the EASY experience suggests that outcomes can be improved in terms of negative symptoms, and suicide rates, with a well-structured early intervention programme without changing the DUP. With EASY, these improvements have been maintained for at least two years, after which patients in the programme went through a "step-down" process (i.e., gradual withdrawal from intensive intervention) and were eventually transferred back to conventional general psychiatry clinics for continuing care if required.

A number of important questions remain to be answered, especially whether the improved outcomes can be sustained beyond the two-year period. This question is now being explored in the JCEP project, comparing patients receiving two-year versus four-year intervention. Optimal development and fine-tuning of psychosocial care is an area of ceaseless innovation and refinement. Further improvement in relapse management is another major issue in first-episode services. The development of at-risk mental state intervention has been an area of intense studies elsewhere (e.g., Broome et al., 2005; Yung et al., 2005), but has not yet been introduced to Hong Kong because of limited resources and pending more clarification and experiences in the risk-benefit issues to guide prioritization. Finally, patients' subjective adaptation to the diagnosis of psychosis and its associated stigmatization is also recognized as an important source of severe difficulty.

References

Broome, M. R., Woolley, J. B., Johns, L. C., Valmaggia, L. R., Tabraham, P., Gafoor, R., Bramon, E., McGuire, P. K. (2005). Outreach and support in south London (OASIS): Implementation of a clinical service for prodromal psychosis and the at risk mental state. *European Psychiatry, 20*(5–6), 372–378. doi: 10.1016/j.eurpsy.2005.02.001

Chang, W. C., Pang, S. L., Chung, D. W., & Chan, S. S. (2009). Five-year stability of ICD-10 diagnoses among Chinese patients presented with first-episode psychosis in Hong Kong. *Schizophrenia Research, 115*(2–3), 351–357. doi: 10.1016/j.schres.2009.09.037

Chee, C. Y., Ng, T. P., & Kua, E. H. (2005). Comparing the stigma of mental illness in a general hospital with a state mental hospital: A Singapore study. *Social Psychiatry and Psychiatric Epidemiology, 40*(8), 648–653. doi: 10.1007/s00127-005-0932-z

Chen, E. Y.-H., Dunn, E. L.-W., Miao, M. Y.-K., Yeung, W.-S., Wong, C.-K., Chan, W.-F., et al. (2005). The impact of family experience on the duration of untreated psychosis (DUP) in Hong Kong. *Social Psychiatry and Psychiatric Epidemiology, 40*(5), 350–356. doi: 10.1007/s00127-005-0908-z

Chen, E. Y., Tang, J. Y., Hui, C. L., Chiu, C. P., Lam, M. M., Law, C. W., et al. (2011). Three-year outcome of phase-specific early intervention for first-episode psychosis: A cohort study in Hong Kong. *Early Intervention in Psychiatry*. doi: 10.1111/j.1751-7893.2011.00279.x

Chiu, C. P., Lam, M. M., Chan, S. K., Chung, D. W., Hung, S. F., Tang, J. Y., et al. (2010). Naming psychosis: The Hong Kong experience. *Early Intervention in Psychiatry, 4*(4), 270–274. doi: 10.1111/j.1751-7893.2010.00203.x

Hui, C. L. M., Wong, G. H. Y., Lam, Y. K., Chow, P. P. L., & Chen, E. Y. H. (2008). Patient-clinician communication and needs identification for outpatients with schizophrenia in Hong Kong: Role of the 2-COM instrument. *Hong Kong Journal of Psychiatry, 18*(2), 69–75.

Krstev, H., Carbone, S., Harrigan, S. M., Curry, C., Elkins, K., & McGorry, P. D. (2004). Early intervention in first-episode psychosis: The impact of a community development campaign. *Social Psychiatry and Psychiatric Epidemiology, 39*(9), 711–719. doi: 10.1007/s00127-004-0798-5

Lam, L. C., Chan, C. K., & Chen, E. Y. (1996). Insight and general public attitude on psychotic experiences in Hong Kong. *International Journal of Social Psychiatry, 42*(1), 10–17.

Larsen, T. K., Friis, S., Haahr, U., Joa, I., Johannessen, J. O., Melle, I., et al. (2001). Early detection and intervention in first-episode schizophrenia: A critical review. *Acta Psychiatrica Scandinavica, 103*(5), 323–334. doi: acp131 [pii]

Law, C. W., Chen, E. Y., Cheung, E. F., Chan, R. C., Wong, J. G., Lam, C. L., et al. (2005). Impact of untreated psychosis on quality of life in patients with first-episode schizophrenia. *Quality of Life Research, 14*(8), 1803–1811. doi: 10.1007/s11136-005-3236-6

McGorry, P. D., & Yung, A. R. (2003). Early intervention in psychosis: An overdue reform. *The Australian and New Zealand Journal of Psychiatry, 37*(4), 393–398. doi: 1192 [pii]

So, S., Wong, C. W., & Chong, H. C. (Eds.). (2002). *Psychological Intervention Programme for Early Psychosis (PIPE) Handbook for EASY Service*. Hong Kong: Early Assessment Service for Young People with Psychosis.

Sugiura, T., Sakamoto, S., Tanaka, E., Tomoda, A., & Kitamura, T. (2001). Labeling effect of Seishin-Bunretsu-Byou, the Japanse translation for schizophrenia: An argument for relabeling. *International Journal of Social Psychiatry, 47*(2), 43.

Wong, K. K., Chan, S. K., Lam, M. M., Hui, C. L., Hung, S. F., Tay, M., et al. (2011). Cost-effectiveness of an early assessment service for young people with early psychosis in Hong Kong. *The Australian and New Zealand Journal of Psychiatry, 45*(8), 673–680. doi: 10.3109/00048674.2011.586329

Yung, A. R., Yuen, H. P., McGorry, P. D., Philips, L. J., Kelly, D., Dell'Olio, M., Francey, S. M., Cosgrave, E. M., Killackey, E., Stanford, C., Godfrey, K., Buckby, J. (2005). Mapping the onset of psychosis: The comprehensive assessment of at-risk mental states. *Australian and New Zealand Journal of Psychiatry, 39*(11–12), 964–971. doi: 10.1111/j.1440-1614.2005.01714.x

3

Overview of Early Psychosis Service Development in Singapore: The EPIP Story

Yee Huei Yong and Swapna Verma

A study of Singaporean patients with first-episode psychosis found that the Duration of Untreated Psychosis (DUP) ranged from 0.1 to 336 months, with a mean of 32.6 months and a median of 12 months (Chong, Mythily, & Verma, 2005). A long DUP is associated with greater disabilities, long and more frequent hospitalizations, disruption in family, suicides, and higher health care costs.

There may be several factors that contribute to a long DUP, including: ignorance, stigma, denial, lack of motivation, absence of information about early psychosis, and lack of access to appropriate intervention. In Singapore, the manifestations of psychosis are often attributed to supernatural causes: around 24% of patients with first-episode psychosis had sought help from traditional healers at the first onset of symptoms (Chong et al., 2005). The alarmingly long DUP in Singapore and the possible dire consequences were the impetus for establishing the Early Psychosis Intervention Programme (EPIP).

EPIP was initiated in April 2001 under the auspices of the Ministry of Health, Singapore. The aims of EPIP are to:

- raise awareness of and reduce stigma associated with psychosis
- establish links with primary health care providers and collaborate in the detection, referral, and management of those with psychosis
- improve the outcome of EPIP patients and reduce the burden of care on their families

Our Strategies

Public education

To reach out to the public, EPIP has engaged a multiplicity of approaches: media (radio shows, TV documentary dramas, newspapers, and magazines), an easy-to-read book on psychosis, posters in train stations, public forums, art exhibitions, and a website (www.epip.org.sg).

One of the outreach partners is Silver Ribbon Singapore (SRS). SRS is a not-for-profit organization aiming to promote positive attitudes towards mental health within the community. In conjunction with SRS, EPIP launched *A View from the Other Side*, a video on psychosis co-written and produced by students from Singapore Polytechnic during an outreach event. Other collaborations included a rock concert, a film screening, public talks, and a walkathon.

EPIP also collaborates closely with the Singapore Health Promotion Board in various health promotion events for young people. In particular, it has close work relationships with the team from *Audible Hearts*, a youth-led online peer support service.

Working with primary health care providers

Singapore Armed Forces (SAF)

Singapore has a conscript army for males aged between 18 to 23 years old. EPIP has established a system to facilitate referrals and co-manage EPIP patients from the SAF. It also holds regular sessions with the SAF psychiatrists to discuss patient management.

General practitioners (GPs)

The EPIP–GP Partnership Programme was initiated to involve GPs in the care and management of stable patients and right-site the care within the community.

School counsellors

Counsellors from post-secondary educational institutes function as EPIP's "eyes" and refer cases to EPIP. If a student is accepted to the programme, counsellors will subsequently work collaboratively with EPIP to manage him or her. Ongoing networking and booster training sessions with these counsellors ensure ongoing education and collaboration.

Clinical services

Case management

EPIP began its work by adopting a holistic framework where treatment included more than medications, such as addressing social or psychological concerns of patients and their families. This marked a significant transition from the traditional approach where patients were seen only by a doctor when they came for their appointments in the hospital. With EPIP, the case manager is a central point of contact for each patient and plays various roles, such as individual and family counsellor, broker, mentor, and mediator, to aid the patient through recovery. Thus, these extensive services can range from helping the patient to find lodgings, providing psychoeducation on the illness, to referring the patient to various resources available in Singapore. Case managers see their patients when they come for their medical appointments, make regular phone contacts with them, and make home visits when necessary. Mainly, case managers offer support to the patients especially when they are going through stressful periods, such as during exams or job-seeking. When necessary, case managers also work systemically, engaging patients and their families in counselling sessions. In the event that a patient is assessed to benefit from structured in-depth psychotherapy, he or she will be referred to a psychologist. Referral is also made for assessment of any cognitive impairment. As a result, EPIP is now recognized as a leader in psychiatric case management and carries out training and official attachments for other mental health professionals.

EPIP Active Programme

The EPIP Active Programme was officially launched in February 2005 with initial support from Johnson & Johnson as part of *Give2Asia*, their global philanthropic initiative. The Active Programme is conducted in a drop-in centre called Club EPIP (see Chapter 19, "Community Psychosocial Intervention in Early Psychosis"). The Club provides a relaxed, warm, and comfortable environment for assessment, rehabilitation, and discussion on reintegrating patients back to school or work. The Club provides a chance for inpatients to interact outside a ward environment and prepares them for transition before discharge. Outpatients also benefit from coming to the Club to interact with other patients and engage in activities during the transition period before going back to school or workplace. The various activities conducted at the Club improve patients' social interaction skills and encourage them to support one another. They also help patients create their own support network while coping with their illnesses.

Initially, social and recreational activities were conducted by administrative support personnel and case managers, and included sports, personal grooming, and artwork. But recognizing the usefulness of therapy through activities, an occupational therapist joined the team in 2007. Group-based activities continue to be carried out for patients by the occupational therapist with the assistance of an assistant. On top of group-based activities, the occupational therapist also conducts other assessments, such as the patient's ability to take care of daily needs, his or her physical functioning, and cognitive functioning. When necessary, the occupational therapist also conducts onsite work assessments. The EPIP Active Programme recognizes that recovery does not mean merely being free of psychotic symptoms, but integration back into society with meaningful lives is equally important.

Patients and families

In EPIP, patients and their families are actively involved in some of the programmes, facilitate support groups, and contribute to a quarterly newsletter. One example is EPIP Day, which was launched in 2007. EPIP Day is an annual event honouring exceptional, promising, and inspirational people. Through this event, EPIP acknowledge and award clients for their efforts towards recovery as well as caregivers for their tireless contributions. In addition, this is an occasion to thank volunteers, various organizations and hospital management for their continuous support. One of the highlights of the programme is having clients share their personal journeys of struggle and recovery.

EPIP Voice is a quarterly newsletter that is distributed to all EPIP patients and their families, which reports various activities at Club EPIP, new programmes at the hospital, and other youth-related topics such as personal growth and interpersonal relationship. Patients are welcome to contribute articles, creating a chance for them to improve their writing skills while creating a sense of ownership.

In 2004, EPIP started its first English caregivers' workshop which aims to equip caregivers with an understanding of the illness and treatment, psychosocial interventions, their role and ways of looking after themselves, preventing relapse, and managing crises. The workshop also informs carers of community resources and ways to improve communication between patients and their family. As the number of EPIP patients grew, a Chinese-language version of the workshop was added. Over time this workshop has created a platform for families to share their experiences and support each other. For example, in 2010, a caregiver of a patient in our programme shared with other families her journey with her son and how she coped with his illness.

New initiatives

In 2007, EPIP became a part of the Ministry of Health's National Mental Health Programme. This five-year blueprint looks at mental health promotion, integrated mental health care, development of mental health manpower, and research on a national level. With this additional support and funding from the Ministry, EPIP launched two new initiatives.

Support for the Wellness Achievement Programme (SWAP)

SWAP, launched in April 2008, is a service that promotes early detection and provides intervention for distressed youths who present with prodromal symptoms or at-risk mental states. As not all individuals with at-risk mental state eventually develop full-blown psychosis, participants in SWAP are not given antipsychotic medications. Instead, case managers follow up closely each person using psychosocial interventions. Before SWAP was established, several factors were taken into consideration to create a less stigmatizing environment for youths to seek assessment, including the name and location of the clinic. The name "SWAP" was finally chosen as it is non-labelling and has no direct reference to mental health or psychiatric services. A neighbourhood polyclinic setting was chosen so as to improve accessibility and encourage more individuals in distress to seek for necessary assessment and treatment.

Youth Mental Health Outreach: Community Health Assessment Team (CHAT)

In an ongoing attempt to encourage youths to seek help early, barriers to early help-seeking were identified. These included unnecessary obstacles such as long-waiting times and cumbersome referral processes, stigma of seeking assessment and treatment on mental health problems, and a gap in the provision of mental health assessment services for youths in post-secondary education.

Under the funding of the Ministry of Health, Singapore, EPIP launched the Community Health Assessment Team (CHAT) programme in April 2009 with the aim to promote awareness of youth mental health issues, to increase accessibility and use of mental health services in this population, and to streamline referral process for youths to access mental health services. For distressed youths, CHAT seeks to intervene before severe symptoms and deterioration in functioning become entrenched, which may otherwise lead to enduring disability such as school failure and impaired unemployment.

The CHAT hub is strategically located at *SCAPE in Orchard Road, a place where youths often hang out after school. The location is an important consideration as it provides the pool of youths that CHAT aims to serve. Also, by being situated in this prime location associated with leisure and fun activities, EPIP trusts that youths will be more forthcoming when seeking mental health information and services. The hub is designed as a youth-friendly place, with bright colours and a functional layout, for not just conducting assessment and training, but also for use as a resource centre and a place where youths can meet with the CHAT team to discuss youth-related projects. Given that the medium to reach out and influence youths is important, CHAT set up its own youth website and Facebook page. With the availability of such popular social media, youth can readily access mental health information in a fun and light-hearted way.

CHAT also liaises with various education institutions, encouraging school counsellors to refer students with possible mental health problems to the hub for a free assessment provided by a doctor and a youth support worker. The team's impression of the problem, recommendations, and suggestions are then communicated to the counsellor. CHAT also trains school student leaders to equip them with skills needed to look out for peers who may be in distress and need early assessment.

Conclusion

The journey for a young person struck with a mental illness is not an easy one and is often a frightening process. Many times, a young person with first-episode psychosis denies the illness and any uncertainty about the future. The process is also tough for family members who take care of them. Thus, patient care instilled with hope is important. This early phase is also crucial to psychoeducate patients that they can recover if they manage their illness and take appropriate steps in preventing a relapse. Throughout the years, mental health services have also evolved, from focusing mainly on medical treatment to a more holistic intervention. EPIP has moved away from the traditional approach of seeing the patient in the clinic or hospital to engaging the patient via phone calls or less formal meet-ups. This method allows problems to be identified early and appropriate intervention put in place before problems worsen. EPIP also shifts the focus away from just treating an illness symptomatically to looking at how environmental systems perpetuate illness. Youth outreach is an important component of promoting awareness of mental health, encouraging youth to come forward for earlier treatment.

References

Chong, S. A., Mythily, S., & Lum, A., Chan, Y. H., & McGorry, P. (2005). Determinants of duration of untreated psychosis and the pathway to care in Singapore. *International Journal of Social Psychiatry, 51*(1), 55–62.

Chong, S. A., Mythily, S., & Verma, S. (2005). Reducing the duration of untreated psychosis and changing help-seeking behaviour in Singapore. *Social Psychiatry and Psychiatric Epidemiology, 40*(8), 619–621. doi: 10.1007/s00127-005-0948–4

4

Early Psychosis Intervention in an Urban Japanese Setting: Overview of Early Psychosis Services in Japan

Masafumi Mizuno, Takahiro Nemoto, and Naohisa Tsujino

Historical Background of Psychiatric Services in Japan

For decades, Japanese psychiatric services have been predominantly hospital-based. Many psychiatrists who are more oriented to psychosocial or integrated approaches have been struggling with this conservative system and trying to achieve a transition to community-based psychiatry. However, to date, there have few profound changes. The number of psychiatric inpatients is still large, and most admissions are long-term.

In Japan, "mental disorder" is usually taken to mean "depression" or "adjustment disorder". However, the real world of psychiatric conditions in this country is more serious, with the psychiatric wards having some 300,000 beds and around 30,000 suicides occurring every year. What lies between these two "realities" is a somewhat shadowy world that traps many patients and even professionals in the psychiatry field.

The number of mental hospitals in Japan increased during the rapid economic growth post-World War II, during comprehensive renewal of the nation's infrastructure. Since then, even more mental hospitals have been built and, fuelled by the lack of social acceptance, more and more psychiatric patients have been institutionalized and forced into social isolation. Thus, the current biggest task for psychiatry in Japan is deinstitutionalization.

There has been a slight decline in the number of psychiatric beds since 1994. However, the number is still high compared with other developed countries, being 2.9 per 1,000 people in Japan versus 0.9 in the UK and 0.5 in the US. Such extreme reliance on hospital-based psychiatry is a barrier to the development of community-based psychiatry. The total number of inpatients in Japanese psychiatric wards was about 332,000 in June 2008. Several nationwide surveys have shown that approximately 20% to 40% of these patients could be discharged if appropriate support services were available. These cases are called "social admissions", as it is the deficiency of social support services that forces the patient into hospital. Despite the challenges, some innovative hospitals have attempted to promote a transition to community-based psychiatry through their own endeavours.

The difficulties faced by innovative hospitals are related to characteristics of the Japanese national health system and laws regarding psychiatric hospitals. In Japan, all citizens are covered by a national health plan and have access to a wide range of medical resources, for which they pay only 10%–30% of the actual cost, while the remaining cost is covered by the national health insurance scheme. Thus, a nominal fee is paid for each service and these fees are regulated by a national uniform reimbursement schedule that does not favour community-based psychiatry. Even though there have been gradual improvements over the last ten years, including the creation of a new category for nurses visiting patients in their home (outreach activities) and a decrease in the payments for inpatients as the length of hospital stay increases, however, there is still no category for early intervention in the national health reimbursement schedule. This slow and incomplete transition to community-based psychiatry leaves Japan a long way from being an "inclusive society" and remains a reason for stigmatizing patients with schizophrenia. As for the legal system, the Medical Care Act defines the minimum number of psychiatrists required by psychiatric hospitals as one per forty-eight inpatients, which is only one-third that of the number for general hospitals, while one nurse is needed per four inpatients (versus one per three inpatients in general hospitals).

Despite these conditions, in keeping with the trend towards early intervention and the raising of several issues regarding mental health services, the Japanese Ministry of Health, Welfare, and Labour (MHWL) has injected research funds into early intervention by providing a Health Labour Sciences Research Grant to Masafumi Mizuno (principal investigator). According to the results obtained so far, the mean duration of untreated psychosis (DUP) was 17.6 months at seven university hospitals, where people could present for assistance without much stigmatization. The DUP would probably be longer if data from conventional psychiatric hospitals were included, especially those in rural areas where stigma associated with mental illness is stronger. Unexpectedly, about 10% of patients with a first episode of schizophrenia on the first day of consulting a psychiatrist had already attempted suicide by a potentially lethal method. This could mean that quite a number of suicides are due to untreated psychosis in Japan. Regrettably, DUP is relatively long, even though Japan is an advanced country with abundant medical resources, including a public health insurance system for all citizens. Recently, the MHWL has started a website for young adolescents to inform them about the importance of early intervention for mental illness (www.mhlw.go.jp/kokoro/youth/).

According to the Medical Care Act, from 2013, mental illness will be added to the list of four conventional designated illnesses, i.e. cancer, stroke, acute myocardial infarction, and diabetes mellitus, for which prefectures have to prepare health care plans. The numbers of patients with mental illness is increasing up to 3.2 million, and the number exceeds cancers (1.5 million) and diabetes mellitus (2.4 million). This reform aims to supply broader and continuous medical services including prevention and early treatment. Following this implementation of the medical care planning, numerical targets will be set to check whether the plans prepared by the prefectures are successful. Data concerning the numerical targets will be collected continuously. The introduction of health care planning for mental illnesses will provide a valuable opportunity for psychiatric care professionals to reform the psychiatric care system and improving the quality of care.

Japanese Society for Prevention and Early Intervention in Psychiatry (JSEIP)

The JSEIP (www.jseip.jp) is an organization for people involved in the study and treatment of psychiatric disorders in Japan. This group provides a forum for members to promote practice and research, based on medical ethics, into the prevention of psychiatric disorders, to arrange conferences and professional meetings regarding the prevention of psychiatric disorders, to facilitate research (including multicentre trials), and enhance other efforts to achieve end goals. The JSEIP was inaugurated in March 1996 in Okinawa, following the first symposium on primary prevention of schizophrenia held at the 16th meeting of the Japanese Society of Social Psychiatry.

In 2007, the 10th annual academic conference was held in Yokohama emphasized multicentre research on early psychosis in Japan. The JSEIP has more than 300 members.

Il Bosco

A representative early intervention facility for young people is "Il Bosco" (www.lab.toho-u.ac.jp/med/omori/mentalhealth/), where the authors and their colleagues work. Founded in May 2007 at the Toho University Omori Medical Centre in Tokyo, the DUP of the hospital catchment area is longer (mean, 30 months) compared with other areas of Tokyo. The unit is run according to an optimal treatment project (OTP), employing a multidisciplinary team approach that utilizes cognitive remediation-oriented methods advocated by Ian R. Falloon (1992). The service model includes early detection and intervention, repeated assessment, and psychoeducation.

Treatment strategies consist of optimal pharmacotherapy based on atypical neuroleptics, cognitive function training, cognitive behavioural therapy, and job coaching as the final treatment programme. The cognitive function training aims to stimulate divergent thinking and in the main, is computer-based. Both patients with chronic schizophrenia and those with their first-episode schizophrenia (FES) show cognitive impairments affecting a wide range of domains. People with an at-risk mental state (ARMS) also exhibit cognitive deficits, although they usually demonstrate superior performance compared with schizophrenic patients. Since cognitive impairment significantly influences social functioning, cognitive intervention at the early stage of schizophrenia is often preferable. This cognitive training programme targets divergent thinking deficits because previous interventions for divergent thinking have been proven to significantly improve negative symptoms and social functioning in patients with schizophrenia (Nemoto et al., 2009). Cognitive intervention such as this may maximize the chance for functional recovery and such intervention may minimize the risk of future progression in a subset of people with ARMS because divergent thinking is critical for generating solutions to various social problems and for navigating the complexities of social interactions.

At Il Bosco, the staff ratios are higher than those typically found at day care services for chronic patients, which are restricted by the health insurance system to three professionals (one nurse, one occupational therapist, and one social worker or clinical psychologist). The additional staffing at Il Bosco is made possible by the parent hospital plus a research grant from the government. Details of Il Bosco are shown in Table 4.1.

The clients are restricted to ARMS patients or first-episode schizophrenia patients between the ages of 15 and 30 years. Four years have passed since the

Table 4.1
Characteristics of "Il Bosco"

Office area	132 m^2
Opening hours	9:00 am to 5:00 pm
Professional staff*	5.5 (1 psychiatrist, 1 resident, 1 occupational therapist, 1 nurse, 1 social worker 1, and a part-time clinical psychologist)
Non-professional staff	1.5 (1 part-time administrator, 1 educator)

* Note: Each full-time member (working 5 days a week) is counted as 1.

opening of Il Bosco, and so far 112 patients (62 women and 50 men; mean age 20.4 ± 3.5 years) have been registered. Many patients have improved through participation in the rehabilitation programme that focuses on social cognition, and have returned to their former workplace or school. Some patients have shown dramatic improvement of negative symptoms and global functioning, as assessed by the Global Assessment of Functioning (GAF) scale. The attendance rate is better than that of the previous standard day care service, which had no age limit. The team is currently developing new programmes for cognitive rehabilitation and remediation, as well as a psychoeducation website for early psychosis. As of June 2011, a total of 64 clients (57%) have returned to school or to the same level of employment as pre-illness.

Tokyo Youth Club

Minato Net 21, a non-profit organization in Japan, is the Tokyo centre of the Optimal Treatment Project, an international project advocated by the late Ian Falloon that aims to collect data and develop effective evidence-based treatment strategies for mental illness.

Minato Net 21 has designed a website for the Tokyo Youth Club (www.tokyo-yc.org/) to provide the latest information on mental health. The aim is early detection and intervention to prevent the onset of psychosis, as part of the strategies of the Optimal Treatment Project. The website gives general information about schizophrenia, including its prodromal signs and pathology, as well as the latest biopsychosocial treatment. The site stresses the importance of early intervention for achieving a good prognosis. This project has been named "project DUP zero", reflecting the goal of shortening DUP. A revised version of the self-administered "Yale University PRIME Screening Test" has been translated into Japanese (Kobayashi et al., 2008), so that people who visit the website can take the screening test. And if they match the criteria and feel that they need help, they can select one of the collaborating medical facilities for an initial consultation. Also, emails sent to the site are answered directly and referral is provided to an appropriate clinic or hospital when required. Information is also available for family members because older people continue to have a strong prejudice against psychiatric care and may not support their child's wish to consult a psychiatrist.

The home page contains animations and friendly logos targeting teenagers and young adults who may be at risk. The goal of the website is to promote knowledge of mental health among young people and to help create pathways to professional consultation, thus either preventing the onset of psychosis or reducing the DUP to improve the prognosis.

Other Leading Centres for Early Intervention in Japan

In addition to this service, there are several leading centres for early intervention research and practice in Japan. Most of them are driven by university departments of psychiatry with respect to both research and clinical activities. The common aims of these services are: (1) to provide young people suspected to be at risk with opportunities of receiving assessment by specialists and specific intervention, (2) to reduce delay in accessing evidence-based treatment for persons who already have psychosis, especially a first episode of schizophrenia, and (3) to develop innovative and optimized approaches for diagnosing and treating people at risk of psychosis. Each centre also has its own research projects, with some contributing to the development of early access and intervention systems, while others focusing on elucidation of the biological basis of schizophrenia (Table 4.2).

Research and Education for Specialists

Research has focused on both the biological and psychosocial aspects of early schizophrenia. Studies have demonstrated the anatomical basis of the schizophrenia spectrum in the brain (Suzuki et al., 2005), the effect of DUP on brain morphology (Takahashi et al., 2007), and the applicability of structural brain imaging to the objective diagnosis of schizophrenia (Kawasaki et al., 2007). The

Table 4.2
Leading research and clinical centres in Japan

Centre	Location
Consultation and Support Service in Toyama (CAST) www.med.u-toyama.ac.jp/neuropsychiatry/index-kokoro.html	Toyama city
Il Bosco, Toho University Omori Medical Center www.lab.toho-u.ac.jp/med/omori/mentalhealth/	Ota City, Tokyo
Risk Unit in the University of Tokyo Hospital http://plaza.umin.ac.jp/arms-ut/	Bunkyo City, Tokyo
Sendai At-Risk Mental State and First Episode Service (SAFE) http://safe-youthcentre.jp/	Sendai City
Tokyo Youth Club www.tokyo-yc.org/	Minato City, Tokyo
Youth Mental Support Center Mie (YMSC MIE) www.pref.mie.lg.jp/KOKOROHP/HP/souki/index.htm	Tsu City
Youth Mental Support Center in Matsuzawa (WAKABA) www.byouin.metro.tokyo.jp/matsuzawa/wakaba/index.html	Setagaya City, Tokyo

influence of DUP on brain function has also been investigated (Nishii et al., 2010; Yamazawa et al., 2008). Development of screening methods for ARMS (Kobayashi et al., 2008), assessment of ARMS (Miyakoshi et al., 2009), and psychopathological studies on psychosis-like experiences have been reported (Kinoshita et al., 2011; Nishida et al., 2010), contributing to early intervention and supports for adolescents in Japan. Both comprehensive and pharmacological approaches (Kobayashi et al., 2009) to treatment have been investigated. Moreover, several important English monographs about early intervention in psychiatry by leading researchers in this field have been translated into Japanese (Jackson & McGorry, 2009; McGlashan, Walsh, & Woods, 2010; McGorry & Jackson, 1999).

Conclusion

The development of early intervention services is expected to provide a breakthrough in the treatment of psychosis in Japan, including reduction of prejudice, prevention of suicide among young persons, and the promotion of general knowledge about mental health. There are several common or similar aspects, including the service system, community attitudes to psychiatric illness (including prejudice), and dependence on pharmacotherapy, among Asian countries. One of the possible solutions is coexistence, which has traditionally been practised in East Asia including old Japan.

References

Falloon, I. R. (1992). Early intervention for first episodes of schizophrenia: A preliminary exploration. *Psychiatry, 55*(1), 4–15.

Jackson, H. J., & McGorry, P. D. (2009). *The Recognition and Management of Early Psychosis: A Preventive Approach* (2nd ed.). Cambridge, UK; New York: Cambridge University Press.

Kawasaki, Y., Suzuki, M., Kherif, F., Takahashi, T., Zhou, S. Y., Nakamura, K., et al. (2007). Multivariate voxel-based morphometry successfully differentiates schizophrenia patients from healthy controls. *Neuroimage, 34*(1), 235–242. doi: S1053-8119(06)00840-8 [pii]10.1016/j.neuroimage.2006.08.018

Kinoshita, Y., Shimodera, S., Nishida, A., Kinoshita, K., Watanabe, N., Oshima, N., et al. (2011). Psychotic-like experiences are associated with violent behavior in adolescents. *Schizophrenia Research, 126*(1–3), 245–251. doi: S0920-9964(10)01499-4 [pii]10.1016/j.schres.2010.08.028

Kobayashi, H., Morita, K., Takeshi, K., Koshikawa, H., Yamazawa, R., Kashima, H., et al. (2009). Effects of aripiprazole on insight and subjective experience in individuals with an at-risk mental state. *Journal of Clinical Psychopharmacology, 29*(5), 421–425. doi: 10.1097/JCP.0b013e3181b2fe2200004714-200910000-00003 [pii]

Kobayashi, H., Nemoto, T., Koshikawa, H., Osono, Y., Yamazawa, R., Murakami, M., et al. (2008). A self-reported instrument for prodromal symptoms of psychosis: Testing the clinical validity of the PRIME Screen-Revised (PS-R) in a Japanese population. *Schizophrenia Research, 106*(2–3), 356–362. doi: S0920-9964(08)00380-0 [pii]10.1016/j.schres.2008.08.018

McGlashan, T. H., Walsh, B., & Woods, S. (2010). *The Psychosis-Risk Syndrome: Handbook for Diagnosis and Follow-Up*. New York: Oxford University Press.

McGorry, P. D., & Jackson, H. J. (1999). *The Recognition and Management of Early Psychosis: A Preventive Approach*. New York: Cambridge University Press.

Miyakoshi, T., Matsumoto, K., Ito, F., Ohmuro, N., & Matsuoka, H. (2009). Application of the Comprehensive Assessment of At-Risk Mental States (CAARMS) to the Japanese population: Reliability and validity of the Japanese version of the CAARMS. *Early Intervention in Psychiatry, 3*(2), 123–130. doi: 10.1111/j.1751-7893.2009.00118.x

Nemoto, T., Yamazawa, R., Kobayashi, H., Fujita, N., Chino, B., Fujii, C., et al. (2009). Cognitive training for divergent thinking in schizophrenia: A pilot study. *Prog Neuropsychopharmacological Biology in Psychiatry, 33*(8), 1533–1536. doi: S0278-5846(09)00285-1 [pii]10.1016/j.pnpbp.2009.08.015

Nishida, A., Sasaki, T., Nishimura, Y., Tanii, H., Hara, N., Inoue, K., et al. (2010). Psychotic-like experiences are associated with suicidal feelings and deliberate self-harm behaviors in adolescents aged 12–15 years. *Acta Psychiatrica Scandinavica, 121*(4), 301–307. doi: ACP1439 [pii]10.1111/j.1600–0447.2009.01439.x

Nishii, H., Yamazawa, R., Shimodera, S., Suzuki, M., Hasegawa, T., & Mizuno, M. (2010). Clinical and social determinants of a longer duration of untreated psychosis of schizophrenia in a Japanese population. *Early Intervention in Psychiatry, 4*(2), 182–188. doi: EIP179 [pii]10.1111/j.1751–7893.2010.00179.x

Suzuki, M., Zhou, S. Y., Takahashi, T., Hagino, H., Kawasaki, Y., Niu, L., et al. (2005). Differential contributions of prefrontal and temporolimbic pathology to mechanisms of psychosis. *Brain, 128*(Pt 9), 2109–2122. doi: awh554 [pii]10.1093/brain/awh554

Takahashi, T., Suzuki, M., Tanino, R., Zhou, S. Y., Hagino, H., Niu, L., et al. (2007). Volume reduction of the left planum temporale gray matter associated with long duration of untreated psychosis in schizophrenia: A preliminary report. *Psychiatry Research, 154*(3), 209–219. doi: S0925–4927(06)00157–0 [pii]10.1016/j.pscychresns.2006.10.001

Yamazawa, R., Nemoto, T., Kobayashi, H., Chino, B., Kashima, H., & Mizuno, M. (2008). Association between duration of untreated psychosis, premorbid functioning, and cognitive performance and the outcome of first-episode schizophrenia in Japanese patients: Prospective study. *Australian and New Zealand Journal of Psychiatry, 42*(2), 159–165. doi: 789607005 [pii]10.1080/00048670701787537

5
Overview of the Development of Services for Early Psychosis in Korea

Young-chul Chung, Guang-biao Huang, and Keun-Young Oh

An old Chinese book of traditional medicine offered the following advice to practitioners: "Do not treat a disease that has already been, treat before it starts (不治已病，治未病)". Although well established in the context of serious physical illnesses, the strategy of early intervention has been ignored for many decades with respect to psychotic disorders due to pessimism, stigma, and neglect regarding the treatment of conditions such as schizophrenia. Recently, however, the notion of early intervention in psychotic disorders has generated significant interest and optimism in many countries. To this end, the effective identification and intervention in early psychosis require a coordinated process from a diverse spectrum of socio-clinical services. Within this context, this chapter describes issues related to services for early psychosis in Korea, such as the role of community psychiatry and clinical networks, the development of optimal psychosocial treatments, renaming the disorder, and sociopolitical considerations.

Background

The lifetime prevalence and incidence of schizophrenia range from 0.30% to 0.66% and 10.2 to 22.0 per 100,000 person-years, respectively (McGrath et al., 2008). A systematic review of all reported studies of the prevalence and incidence of subclinical psychotic experiences found a overall median prevalence rate of 5.3% and a median incidence rate of 3.1% (van Os et al., 2009). The 2000 Global Burden of Disease study reported that 23,182 deaths worldwide were related to schizophrenia, a figure higher than that for unipolar depressive disorders (12,044) (Ustun et al., 2004). Moreover, active psychosis is the third most disabling health condition in the world, following only quadriplegia and dementia in terms of its impact (Ustun et al., 1999). Not surprisingly, improving the outcomes of patients with schizophrenia remains a primary mission of psychiatry. To accomplish this goal, two key philosophical questions must be asked: (1) Can early intervention techniques really prevent or decrease the incidence of schizophrenia in those at high risk for psychosis; and (2) can optimal biopsychosocial treatment during the critical period of five years following the onset of psychosis really stop the progression of the illness?

At present, these questions remain unanswered because schizophrenia is a highly heterogeneous disease characterized by multiple aetiological factors and varied outcomes. Irrespective of the current state of data in this domain, the pursuit of answers to these two questions remains of paramount importance. Indeed, this mission requires an evangelical spirit, given that strong convictions and a readiness to endure prejudice and hardships are required for this task. This spirit lies at the core of the early psychosis movement.

Major figures in psychiatry have historically emphasized the importance of the early identification of psychosis. Kraepelin (1987) noted that "it is of the greatest importance to diagnose cases of *dementia praecox* with certainty and at an early stage". Sullivan (1994) wrote, "I feel certain that many incipient cases might be arrested before the efficient contact with reality is completely suspended, and a long stay in institutions made necessary." In modern times, Falloon (1992) engaged in pioneering work to decrease the incidence of schizophrenia by educating family practitioners to recognize prodromal symptoms. This pioneering spirit was later embodied by McGorry (1996), who catalysed the worldwide early psychosis movement. Following the publication of several key papers by McGorry and colleagues in the *Schizophrenia Bulletin* (McGlashan & Johannessen, 1996; McGorry et al., 1996; Yung & McGorry, 1996), early intervention in psychotic disorders has generated significant interest and optimism in many countries and prompted policy-makers to place a high priority on this effort. Currently, nearly 200 early intervention centres operate worldwide.

This chapter introduces several key trends and situations relevant to the early psychosis movement in Korea, namely (1) an increasing emphasis on community psychiatry including screening and early detection; (2) optimal psychosocial treatment during the critical period; and (3) renaming schizophrenia.

The Role of Community Psychiatry in the Screening and Early Detection of Psychosis

Since the enactment of mental health legislation in 1995, the number of mental health centres in Korea has steadily increased and stands at 164 in 2011. The initial primary services offered by these centres involved registering patients, providing day treatment, and managing the cases of patients with chronic schizophrenia. Recently, however, the major focus of mental health centres has shifted from rehabilitation to early intervention. The annual guidelines issued by the Ministry of Education, Science and Technology (MEST) recommend to operate one centre per 200,000 population.

In the service of preventing mental illness and promoting mental health, these centres engage in a variety of activities such as awareness campaigns, lectures on mental health for the general public, mental health workshops for school health teachers and counsellors, free online counselling, outreach counselling, school mental health projects.

Given that adolescence and the early 20s constitute the most common ages for the onset of mental illness (Lee et al., 2001), school mental health projects have been of particular importance in prevention and early detection. These projects began in 2002 and are now actively pursued in 52 mental health centres nationwide. In brief, each local mental health centre (1) seeks to engage in partnerships with schools interested in promoting mental health of students as well as in operating Wee Education Emotion (WEE) centres organized by the Ministry of Education, Science and Technology (MEST) to provide one-stop counselling services for students; (2) administers secondary screening tests such as the Child Behavior Checklist (CBCL) (Achenbach & Edelbrock, 1983), the Youth Self-Report (YSR) (Achenbach, 1991), or the Beck Depression Inventory (BDI; Beck et al., 1961) to those who score high on primary screening tests such as the Child Problems Screening Questionnaire (CPSQ) (Ahn, 2007) or the Adolescent Mental Health and Problem-behaviour Questionnaire (AMPQ) (Ahn, 2007) conducted by the MEST; (3) provides psychiatrists to conduct in-depth diagnostic interviews with students who obtain scores indicative of psychopathology on the screening tests; and (4) refers those diagnosed with a mental disorder to a hospital or private clinic and those diagnosed with subsyndromal, borderline, or high-risk characteristics to school-based interventions such as individual counselling or group programmes. Recently, some local schools in Seoul refused to participate in the screening project because of stigma issues. Nevertheless, as the ever-increasing rates of suicide, school violence, and bullying are becoming serious social issues in Korea, most schools and parents do not oppose screening project per se. It should be kept in mind that special attention should be paid to not causing unintentional damage during treatment, and to avoiding unnecessary conflicts with parents.

Use of the aforementioned standard measures and more specialized screening instruments in the early detection of individuals at high risk for psychosis remains important. Thus, the Eppendorf Schizophrenia Inventory (ESI; Mass, Haasen, & Borgart, 2005) was standardized for this purpose in Korea (Kwon, Chung, & Lee, 2006). Several centres have posted the ESI on their websites and used this instrument in school mental health projects. According to a large-scale school-based survey, the rate at which subjects scored at or greater than the cut-off level on the ESI (29 is the suggested score for detecting individuals at high risk for psychosis) was 6.55% (78/1,190) (Chung et al., 2012). Of those with this score, only 15 (1.26%) were identified as being at high risk for psychosis based on the Comprehensive Assessment of At-Risk Mental States (CAARMS; Yung et al., 2005). Additionally, the Peters Delusions Inventory (PDI; Peters, Joseph, & Garety, 1999), used to measure delusional ideations in general populations, has been standardized by Jung et al. (2008). In the absence of a universally accepted instrument for identification of the at-risk mental state population, the application of PDI to screening was explored in Korea. The PDI is a widely used scale to capture subclinical psychotic experience with good sensitivity for subclinical delusional ideations. Based on item response theory, the PDI-21 and the Korean version of the Magical Ideation Scale (Choi & Yang, 1997) have been shown to complement each other with different thresholds in assessing the delusional ideation of Korean non-clinical adolescents (Kim et al., 2011). Several questionnaires useful for the mass screening of early detection for individuals at a high risk for psychosis are summarized in Table 5.1.

In 2008, the MEST joined the school mental health project to support all efforts to attend to mental health issues during childhood and adolescence. Since 2008, the MEST has assumed the role of conducting primary mass screening tests while mental health centres have continued to care for those referred for treatment on the basis of these tests. At the community mental health centre, short-term (4–6 sessions) counselling or psychotherapy is provided if the intensity of distress and functional impairment is not severe. If the condition is assessed to be severe, individuals will be referred to hospital services. This cooperative system represents a collaborative model in which

Table 5.1
Summary of results from self-administered questionnaires used for mass screenings to identify individuals at high risk for psychosis

Questionnaire	Structure	Related findings
ESI (Mass 2000; Mass et al., 2005)	40 items, four subdomains (attentional and speech impairment, auditory uncertainty, ideas of reference, and deviant perceptions)	• Confirmed reliability and diagnostic validity for schizophrenia • The cutoff for the Korean version was 29
PQ (Loewy et al., 2005; Loewy & Cannon 2008)	92-item self-report screening measure, four major subscales (positive symptoms, negative symptoms, disorganized symptoms, and general symptoms)	• Shows good validity in detecting individuals with prodromal and psychotic symptoms • Brief version (25-item) (Loewy & Cannon, 2008) might be a more useful screening test
CAPE (Konings et al., 2006)	42-item instrument based primarily on the 21-item Delusions Inventory developed by Peters et al. (2004) (three dimensions: positive, negative, and depressive)	• Appears to be stable, reliable, and valid for detecting psychotic experiences in the general population
PDI (E. Peters et al., 2004; E. R. Peters et al., 1999)	• Originally 40 items (PDI-40); the new version contains 21 items (PDI-21) • Self-report measure that assesses multidimensionality of delusional ideations in normal population	• To differentiate deluded group from healthy adults, dimensions of delusional ideations, such as distress, preoccupation and conviction are more important than the content of belief alone
Y-PARQ-B (Ord et al., 2004)	24-item measure derived from the 24 most discriminating questions on the CAARMS	• A score greater than the cutoff of 11 shows good sensitivity and specificity for prodromal attenuated psychotic symptoms

Abbreviations: CAPE, Community Assessment of Psychic Experiences; CAARMS, Comprehensive Assessment of At-Risk Mental States; ESI, Eppendorf Schizophrenia Inventory; PDI, Peters et al., Delusions Inventory; PQ-B, Prodromal Questionnaire, Brief Version; Y-PARQ-B, Abbreviated Youth Psychosis At-Risk Questionnaire.

two governmental organizations, the MEST and the Ministry for Health and Welfare (MW), collaborate in an effort to achieve the same goal. However, the MEST uses a general screening test rather than measures specifically designed to detect particular mental disorders, which decreases the precision of the screening process and may not be the most aligned development in progressing early detection.

The recent increase in metropolitan centres for mental health is another main trend in community psychiatry in Korea. Six metropolitan centres are currently in operation, and a primary objective pursued by these centres involves the identification and treatment of early psychosis. In 2009, the Seoul Mental Health Centre proposed a clinical consortium involving a partnership with several university hospitals and private clinics in Seoul to promote the early detection and optimal psychosocial intervention for those at risk for psychosis and for patients experiencing their first episode of psychosis. Additionally, the Seoul Mental Health Centre recently developed the Social Treatment for Early Psychosis (STEP) programme, which includes a CD (content downloadable at http://semis.blutouch.net/page/page51.php). More efficient networks and more diverse programmes will emerge as the number of metropolitan centres increases.

Furthermore, in 2011, the MW announced a nationwide community service investment plan that includes the complete range of services needed by individuals with mental illness. Total care service, a concept driven by assertive community treatment, provides counselling, crisis intervention, medication management, and support in pursuit of social adaptation and employment. This approach, which involves the provision of services at least four times per week, is expected to enhance the quality of case management by decreasing the current caseload in community mental health centres from approximately 1:50 to about 1:20.

Korean Network of Early Psychosis

The Korean Network of Early Psychosis (K-NEP) was organized in 2005 initially with 13 centres participating. With the help of an unrestricted educational funding from the Janssen Pharmaceutical Company in Korea, K-NEP launched several important projects aimed at facilitating the activities and goals of the early psychosis movement. First, the current self-administered questionnaires and interview tools addressing psychosis were thoroughly reviewed to identify valid, reliable, and simple instruments that might be useful for detecting early psychosis. The ESI and the Early Recognition Inventory retrospective assessment of the onset and course of schizophrenia and other psychoses (ERIroas) checklist/interview (Hafner et al., 2004) were among those reviewed. The CAARMS (Yung et al., 2005), a semi-structured interview for identifying individuals at high risk for psychosis, was translated into Korean and a DVD providing CAARMS training was translated and dubbed. In 2009, a manual for the Korean version of CAARMS, several case studies of individuals at high risk for psychosis, and a set of practical tips and cautions relevant to this assessment were published by K-NEP and the Gyeonggi Metropolitan Centre of Mental Health. Additionally, K-NEP conducted a one-year prospective multicentre study on the progress of those at high risk for psychosis.

Optimal Psychosocial Treatment during the Critical Period

The concept of a critical period in the development of psychosis was proposed by Birchwood et al. (1998). Previous studies have identified the initial stages of psychosis in which patients are most vulnerable in terms of overall course of schizophrenia; the first five years after the initial presentation of psychotic symptoms were thus defined as the critical period. The literature indicated that the cumulative first-relapse rate was 81.9 % within five years after initial recovery from the first episode of schizophrenia (Robinson et al., 1999) and that more than 60% of those with schizophrenia who committed suicide did so within six years after their first hospitalization (Westermeyer, Harrow, & Marengo, 1991). Additionally, the ongoing changes in the brain of schizophrenic patients tended to occur during the initial years following the diagnosis (Ho et al., 2003). Hence, optimal psychosocial treatment, in addition to pharmacological therapy, must be provided to patients experiencing their first episodes of schizophrenia to prevent further deterioration and to help them return to their previous level of functioning.

Recently, there has been a growing interest in psychosocial intervention as a means of facilitating recovery or remission from the first episode of psychosis and early schizophrenia when the duration of illness is less than five years. A pilot study evaluating the effectiveness of individual cognitive-behavioural therapy (CBT) in the treatment of early psychosis indicated that CBT and supportive psychoeducation were acceptable treatments for inpatients with recent-onset acute psychosis (Haddock et al., 1999). Following this study, several randomized controlled trials of CBT for those with early schizophrenia or first-episode psychosis found several beneficial effects of this treatment in symptom reduction, adaptation to illness, and functioning (Jackson et al., 2008; Jolley et al., 2003; Lewis et al., 2002; Tarrier et al., 2004; Wang et al., 2003). However, some studies have not found individual CBT to be effective in reducing rates of relapse or rehospitalization (Jackson et al., 1998; Jackson et al., 2001; Jolley et al., 2003). In addition to individual CBT, multidimensional interventions that incorporate a variety of treatment modalities (e.g., pharmacological treatment, supportive therapy, case management, assertive community treatment, social skills training, family psychoeducation) are provided to individuals experiencing first-episode psychosis and encouraging results, primarily in reference to 1-year outcomes, were observed (Addington et al, 2003; Larsen et al., 2001; Nordentoft et al., 2002).

Nevertheless, treatment for schizophrenia has become increasingly biologically oriented, relying primarily on pharmacotherapy. Even though the Psychiatry Board examination in Korea requires applicants to submit interview notes for a single case where psychotherapy was performed for at least 12 sessions, these cases are usually patients with mood disorders, anxiety disorders, or personality problems. Sadly, there has been little expression of interest in psychosocial intervention for schizophrenia. In this particular climate, it is encouraging to note that the Korean Academy of Schizophrenia (KAS) published *Psychosocial Intervention for Patients with Schizophrenia in the Critical Period* (Chung et al., 2008), which promotes alternative treatment regimens. In 2009, the KAS organized a successful workshop that attracted about 90 attendees on using CBT interventions for the treatment of psychosis. Similarly, in 2008, the MW supported a two-year study on the "Development and Application of a Group Cognitive-Behavioural Therapy Program for Schizophrenic Patients in the Critical Period" (Chung, 2008) as a research and development project for health, medicine, and technology.

In an ultra-high-risk research clinic called Clinic FORYOU of the Green Program for Recognition and Prevention of Early Psychosis (GRAPE), the clinical efficacy of individual cognitive therapy in reducing psychiatric symptoms has been recently demonstrated in ultra-high-risk patients (Kim et al., 2011), and a book titled *GRAPE Cognitive Therapy: Manual for Therapists* has been published (Lee et al., 2010) detailing the procedure. The key concepts of the GRAPE programme involve the stress–vulnerability model, resilience, and normalization.

Practitioners hope that the government will increase its support for the development of diverse psychosocial treatment programmes that target patients with schizophrenia during the critical period of this disorder. To encourage more wide-ranging interest in using CBT to treat early psychosis calls for an appropriate fee structure for CBT within the medical insurance system. Currently, CBT is not covered by medical insurance in Korea and the fees for these services can legally be set at the discretion of each hospital. More active research is essential for any expansion of interest in this area.

Renaming Schizophrenia: Pros and Cons

Stigmatization remains a significant problem for individuals with mental illness, especially schizophrenia. The term "schizophrenia" comes from the Greek words *schizein* and *phren*, meaning "to split" and "mind". Countries that use the Chinese writing system translate schizophrenia as "mind-split disease" (精神分裂症). Hence, a greater negative connotation accompanies this label in Asian than in Western countries. Indeed, most people in Western countries do not speak Greek and are thereby shielded from the implications of the semantic origins of the term. Given the consensus that the term schizophrenia is a source of stigma, the Japanese Society of Psychiatry and Neurology (JSPN) changed the label *seishin bunretsu byo* (mind-split disease) to *togo shitcho sho* (integration disorder; 統合失調症) in 2002.

Influenced by this Japanese movement, the KAS has been actively engaged in changing the name of this condition to one that is more scientifically accurate and socially acceptable. In 2007, the stigma associated with the term schizophrenia was initially discussed at the summer workshop organized by the KAS under the symposium title of "Is it necessary to change the term schizophrenia?" Since that time, similar issues have been repeatedly addressed at academic conferences and workshops. In 2008, *Beautiful Companion*, an online society consisting of family members of patients with schizophrenia, initiated a signature campaign in favour of renaming schizophrenia. This group sent a 3,000-signature petition to the MW and the National Human Rights Commission. This heightened awareness prompted the KAS to take two important actions: (1) to initiate two KAS-sponsored studies on the renaming issue; and (2) to organize the Name Revision Committee for schizophrenia. Two KAS-sponsored studies, "Renaming schizophrenia in Korea" (Park & Chung, 2008) and "Study of the stigma attached to psychosis by the major media sources" (Kim et al., 2011) resulted from these actions. The major findings of the first study showed that 54% of patients, 69.9% of family members, 68.3% of the general public, and 67.3% of psychiatrists favoured renaming schizophrenia although the proposed revised names varied.

A 2009 report emanating from this study and supported by Seoul National Hospital addressed the issues of stigma and renaming (Chung et al., 2009). This particular study emerged from an international collaboration between Korea and Japan and indicated that: (1) a total of 37% of patients, 67% of family members, 57% of psychiatrists, and 71% of lay people favoured renaming schizophrenia; (2) when asked "What is the most desirable alternative name for schizophrenia?", patients and family members preferred "thought–perception sensitivity disorder" and "thought–emotion confusion disorder", whereas psychiatric residents and psychiatrists preferred "hyperdopaminergic state", "dopamine dysregulation", or "integration disorder"; and (3) in terms of academic validity, therapeutic usefulness, and dissipation of social stigma, hyperdopaminergic state ranked highest among the combined sample of psychiatric residents and psychiatrists. In Japan, 89% of psychiatrists reported that they had used "integration disorder" to discuss this condition with diagnosed patients and family members, but that 59% of patients, 53% of family members, and 59% of psychiatrists noted that this term was difficult to understand.

The Name Revision Committee sought detailed discussions of the strengths and weaknesses of each candidate name, establishment of principles and a roadmap for revising the name and scrutinizing the medical–legal issues stemming from this change. The committee recently announced that the following principles would be used as guidelines for renaming schizophrenia: that the new name should have sound scientific validity, social utility in terms of dispelling stigma, and medical utility in relation to biopsychosocial treatment. The most recent name, "attunement (調絃) disorder", was proposed by a scholar of Korean literature and extensively discussed in the committee. This label initially sounded quite metaphorical and metaphysical, rendering it difficult to understand at first. However, it includes two key pathogenic mechanisms of schizophrenia: sensitization and the loosening of associations. When a violin string is too tight, the sound becomes high pitched. This may be compared to the state of mind characterized by hypersensitivity and paranoia. When a string is too loose, the sound becomes dull. This may be compared to the state of mind characterized by negativism or disorganization. In this sense, attunement disorder is not only comprehensive and scientifically, it is also refreshing. The pros and cons of proposed candidate names are summarized in Table 5.2.

Recently, the KAS surveyed preferences for candidate names to full members of the KAS and attendees at the 2010 KAS Fall conference. Based on the survey results and the general consensus within the name-revision committee, a final agreement selected "attunement disorder" as the new diagnostic term for schizophrenia. At a second Asian workshop on schizophrenia in Seoul in 2011, the new name was announced. Irrespective of the choice of new name, real success in dissolving the stigma is possible only when social, cultural, and political considerations accompany the renaming movement.

Table 5.2
Pros and cons of proposed candidate names

Candidate names	**Pros**	**Cons**
Attunement Disorder	• Good scientific validity • Very comprehensive, incorporating both positive (sensitizing) and negative (loosening) symptoms • Lesser chance of being mocked due to its particular implications and connotations	• Too metaphorical and metaphysical • Similar to Integration Disorder used in Japan • Less useful for psychoeducation about pharmacotherapy
Integration Disorder	• Good scientific validity • The word "integration" has a positive symbolic meaning • Used successfully in Japan	• The phonetic sound of the Korean word for "dysregulation" often denotes "malnutrition" • Meaning is difficult to understand • More stigmatizing when it refers to the breakdown of a whole personality
Dopamine Dysregulation	• Strong scientific validity • Relieves family members of guilt • Greater utility for psychoeducation about pharmacotherapy and improving drug compliance • Greater chance of airing in mass media	• Narrow conceptualization focusing only on biological aspects • Neurotransmitters other than dopamine are also important • Neglects psychosocial factors

(continued on p. 58)

Table 5.2 (continued)

Candidate names	**Pros**	**Cons**
Bleuler's Disease	• Another eponymous marker for a founder of schizophrenia • Successful precedents like Hansen's disease	• People will soon find out that it is just another name for schizophrenia • Splitting, a key pathogenetic mechanism of schizophrenia, is not as valid as it used to be • The word "broiler", which sounds similar to Bleuler, refers to the meat of young chickens
Thought and Perception Sensitivity Disorder	• Good scientific validity (for example, dopamine sensitization) • Because of universality of sensitivity, more acceptable and less stigmatizing • Greater utility for cognitive therapy and psychoeducation about pharmacotherapy • Greater chance of airing in mass media	• Sounds stiff • Long name and difficult to understand at first • Excludes mood symptoms • Sensitivity often regarded as reflective of mild symptoms, possibly discouraging treatment
Thought-Loosening Disorder	• Good scientific validity (for example, disconnection hypothesis) • Cardinal symptom among 4 A symptoms • Explains the phenomenon of cognitive deficits and loss of reality testing	• Not a common and representative symptom • Connotation of loosening is negative • Discouraging name because it is often associated with grave outcome • Less useful for psychoeducation about pharmacotherapy

Conclusion

The early psychosis movement should not be confined to simply expanding academic interest in this domain. To be successful, any change must incorporate multiple issues and constituencies, including those related to community psychiatry, renaming the disorder, the development of optimal psychosocial treatment for the critical period, sociopolitical considerations, and so on. Most importantly, optimism that early interventions could yield better outcomes should serve as the driving force for this movement. In essence, becoming an evangelical advocate of the early psychosis movement means being able to answer the two key philosophical questions posed at the beginning of this chapter with a definite "YES".

References

Achenbach, T. M. (1991). *Manual for the Youth Self-Report and 1991 Profile*. Burlington, VT: University of Vermont, Department of Psychiatry.

Achenbach, T. M., & Edelbrock, C. S. (1983). *Manual for the Child Behavior Checklist and Revised Child Behavior Profile*. Burlington, VT: University of Vermont, Department of Psychiatry.

Addington, J., Coldham, E. L., Jones, B., Ko, T., & Addington, D. (2003). The first episode of psychosis: The experience of relatives. *Acta Psychiatrica Scandinavica, 108*(4), 285–289.

Ahn, D. H. (2007). *Development of the Adolescent Mental Health and Problem-Behavior Questionnaire*. Korea: Ministry for Health, Welfare and Family Affairs.

Beck, A. T., Ward, C. H., Mendelson, M., Mock, J., & Erbaugh, J. (1961). An inventory for measuring depression. *Archives of General Psychiatry, 4*, 561–571.

Birchwood, M., Todd, P., & Jackson, C. (1998). Early intervention in psychosis: The critical period hypothesis. [Review]. *The British Journal of Psychiatry. Supplement, 172*(33), 53–59.

Choi, M. G., & Yang, I. H. (1997). MMPI response study on psychosis proneness group. *Journal of Educational Psychology, 11*, 255–289.

Chung, Y. C. (2008). *The Development and Application of a Group Cognitive-Behavioral Therapy Program for Schizophrenic Patients in the Critical Period (A080667)*. Korea: Research and Development Projects for Health, Medicine, and Technology.

Chung, Y. C., Kang, N. I., Im, Y. J., Kim, S. W., Cho, I. H., Lee, Y. M., et al. (2012). Validation of the Korean version of the Eppendorf Schizophrenia Inventory as a screening measure to detect adolescents at ultra-high risk for psychosis. *Early Intervention in Psychiatry*. doi: 10.1111/j.1751–7893.2012.00363.x

Chung, Y. C., Kim, C. E., Han, C. H., Li, C. R., Shim, J. C., & Hwang, T. Y. (2008). *Psychosocial Intervention for Patients with Schizophrenia in the Critical Period.* Korea: Hakjisa.

Chung, Y. C., Lee, C. H., Mizuno, M., Kim, S. W., Kim, J. H., Han, S. W., et al. (2009). *A Report of the Study on the Stigma and Renaming Issue for "Schizophrenia": Academic Research Project by Seoul National Hospital.* Seoul: Seoul National Hospital.

Falloon, I. R. (1992). Early intervention for first episodes of schizophrenia: A preliminary exploration. *Psychiatry, 55*(1), 4–15.

Haddock, G., Tarrier, N., Morrison, A. P., Hopkins, R., Drake, R., & Lewis, S. (1999). A pilot study evaluating the effectiveness of individual inpatient cognitive-behavioural therapy in early psychosis. [Clinical Trial Controlled Clinical Trial]. *Social Psychiatry and Psychiatric Epidemiology, 34*(5), 254–258.

Hafner, H., Maurer, K., Ruhrmann, S., Bechdolf, A., Klosterkotter, J., Wagner, M., et al. (2004). Early detection and secondary prevention of psychosis: Facts and visions. [Research Support, Non-U.S. Government Review]. *European Archives of Psychiatry and Clinical Neuroscience, 254*(2), 117–128. doi: 10.1007/s00406-004-0508-z

Ho, B. C., Alicata, D., Ward, J., Moser, D. J., O'Leary, D. S., Arndt, S., et al. (2003). Untreated initial psychosis: relation to cognitive deficits and brain morphology in first-episode schizophrenia. *American Journal of Psychiatry, 160*(1), 142–148.

Jackson, H., McGorry, P., Edwards, J., Hulbert, C., Henry, L., Francey, S., et al. (1998). Cognitively-oriented psychotherapy for early psychosis (COPE). Preliminary results. [Clinical Trial Research Support, Non-U.S. Government]. *The British Journal of Psychiatry. Supplement, 172*(33), 93–100.

Jackson, H., McGorry, P., Henry, L., Edwards, J., Hulbert, C., Harrigan, S., et al. (2001). Cognitively oriented psychotherapy for early psychosis (COPE): A 1-year follow-up. [Clinical Trial Research Support, Non-U.S. Government]. *The British Journal of Clinical Psychology/The British Psychological Society, 40*(Pt 1), 57–70.

Jackson, H. J., McGorry, P. D., Killackey, E., Bendall, S., Allott, K., Dudgeon, P., et al. (2008). Acute-phase and 1-year follow-up results of a randomized controlled trial of CBT versus Befriending for first-episode psychosis: The ACE project. [Comparative Study Randomized Controlled Trial Research Support, Non-U.S. Government]. *Psychological Medicine, 38*(5), 725–735. doi: 10.1017/S0033291707002061

Jolley, S., Garety, P., Craig, T., Dunn, G., White, J., & Aitken, M. (2003). Cognitive therapy in early psychosis: A pilot randomized controlled trial. *Behavioural Cognitive Psychotherapy, 31*, 473–478.

Jung, H. Y., Chang, J. S., Yi, J. S., Hwang, S., Shin, H. K., Kim, J. H., et al. (2008). Measuring psychosis proneness in a nonclinical Korean population: Is the Peters et al Delusions Inventory useful for assessing high-risk individuals? [Research Support, Non-U.S. Government]. *Comprehensive Psychiatry, 49*(2), 202–210. doi: 10.1016/j.comppsych.2007.08.011

Kim, K. R., Lee, S. Y., Kang, J. I., Kim, B. R., Choi, S. H., Park, J. Y., et al. (2011). Clinical efficacy of individual cognitive therapy in reducing psychiatric symptoms in people at ultra-high risk for psychosis. [Clinical Trial Research Support, Non-U.S. Government]. *Early Intervention in Psychiatry, 5*(2), 174–178. doi: 10.1111/j.1751-7893.2011.00267.x

Konings, M., Bak, M., Hanssen, M., van Os, J., & Krabbendam, L. (2006). Validity and reliability of the CAPE: A self-report instrument for the measurement of psychotic experiences in the general population. [Comparative Study Research Support, Non-U.S. Government]. *Acta Psychiatrica Scandinavica, 114*(1), 55–61. doi: 10.1111/j.1600-0447.2005.00741.x

Kraepelin, E. (1987). Dementia praecox. In *The Clinical Roots of the Schizophrenia Concept*, edited by J. Cutting and M. Shepherd, 13–24. Cambridge: Cambridge University Press.

Kwon, J. S., Chung, Y. C., & Lee, Y. M. (2006). *Standardization of the Eppendorf schizophrenia inventory*. Korea: The Korea Institute for Health and Social Affairs.

Larsen, T. K., Friis, S., Haahr, U., Joa, I., Johannessen, J. O., Melle, I., et al. (2001). Early detection and intervention in first-episode schizophrenia: A critical review. *Acta Psychiatrica Scandinavica, 103*(5), 323–334. doi: acp131 [pii]

Lee, C. G., Park, G. G., Jo, M. J., Chung, E. K., Kim, J. G., & Kim, S. W. (2001). *The Epidemiological Survey of Psychiatric Illness in Korea: A Study Report of the Ministry of Health and Welfare*. Korea: Ministry of Health and Welfare.

Lee, S. Y., Kim, K. R., Kang, J. I., Kim, B., Choi, S. H., Park, J. Y., et al. (2010). *GRAPE Cognitive Therapy: Manual for Therapists*. Seoul: Hakjisa.

Lewis, S., Tarrier, N., Haddock, G., Bentall, R., Kinderman, P., Kingdon, D., et al. (2002). Randomised controlled trial of cognitive-behavioural therapy in early schizophrenia: Acute-phase outcomes. [Clinical Trial Randomized Controlled Trial Research Support, Non-U.S. Government]. *The British Journal of Psychiatry. Supplement, 43*, s91–97.

Loewy, R. L., Bearden, C. E., Johnson, J. K., Raine, A., & Cannon, T. D. (2005). The Prodromal Questionnaire (PQ): Preliminary validation of a self-report screening measure for prodromal and psychotic syndromes. [Validation Studies]. *Schizophrenia Research, 79*(1), 117–125.

Loewy, R. L., & Cannon, T. D. (2008). *The Prodromal Questionnaire, Brief Version (PQ-B)*: University of California.

Mass, R. (2000). Characteristic subjective experiences of schizophrenia. [Comparative Study Research Support, Non-U.S. Government]. *Schizophrenia Bulletin, 26*(4), 921–931.

Mass, R., Haasen, C., & Borgart, E. J. (2005). Abnormal subjective experiences of schizophrenia: Evaluation of the Eppendorf Schizophrenia Inventory. [Validation Studies]. *Psychiatry Research, 135*(2), 91–101. doi: 10.1016/j.psychres.2004.08.011

McGlashan, T. H., & Johannessen, J. O. (1996). Early detection and intervention with schizophrenia: Rationale. *Schizophrenia Bulletin, 22*(2), 201–222.

McGorry, P. D., Edwards, J., Mihalopoulos, C., Harrigan, S. M., & Jackson, H. J. (1996). EPPIC: An evolving system of early detection and optimal management. *Schizophrenia Bulletin, 22*(2), 305–326.

McGrath, J., Saha, S., Chant, D., & Welham, J. (2008). Schizophrenia: A concise overview of incidence, prevalence, and mortality. [Research Support, Non-U.S. Government Review]. *Epidemiologic Reviews, 30*, 67–76. doi: 10.1093/epirev/mxn001

Nordentoft, M., Jeppesen, P., Abel, M., Kassow, P., Petersen, L., Thorup, A., et al. (2002). OPUS study: Suicidal behaviour, suicidal ideation and hopelessness among patients with first-episode psychosis. One-year follow-up of a randomised controlled trial. [Clinical Trial Randomized Controlled Trial Research Support, Non-U.S. Government]. *The British Journal of Psychiatry. Supplement, 43*, s98–106.

Ord, L. M., Myles-Worsley, M., Blailes, F., & Ngiralmau, H. (2004). Screening for prodromal adolescents in an isolated high-risk population. [Letter Research Support, Non-U.S. Government]. *Schizophrenia Research, 71*(2–3), 507–508. doi: 10.1016/j.schres.2004.03.014

Park, J. I., & Chung, Y. C. (2008). Renaming the term "schizophrenia" in Korea. *Korean Journal of Schizophrenia Research, 11*(2), 107–117.

Peters, E,, Joseph, S., Day, S., & Garety, P. (2004). Measuring delusional ideation: The 21-item Peters et al. Delusions Inventory (PDI). *Schizophrenia Bulletin, 30*(4), 1005–1022.

Peters, E. R., Joseph, S. A., & Garety, P. A. (1999). Measurement of delusional ideation in the normal population: Introducing the PDI (Peters et al. Delusions Inventory). *Schizophrenia Bulletin, 25*(3), 553–576.

Robinson, D., Woerner, M. G., Alvir, J. M., Bilder, R., Goldman, R., Geisler, S., et al. (1999). Predictors of relapse following response from a first episode of schizophrenia or schizoaffective disorder. [Research Support, Non-U.S. Government Research Support, U.S. Government, P.H.S.]. *Archives of General Psychiatry, 56*(3), 241–247.

Sullivan, H. S. (1994). The onset of schizophrenia. 1927. [Biography Classical Article Historical Article Portraits]. *The American Journal of Psychiatry, 151*(6 Suppl), 134–139.

Tarrier, N., Lewis, S., Haddock, G., Bentall, R., Drake, R., Kinderman, P., et al. (2004). Cognitive-behavioural therapy in first-episode and early schizophrenia: 18-month follow-up of a randomised controlled trial. [Clinical Trial Multicenter Study Randomized Controlled Trial Research Support, Non-U.S. Government]. *The British Journal of Psychiatry: The Journal of Mental Science, 184*, 231–239.

Ustun, T. B., Ayuso-Mateos, J. L., Chatterji, S., Mathers, C., & Murray, C. J. (2004). Global burden of depressive disorders in the year 2000. [Multicenter Study Research Support, Non-U.S. Government Research Support, U.S. Government, P.H.S.]. *The British Journal of Psychiatry: The Journal of Mental Science, 184*, 386–392.

Ustun, T. B., Rehm, J., Chatterji, S., Saxena, S., Trotter, R., Room, R., et al. (1999). Multiple-informant ranking of the disabling effects of different health conditions in 14 countries. WHO/NIH Joint Project CAR Study Group. [Comparative Study Research Support, Non-U.S. Government Research Support, U.S. Government, P.H.S.]. *Lancet, 354*(9173), 111–115.

van Os, J., Linscott, R. J., Myin-Germeys, I., Delespaul, P., & Krabbendam, L. (2009). A systematic review and meta-analysis of the psychosis continuum: Evidence for a psychosis proneness-persistence-impairment model of psychotic disorder. [Meta-Analysis Review]. *Psychological Medicine, 39*(2), 179–195. doi: 10.1017/S00332917080038

Wang, C., Li, Y., Zhao, Z., Pan, M., Feng, Y., Sun, F., et al. (2003). Controlled study on long-term effect of cognitive behavior intervention on first episode schizophrenia. *Chinese Mental Health, 17*, 200–202.

Westermeyer, J. F., Harrow, M., & Marengo, J. T. (1991). Risk for suicide in schizophrenia and other psychotic and nonpsychotic disorders. [Comparative Study Research Support, Non-U.S. Government Research Support, U.S. Government, P.H.S.]. *The Journal of Nervous and Mental Disease, 179*(5), 259–266.

Yung, A. R., & McGorry, P. D. (1996). The prodromal phase of first-episode psychosis: Past and current conceptualizations. *Schizophrenia Bulletin, 22*(2), 353–370.

Yung, A. R., Yuen, H. P., McGorry, P. D., Phillips, L. J., Kelly, D., Dell'Olio, M., et al. (2005). Mapping the onset of psychosis: The comprehensive assessment of at-risk mental states. [Comparative Study]. *The Australian and New Zealand Journal of Psychiatry, 39*(11–12), 964–971. doi: 10.1111/j.1440-1614.2005.01714.x

Part II

Public Awareness and Early Detection in Cultural Context

6

Factors Affecting the Duration of Untreated Psychosis in Hong Kong

Eric Yu-hai Chen

A reduction in the duration of untreated psychosis (DUP), defined as the time-lapse between onset of psychotic symptoms and initiation of treatment, is a key target of early intervention for psychotic disorders (Harrigan, McGorry, & Krstev, 2003; McGlashan & Johannessen, 1996; McGorry, 2000). Many early intervention programmes aim at DUP reduction, considering it a measurable and achievable goal (Johannessen, 1998; Malla et al., 2003).

At present, the body of knowledge on DUP has largely been focusing on its relationship with clinical outcomes (Altamura et al., 2001; Amminger et al., 2002; Black et al., 2001). Meta-analyses have provided solid evidence for its role in predicting outcomes (Marshall et al., 2005; Perkins et al., 2005). Yet, given the pivotal role of DUP in early intervention, it should be equally important to identify the factors that may influence DUP. These may include premorbid features, clinical profile, and the sociocultural context of the illness. In particular, the sociocultural context of the illness and the health care system, which includes cultural, family, and service delivery factors, are important, as they are potentially modifiable for shortening DUP.

A small number of studies have attempted to look at these issues. Among them, DUP has been linked to clinical features such as poor insight, social withdrawal, and isolation (Barnes et al., 2000; Drake et al., 2000; Larsen, Johannessen, & Opjordsmoen, 1998). Skeate et al. (2002) also found that patients with a shorter DUP have more active help-seeking behaviours and made more contact with their general practitioners six years before onset. Furthermore, Moller (2001) suggested that the acute development of a psychotic episode might be associated with a shorter DUP. Most of these previous studies, however, have focused on referral patterns and patient features; factors related to the patient's family have seldom been examined in details. Yet, as the majority of first-episode patients reported that others, rather than themselves, were critical in the initiation of treatment (de Haan et al., 2002), factors that concern caregivers may be important determinants of DUP (see Chapter 17, "Experience of Stigma in Early Psychosis Patients and Caregivers").

In Hong Kong, the relatively lengthy average duration of untreated psychosis (DUP) of over 18 months among first-episode psychosis patients was comparable to that found in many previous studies (Black et al., 2001; Ho et al., 2003; Johannessen, 1998; Kalla et al., 2002; Larsen, McGlashan, & Moe, 1996; Loebel et al., 1992). This chapter will explore features associated with lengthy of DUP, using Hong Kong as an example, but also recognizing that each population might have distinctive determinants of DUP.

Previous Familial Experience

Compared with many other societies, individuals in Hong Kong are more likely to live with their parents. Whether because of space limitations, high property prices, or cultural trends, single-person households only constitute 17.1% of all households in Hong Kong (Census and Statistics Department, 2002), while the figure is 25.7% in the US, 29.5% in Sweden, and 26.3% in Norway (Ness & Ciment, 1999; Russell, 2000). Therefore, among the potential factors that affect DUP, social isolation is expected to be less prominent in Hong Kong. In contrast, response of the family to the patient's symptoms may be relatively critical in determining the length of DUP.

Where the patient resides with family, whether other family members have adequate knowledge of psychosis may be a decisive factor in help-seeking. Findings from previous studies, which suggest that having another ill family member may lead to improved knowledge about the illness (Chung et al., 1997; Lam, Chan, & Chen, 1996), also demonstrate that previous family experience of psychiatric illness has a significant effect on DUP (Chen et al., 2005). Patients with another family member who had already received psychiatric treatment tended to have a shorter DUP (225 days) compared with patients without a family history of psychiatric treatment (645 days).

There are two potential interpretations for this finding. The first is that patients with family history exhibit some biologically determined features that alter the presentation of the illness in a way that leads to a shorter DUP. Although it has been suggested that familial cases of schizophrenia may be characterized by a distinctive profile (such as age of onset or negative symptoms), studies have failed to find a consistent difference between sporadic and familial cases

(Kendler, Karkowski-Shuman, & Walsh, 1996; Roy et al., 1994). Furthermore, some of the suggested features of familial cases, such as increased negative symptoms (Malaspina et al., 2000), would have led to a longer, rather than a shorter, DUP. In Hong Kong, patients with a family history did not differ in terms of demographic and clinical profiles, or in the mode of development of psychosis. Therefore it was considered less likely that any biological characteristics of familial illness would directly contribute to the length of DUP (Chen et al., 2005).

The second interpretation of such findings is that previous family experience of psychiatric illness could influence the future help-seeking behaviours of other family members, possibly through enhancement of knowledge about potential symptoms and their significance. In an earlier study, it was found that among the general public in Hong Kong, awareness of the nature and significance of psychiatric symptoms was related to previous contact with a person with psychiatric problems (Lam et al., 1996). A subsequent study also demonstrated that compared with the general population, caregivers were more knowledgeable about the potential significance of psychotic symptoms (Chung et al., 1997). This effect may be mediated by the acquisition of psychiatric knowledge through taking care of their family members. Previous exposure may, therefore, enable experienced caregivers to arrive at an earlier appraisal of the situation and enable earlier help-seeking in the event of a further family member becoming ill. Although it is also possible that families with previous experience of illness may have a general propensity for more active help-seeking, this is a less likely explanation, as this effect is observed specifically only in families with a previous experience of psychotic disorders.

It is also suggested that previous family experience is particularly important when the onset is insidious, perhaps because the changes are more subtle and difficult to recognize. In contrast, factors that cause delay in seeking help in isolated patients with a poor social network, such as lack of insight and social isolation, appeared to assume a relatively less important role in Hong Kong.

Demographics and DUP

Some previous findings have suggested a lack of relationship between DUP and basic demographic features (Drake et al., 2000), while others found premorbid personality as relating to DUP (Verdoux et al., 2001). In Hong Kong, a relationship between a higher education level and a shorter DUP has been found (Chen et al., 2005). Although less reported in previous studies, this relationship is not unexpected, as educational level is associated with a broad range of factors, such as intelligence level, psychosocial advantage, and access to information. These factors are likely to facilitate a more favourable response towards seeking help. It was also found that neither the age of onset, gender, premorbid adjustment, nor premorbid personality had a significant impact on DUP (Chen et al., 2005). These results may be compared with findings from other Asia-Pacific countries: in a Singapore study, while being unmarried and unemployed was found to be associated with a longer DUP, gender and ethnicity were unrelated (Pek, Mythily, & Chong, 2006). In an Australian cohort, on the other hand, DUP was related to younger age of onset and worse premorbid functioning (Schimmelmann et al., 2008).

Mode of Illness Development

In Hong Kong, another key determinant of DUP was found to be the mode of illness development (Chen et al., 2005). Patients with an acute onset tend to present earlier for treatment than patients with an insidious onset. The potential importance of onset mode has been suggested in other studies (Moller, 2001). Similar findings of a longer DUP among patients with insidious onset have also been found in both Spanish and Finnish samples (Kalla et al., 2002).

This relationship can be understood in terms of the "perceived change over time". Abrupt changes in experience and behaviour are more likely to be considered the result of anomalous processes, and are more likely to trigger help-seeking than insidious changes. In contrast, if the psychotic illness has an insidious onset, there is more room for a process of family adaptation to take place. With adaptation, the patient and the patient's family gradually become desensitized to the presence of abnormal behavioural signals indicative of a psychotic illness, and have less motivation to overcome barriers to seeking help, such as stigmatization, financial expenses, and waiting lists.

In addition, insidious symptoms may be less prominent, and require more knowledge and experience to identify. In support of this view is the finding that the facilitative effect of previous family experience in identifying psychosis appears to be particularly notable in patients with an insidious onset of illness.

Summary

In contrast to some other populations, individuals in Hong Kong are more likely to be living with their families. It is expected that living in the same household would increase family involvement in the detection of psychotic illness and the decision to seek help, so the role of family members may be relatively important in Hong Kong. Findings from Hong Kong could potentially be of interest in similar settings in Asia in which family decision plays a major role in help-seeking. The importance of caregiver exposure, together with the fact that a large proportion of young people live with their families, suggest that one of the primary strategies for an early detection programme in similar populations should be broad-based mental health education that targets potential caregivers in the general population. On the other hand, although it is easier for education programmes to focus on the unambiguous changes typical of acute psychosis, a shift of emphasis towards the signs and symptoms that are associated with insidious presentation could be an important step towards achieving more effective early detection.

References

Altamura, A. C., Bassetti, R., Sassella, F., Salvadori, D., & Mundo, E. (2001). Duration of untreated psychosis as a predictor of outcome in first-episode schizophrenia: A retrospective study. *Schizophrenia Research, 52*(1–2), 29–36. doi: S0920-9964(00)00187-0 [pii]

Amminger, G. P., Edwards, J., Brewer, W. J., Harrigan, S., & McGorry, P. D. (2002). Duration of untreated psychosis and cognitive deterioration in first-episode schizophrenia. *Schizophrenia Research, 54*(3), 223–230. doi: S092099640100278X [pii]

Barnes, T. R., Hutton, S. B., Chapman, M. J., Mutsatsa, S., Puri, B. K., & Joyce, E. M. (2000). West London first-episode study of schizophrenia: Clinical correlates of duration of untreated psychosis. *British Journal of Psychiatry, 177*, 207–211.

Black, K., Peters, L., Rui, Q., Milliken, H., Whitehorn, D., & Kopala, L. C. (2001). Duration of untreated psychosis predicts treatment outcome in an early psychosis program. *Schizophrenia Research, 47*(2–3), 215–222. doi: S0920996400001444 [pii]

Census and Statistics Department. (2002). *Hong Kong 2001 Population Census Main Report*. Hong Kong: The Government of the Hong Kong Special Administrative Region.

Chen, E. Y.-H., Dunn, E. L.-W., Miao, M. Y.-K., Yeung, W.-S., Wong, C.-K., Chan, W.-F., et al. (2005). The impact of family experience on the duration of untreated psychosis (DUP) in Hong Kong. *Social Psychiatry and Psychiatric Epidemiology, 40*(5), 350–356. doi: 10.1007/s00127-005-0908-z

Chung, K. F., Chen, E. Y., Lam, L. C., Chen, R. Y., & Chan, C. K. (1997). How are psychotic symptoms perceived? A comparison between patients, relatives and the general public. *Australian and New Zealand Journal of Psychiatry, 31*(5), 756–761.

de Haan, L., Peters, B., Dingemans, P., Wouters, L., & Linszen, D. (2002). Attitudes of patients toward the first psychotic episode and the start of treatment. *Schizophrenia Bulletin, 28*(3), 431–442.

Drake, R. J., Haley, C. J., Akhtar, S., & Lewis, S. W. (2000). Causes and consequences of duration of untreated psychosis in schizophrenia. *British Journal of Psychiatry, 177*, 511–515.

Harrigan, S. M., McGorry, P. D., & Krstev, H. (2003). Does treatment delay in first-episode psychosis really matter? *Psychological Medicine, 33*(1), 97–110.

Ho, B. C., Alicata, D., Ward, J., Moser, D. J., O'Leary, D. S., Arndt, S., & Andreasen, N. C. (2003). Untreated initial psychosis: Relation to cognitive deficits and brain morphology in first-episode schizophrenia. *American Journal of Psychiatry, 160*(1), 142–148.

Johannessen, J. O. (1998). Early intervention and prevention in schizophrenia: Experiences from a study in Stavanger, Norway. *Seishin Shinkeigaku Zasshi, 100*(8), 511–522.

Kalla, O., Aaltonen, J., Wahlstrom, J., Lehtinen, V., Garcia Cabeza, I., & Gonzalez de Chavez, M. (2002). Duration of untreated psychosis and its correlates in first-episode psychosis in Finland and Spain. *Acta Psychiatrica Scandinavica, 106*(4), 265–275. doi: 2o302 [pii]

Kendler, K. S., Karkowski-Shuman, L., & Walsh, D. (1996). Age at onset in schizophrenia and risk of illness in relatives: Results from the Roscommon Family Study. *British Journal of Psychiatry, 169*(2), 213–218.

Lam, L. C., Chan, C. K., & Chen, E. Y. (1996). Insight and general public attitude on psychotic experiences in Hong Kong. *International Journal of Social Psychiatry, 42*(1), 10–17.

Larsen, T. K., Johannessen, J. O., & Opjordsmoen, S. (1998). First-episode schizophrenia with long duration of untreated psychosis: Pathways to care. *British Journal of Psychiatry. Supplement, 172*(33), 45–52.

Larsen, T. K., McGlashan, T. H., & Moe, L. C. (1996). First-episode schizophrenia: I. Early course parameters. *Schizophrenia Bulletin, 22*(2), 241–256.

Loebel, A. D., Lieberman, J. A., Alvir, J. M., Mayerhoff, D. I., Geisler, S. H., & Szymanski, S. R. (1992). Duration of psychosis and outcome in first-episode schizophrenia. *American Journal of Psychiatry, 149*(9), 1183–1188.

Malaspina, D., Goetz, R. R., Yale, S., Berman, A., Friedman, J. H., Tremeau, F., et al. (2000). Relation of familial schizophrenia to negative symptoms but not to the deficit syndrome. *American Journal of Psychiatry, 157*(6), 994–1003.

Malla, A., Norman, R., McLean, T., Scholten, D., & Townsend, L. (2003). A Canadian programme for early intervention in non-affective psychotic disorders. *Australian and New Zealand Journal of Psychiatry, 37*(4), 407–413. doi: 1194 [pii]

Marshall, M., Lewis, S., Lockwood, A., Drake, R., Jones, P., & Croudace, T. (2005). Association between duration of untreated psychosis and outcome in cohorts of first-episode patients: A systematic review. *Archives of General Psychiatry, 62*(9), 975–983. doi: 62/9/975 [pii]10.1001/archpsyc.62.9.975

McGlashan, T. H., & Johannessen, J. O. (1996). Early detection and intervention with schizophrenia: Rationale. *Schizophrenia Bulletin, 22*(2), 201–222.

McGorry, P. D. (2000). Evaluating the importance of reducing the duration of untreated psychosis. *Australian and New Zealand Journal of Psychiatry, 34 Suppl*, S145–149.

Moller, P. (2001). Duration of untreated psychosis: Are we ignoring the mode of initial development? An extensive naturalistic case study of phenomenal continuity in first-episode schizophrenia. *Psychopathology, 34*(1), 8–14. doi: 49274 [pii]

Ness, I., & Ciment, J. (1999). *The Encyclopedia of Global Population and Demographics.* Armonk, NY: Sharpe Reference.

Pek, E., Mythily, S., & Chong, S. A. (2006). Clinical and social correlates of duration of untreated psychosis in first-episode psychosis patients. *Annals of the Academy of Medicine, Singapore, 35*(1), 24–26.

Perkins, D. O., Gu, H., Boteva, K., & Lieberman, J. A. (2005). Relationship between duration of untreated psychosis and outcome in first-episode schizophrenia: A critical review and meta-analysis. [Meta-Analysis Research Support, N.I.H., Extramural Research Support, Non-U.S. Government Review]. *American Journal of Psychiatry, 162*(10), 1785–1804. doi: 10.1176/appi.ajp.162.10.1785

Roy, M. A., Flaum, M. A., Gupta, S., Jaramillo, L., & Andreasen, N. C. (1994). Epidemiological and clinical correlates of familial and sporadic schizophrenia. *Acta Psychiatrica Scandinavica, 89*(5), 324–328.

Russell, C. (2000). *Demographics of the U.S.* Ithaca: NY: new Strategist Publications, Inc.

Schimmelmann, B. G., Huber, C. G., Lambert, M., Cotton, S., McGorry, P. D., & Conus, P. (2008). Impact of duration of untreated psychosis on pre-treatment, baseline, and outcome characteristics in an epidemiological first-episode psychosis cohort. [Comparative Study Research Support, Non-U.S. Government]. *Journal of Psychiatric Research, 42*(12), 982–990. doi: 10.1016/j.jpsychires.2007.12.001

Skeate, A., Jackson, C., Birchwood, M., & Jones, C. (2002). Duration of untreated psychosis and pathways to care in first-episode psychosis: Investigation of help-seeking behaviour in primary care. *British Journal of Psychiatry. Supplement, 43*, s73–77.

Verdoux, H., Liraud, F., Bergey, C., Assens, F., Abalan, F., & van Os, J. (2001). Is the association between duration of untreated psychosis and outcome confounded? A two-year follow-up study of first-admitted patients. *Schizophrenia Research, 49*(3), 231–241. doi: S0920996400000724 [pii]

7
Public Awareness Approaches in Early Psychosis

Gloria Hoi-yan Wong

Psychosis is a concept surrounded by misunderstanding and stigma. Historically, mental illnesses (in particular schizophrenia) were associated with moral failure, demon-possession, and witchcraft (Miller, 2000). The fear and antipathy against psychosis continues to the present day: the media typically portray an image of a dangerous, violent person with a "split personality". Patients are treated as social outcasts, to be avoided or made fun of.

These misunderstandings, stigma, and discrimination add to the suffering of patients and families struggling to recover from the disease; they also pose major barriers in help-seeking, which impact adversely on patients' outcome (Byrne, 1997). Delays in help-seeking also mean a higher likelihood of publicly displayed symptoms, including those that lead to police intervention or emergency admission, feeding back to the public perception of psychotic patients being dangerous. To break this vicious circle, effective public awareness work is imperative. In many Asian countries, the work of anti-stigma organizations and social campaigns are gaining momentum. With reference to the experience from Hong Kong, this chapter will review the current level of public awareness, the goals of public awareness programmes, the messages to communicate, and the use of various platforms for changing public opinion towards psychosis.

Overview of Public Awareness Campaigns in Hong Kong

Before the establishment of a specialized early intervention service for psychosis, the role of public education in Hong Kong was mainly taken up by local non-governmental organizations (NGOs) that provided services for the mentally ill. Efforts focusing on psychosis were scarce and scattered. The launch of the Early Assessment Service for Young People with Psychosis (EASY) by the Hospital Authority in 2001 marked the beginning of a wave of public education programmes, including mass media activities, talks, and exhibitions. In 2007, the Hong Kong Early Psychosis Intervention Society (EPISO) was formed by a group of volunteers, providing public and professional education in psychosis, with a large-scale campaign entitled "Project Torchlight" commenced in 2009. At about the same time, the University of Hong Kong received support from the Hong Kong Jockey Club Charities Trust to embark on a five-year Jockey Club Early Psychosis (JCEP) project. A major component of JCEP is to enhance public awareness of psychosis, delivering regular and mainly community-based publicity work.

Current Level of Awareness in Hong Kong

A clear picture of the public attitudes and knowledge towards psychosis helps steer public awareness approaches and resources allocation. In 2009, the University of Hong Kong conducted a phone survey in 1,016 Hong Kong residents with support from the Hong Kong Jockey Club Charities Trust.

As can be seen in Figure 7.1, misconceptions about psychosis are common. A 2009 study of 1016 people indicated that 71% of participants still held the idea that psychosis equalled split or multiple personality, a confusion that may have stemmed from the term "schizophrenia" (精神分裂) and sustained through word of mouth and media messaging. The public also believed that a person who had psychosis was strange and annoying, someone who yelled and muttered out loud. Nearly a quarter of people considered that someone with psychosis had low intelligence. Almost half of the respondents thought that anxiety, instead of hallucination or delusion, was the core psychotic symptom (HKU survey reveals misconceptions and lack of awareness towards psychosis, 2009).

In view of these pervasive misconceptions, the social stigma of psychosis remains unsurprisingly common in Hong Kong (Figure 7.2). Half of the respondents thought that patients were being looked down on. The majority thought that patients were dangerous, unpredictable, and disrespected. Importantly, most people would not want to date someone with psychosis, and employers would consider other applicants first during recruitment.

Among the general public, the main source of information on psychosis is the print media and TV. In fact, exposure to news is related to stigmatization: those who have previous exposure to negative news reporting of psychosis express a significantly higher level of resistance in Hong Kong (HKU survey

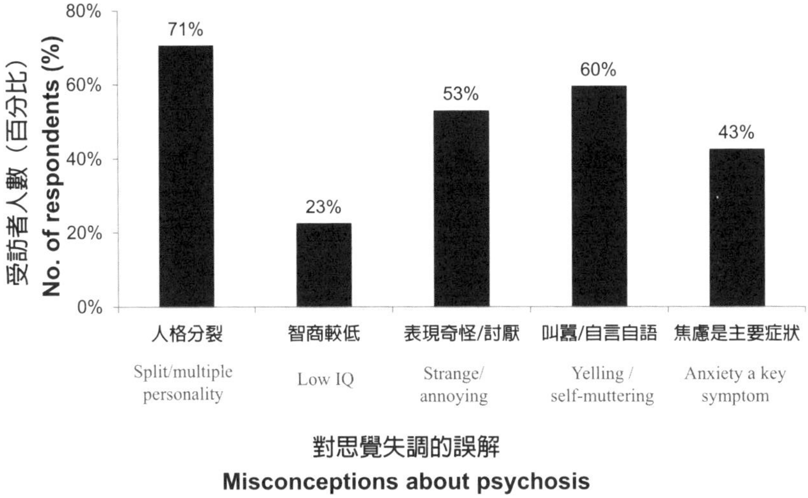

Figure 7.1

Public misconception about psychosis in Hong Kong

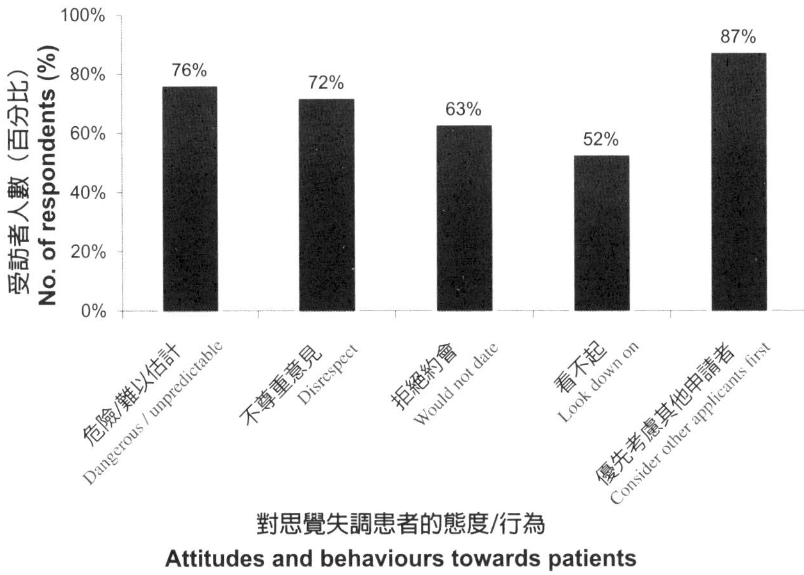

Figure 7.2

Stigmatizing attitudes and behaviours towards psychotic patients in Hong Kong

reveals misconceptions and lack of awareness towards psychosis, 2009). The same has been found in international studies: the amount of TV viewing is related to intolerance towards the mentally ill (Granello & Pauley, 2000) and the desire for social distance from schizophrenia patients (Angermeyer et al., 2005).

A number of key points can be concluded from this research. First, there is still major room for improving public knowledge of psychosis. Second, stigma and negative discrimination towards patients remains the norm in Hong Kong, and strategies to change these attitudes and behaviours are needed. Third, as in most developed communities, mass media play a major role in shaping the stigma connected to psychosis.

Setting Goals: Objectives in Public Awareness Work

Several specific objectives for improved public awareness need to be reached before there is any chance of reducing unnecessary suffering caused by the social stigma. Each of these objectives may require different platforms, messages, and strategies. In Hong Kong, objectives common to many psychosis awareness projects include:

1. To improve the general public's knowledge about psychosis
2. To correct misunderstanding about the characteristics of patients
3. To encourage early detection of the illness
4. To emphasise hope in recovery and the patients' potential to lead a fruitful life

These objectives are inter-related:

- (1) and (2) attempt to address the knowledge aspect in stigmatization directly. These steps would include educating the public about symptoms and signs of psychosis, its causes, treatment, outcomes and course, as well as providing counter-evidence against the misbeliefs that patients are always violent, unpredictable, criminals, spoiled, with problematic personalities.
- By encouraging early detection in (3), which presupposes knowledge of symptoms and treatment regimens, patients' long-term outcomes can be improved. Together with immediate benefits for patients, this step will also reduce the chances of untreated individuals displaying symptoms in public, and reinforcing the public stereotypes about psychosis.
- Public awareness of the possibility of recovery in (4) works a number of ways. Many untreated individuals and their family avoid help-seeking, and

thus hinder treatment efficacy, due to the fear of psychosis being an incurable disease. On the other hand, the public misconception that patients are non-productive members of society is a further major driving force sustaining stigma of psychosis. Once this attitude can be dispelled, any psychological need to stigmatise psychosis could be eased.

As straightforward as these objectives may seem, many issues are involved in prioritizing and realizing them. For example, it is not always easy to strike a balance between painting an over-optimistic image of the disease and stressing on the serious consequences of not getting proper and timely treatment. On the other hand, there are also controversies as to whether improved awareness really reduces stigma. Apparently, the stigma of psychosis may be more deeply rooted than can be explained rationally. Nevertheless, any shift in understanding and cooperation brought about by awareness campaigns has lasting value, compared with the influence on attitudes and behaviours, which tends to fade as quickly as the campaign ends (Evans-Lacko et al., 2010). Having these fruits in mind, the packaging of the message and the strategies used in anti-stigma campaigns can have a decisive effect on their success.

Anti-Stigma Messages and Strategies

Careful planning and design is needed to develop culturally sensitive and effective strategies targeting the root of stigmatizing attitudes and behaviours. Before the launch of the EASY programme, a working group comprising media experts and clinicians was set up to plan public education programmes. Intensive meetings and brainstorming sessions were held before the core messages and strategies were decided, ensuring that they were accurate, effective, and balanced. Likewise, both EPISO and JCEP have a unit focusing on public awareness, with personnel experienced in publicity, event organization, and psychosis work. Conventional public education means and more creative efforts were used effectively as the next section describes.

Renaming and rebranding

In Hong Kong, the new Chinese translation for psychosis (思覺失調) introduced by EASY in 2001 has been valuable in promoting public acceptance of the condition (see Chapter 2, "Early Psychosis Services in an Asian Urban

Setting: EASY and Other Services in Hong Kong). From the launch date, large-scale promotion of the new term (and the new service) included advertisements, radio interviews, road shows, websites, press release, exhibition, public talks, school visits, posters, and distribution of leaflets. Similar movements to revise the translation of schizophrenia have also taken place in other Asian countries such as Japan (integration disorder, *togo shitcho sho*, 統合失調症) (Sato, 2006) and Korea (attunement disorder, 調絃病) (Lee & Kwon, 2011).

With this new term less associated with negative connotations, the stage was set for rebranding and portraying a more positive image for psychosis. The "Project Torchlight" campaign by EPISO played a large part in this work. As implied by the name, the project aims to lead a way out of the darkness to a life filled with hope. To add appeal for young people, two popular singers were appointed as ambassadors and produced a Cantopop song for EPISO. A series of events with celebrity endorsement were organized, including an annual Psychosis Day, walkathon, movie premiere, T-shirt charity sale, charity concert, comedy show, and radio drama. All efforts to attach new, positive associations and images to psychosis through these activities were welcomed, bearing in mind that societal changes would be triggered at a deeper and more subconscious level in the public's mind over time.

Community involvement and gatekeeper training

Although often on a smaller scale, community anti-stigma activities that seek the public's active participation generally effect longer-term changes in knowledge, attitude, and behaviours, and complement all high-profile efforts of big anti-stigma campaigns. JCEP's public awareness efforts focused mainly on the community level. Each year, a territory-wide art and psychosis competition is held, engaging people from all walks of life. Although a different form of art is chosen each year, the short movie and essay competition in 2011 attracted a number of highly creative and touching entries from both the public and secondary school students. Prizes were awarded and as an added incentive, awarded works were showcased in a public exhibition and on JCEP's website.

Gatekeeper training is another key community strategy to achieve the aims of public awareness. This is more in-depth training provided to frontline personnel, such as school teachers, social workers, security guards, police, public service staff (e.g., librarians), and church staff. In Hong Kong, apart from general mental health first aid courses provided by various organizations, JCEP has been organizing specific gatekeeper training about early psychosis, with training materials tailored to the needs of different professionals.

Social networks and online presence

The Internet is the first source of information for many people. Websites are therefore a crucial platform for public awareness. In Hong Kong, EASY, EPISO, and JCEP provide a good deal of information about psychosis on their webpages (www3.ha.org.hk/easy/eng/service.html, www.episo.org, www.jcep.hk), including online self-assessment tools, basic facts on psychosis, useful resources and help-seeking guidelines, as well as patients' stories and artworks. Apart from websites, presence in social networks and mini-blogs (e.g., Facebook, Weibo) and video clips search engines (e.g., YouTube) helps widen the reach of audience, which also allows simple and regular updates.

Media collaboration

The mass media has a pervasive effect on public attitudes and information dissemination. Partnering between the media and professionals on psychosis is an important front for reducing stigma. In Hong Kong, knowledge on psychosis has been promoted through press conferences and TV or radio interviews in news or other informative programmes. These efforts are required on a regular basis for the effects to be sustained.

In the same vein, the media can also seriously undermine years of anti-stigma work. It is not unusual for local tabloids to use emotional wordings (e.g., "psychokiller") with explicit photos or illustrations on the front page when accidents involving psychosis patients occur. At present, no professional guidelines for reporting news related to mental illness or regulations against inferior journalistic practice exist. This is an area where more work is needed, with better communication between the mental health field and media workers.

Direct education

Although knowledge exchange may be less effective in reducing stigma, publicity campaigns are still valuable in promoting helpful attitudes towards early help-seeking and proper management of the disease. Increasing public awareness of the early signs and symptoms of psychosis, local pathways to care, and what to expect during and after treatment are important strategies for removing barriers that lead to delayed treatment and unnecessary suffering in patients and families.

In Hong Kong, basic medical information about psychosis is given to the public by means of educational webpages, pamphlets, exhibitions, and talks by the Hospital Authority, universities, professional bodies (e.g., the Hong Kong College of Psychiatrists), and NGOs. Previously, these educational activities tended to be sporadic but since the introduction of the JCEP project, regular talks and exhibitions are common. JCEP also organizes public talks in collaboration with the Hong Kong Public Libraries, so that the messages can reach a wider population.

The presentation of education materials makes a difference. For example, the use of stories, especially first-person accounts, often increases the relevancy for the readership. More vivid and creative ways that enhance the attractiveness of the educational content are also useful.

Currently, knowledge about psychosis or other mental illness is not included in the education curriculum in Hong Kong. However, schools are an important platform for anti-stigma work, especially among younger age groups, to dispel stereotypes about psychosis before they arise. EPISO launched a school project for secondary school students in 2010. Using drama workshops with talks and a finale performance based on the theme of psychosis, this project has been popular among students and is now in the third round of school tours. Future projects to engage even younger students at primary school may also prove beneficial.

The power of contact

Direct personal contact is a powerful strategy for reducing stigma and discrimination (Pettigrew & Tropp, 2006). The need for stereotypes and the power of media propaganda in forming and reinforcing the stigma of psychosis is, at least partly, a result of a lack of direct contact experience between the public and patients. Most recovered patients would not reveal their medical history in view of the associated heavy stigma, As a result, few members of the public have the opportunity to get to know the real, average recovered patient. This fact places the distorted images portrayed in mass media as the main source of impression for most people.

Social contact in real-world settings where patients and healthy people assume equal status is needed to break the circle. Some overseas programmes (e.g., Like Minds, Like Mine in New Zealand) have already started campaigns that focus on creating contact opportunities and empowerment of patients to face the public. In Hong Kong, this is still challenging, especially in identifying well-recovered patients and families who are not afraid to disclose their situation. However, with increasing momentum of public awareness work, personal contact programmes that facilitate mutual cooperation between patients and healthy individuals can be anticipated. Both JCEP and EPISO have begun to organize volunteer training programmes for patients and carers, and are optimistic that a positive change will soon eventuate.

Choosing the Right Messages

The messages to be delivered need to be carefully designed with cultural sensitivity and tailored to the level of awareness in society. Listed in Table 7.1 are key public awareness messages of JCEP's public awareness programmes. These have been developed specifically to address particular conditions in Hong Kong. For example, it is observed that parents may procrastinate in seeking help due to a "wait-and-see" mentality, hoping that their children's abnormal behaviours will go away while avoiding the possibility that they may have an "incurable" illness that the families cannot handle. Several messages in the JCEP programme target these common attitudes and misconceptions, which are delivered using different strategies mentioned above.

For most campaigns, a slogan that is moving and easy to remember, with a strong highlighting effect. In the UK, a key message of the "Time-to-Change" campaign was "Mental illness is one of our last taboos" (Evans-Lacko et al., 2010). In New Zealand, "Know me before you judge me" was the slogan used in the TV campaign of "Like Minds, Like Mine" in 2003. These examples of precise and powerful messaging persuade minds.

Conclusion

In many Western countries, large-scale anti-stigma initiatives for mental illness are in place. In Asia including Hong Kong, public awareness works are gathering pace. The stigma of psychosis is difficult to tackle and the problem is real. Patients and families are faced with daily misunderstandings and prejudices,

Table 7.1
JCEP's key public awareness messages

1. Psychosis falls within a spectrum of normal experiences • It could happen to anyone—it does not mean that you are free from risk whether you are smart, well-educated, strong-minded, or good-willed • Many everyday conditions can lead to psychotic experiences, e.g., sleep deprivation • Symptoms are common—many people experience them at some point in their life
2. Psychotic disorders are biological conditions that can be treated • It is not so mysterious a condition but just another biological problem, like diabetes or osteoporosis; the only difference is the physical or chemical changes happen to involve the brain (a bodily organ) • The brain can be changed and is constantly changing—psychosis is a state rather than the end of the story • Medical advances are significantly improving the situation
3. Early assessment and treatment helps • Signs of psychosis can be subtle; knowledge, alertness, and timely action of family and friends are what usually help • Assessment is simple and accessible • Delay in assessment and treatment would only make the problem worse and create a domino effect in all aspects of the person's life
4. People with psychosis can lead a positive, fruitful life • A "blessing in disguise"—illness and care experience can be enriching if handled appropriately • People with psychosis have much potential that needs to be recognized (e.g., artistic) • Functional recovery is possible and people can contribute greatly, including professionals and highly skilled workers

living under the threat of being socially excluded and discriminated against. Careful planning with a lot of creativity and clever use of resources is needed in public awareness efforts to genuinely lift the situation and help patients step out of the shadow of stigma.

References

Angermeyer, M. C., Dietrich, S., Pott, D., & Matschinger, H. (2005). Media consumption and desire for social distance towards people with schizophrenia. *European Psychiatry, 20*(3), 246–250. doi: S0924-9338(05)00011-8 [pii]10.1016/j.eurpsy.2004.12.005

Byrne, P. (1997). Psychiatric stigma: Past, passing and to come. *Journal of Research in Social Medicine, 90*(11), 618–621.

Evans-Lacko, S., London, J., Little, K., Henderson, C., & Thornicroft, G. (2010). Evaluation of a brief anti-stigma campaign in Cambridge: Do short-term campaigns work? *BMC Public Health, 10*, 339. doi: 1471-2458-10-339 [pii]10.1186/1471-2458-10-339

Granello, D. H., & Pauley, P. S. (2000). Television viewing habits and their relationship to tolerance toward people with mental illness. *Journal of Mental Health Counseling, 22*(2), 162–175.

HKU survey reveals misconceptions and lack of awareness towards psychosis. (2009). Hong Kong: Li Ka Shing Faculty of Medicine, The University of Hong Kong.

Lee, Y. S., & Kwon, J. S. (2011). The birth of a new Korean term for schizophrenia. Paper presented at the Second Asian Congress on Schizophrenia Research, Korea.

Miller, R. (2000). *Straight Talking About Mental Illness with Emphasis on Schizophrenia: An Educational Guide* (2nd edition). Christchurch: Schizophrenia Fellowship of New Zealand Inc.

Pettigrew, T. F., & Tropp, L. R. (2006). A meta-analytic test of intergroup contact theory. *Journal of Personality and Social Psychology, 90*(5), 751–783. doi: 10.1037/0022–3514.90.5.751

Sato, M. (2006). Renaming schizophrenia: A Japanese perspective. *World Psychiatry, 5*(1), 53–55.

8
Early Psychosis in the Workplace

Eric Yu-hai Chen

At Disease Onset

The workplace: An important setting for early detection

For a person employed full-time and working about 40 hours a week, setting aside the time spent on daily travelling and personal care, on average spends about half of his or her waking time in the workplace. Hence, the workplace is an important setting for detecting and managing early signs of psychosis. People sharing the workplace with the concerned individual form a critical network for early detection.

Given the fact that most people spend so much time in the workplace with a lot of intellectual and social interaction every day, it is not surprising that early signs of psychosis should first present themselves at work. For example, the affected person's interactions with colleagues may change significantly, abilities may decline and unusual responses may manifest and attract workmates' attention.

In an ideal world, people sharing the same workplace are suitable candidates to help identify and refer individuals who show signs of early psychosis to early intervention teams for assessment. If those who notice unusual changes of the individual are well-informed enough to seek help, or at least alert parties that may offer professional advice (e.g., telephone-based assessment system), prompt referrals and early treatment would increase. In this sense, the person's workplace and workmates may be as important as his or her family and friends in detecting psychosis and getting timely help for the condition.

Challenges in the workplace

While the workplace can be an important setting for identifying people with psychosis and for soliciting support and help, it can also be a source of stress that magnifies any problems in these individuals. Before public awareness reaches a level in which the majority in community is informed and concerned about psychosis, it is likely that in reality, colleagues or employers may not be sensitive and considerate enough to assist in the process of early identification and treatment. Worse still, some may even exacerbate the illness with their misunderstanding about the affected person's responses, without being able to see them as arising from a disorder.

Even for individuals who are relatively "healthy" mentally, the workplace can present a number of difficult and ambiguous situations, and this is especially the case for people suffering from early psychosis. The very nature of psychosis often renders its sufferers' levels of impairment in their functioning, which are more readily reflected in work performance. People with early psychosis are also particularly sensitive (and sometimes oversensitive) to the immediate environment around them. They may be easily affected by their coworkers' reactions and behaviours, are particularly vulnerable to office politics, or experience initial impairments in interpersonal interactions. All these factors may contribute to the development of psychosis.

When the problems are not appropriately addressed and treated, the decline in performance and difficulties at work can cause the person to lose his or her job after a period of time. Such a loss and the stress related to this will negatively impact on the illness. Failure to get to the root of the abrupt decline in the person's functioning with professional advice and receiving proper diagnosis and treatment, often results in longer-term unemployment for the person as he or she fails repeatedly in obtaining and sustaining a stable job that complements abilities. The affected person and his or her family are often confused and frustrated as a result. Eventually, many people will lose their confidence as an employee.

Workplace as an Important Setting for Recovery

Many studies have provided evidence for a direct relationship between vocational rehabilitation and treatment outcomes. For example, a study by Fraser, Berger, Killackey, and McGorry (2006) has demonstrated that the psychosocial development of patients, which include aspects of social welfare, physical health, and vocational rehabilitation, leads to an improvement in quality of life. A prospective follow-up study by Salokangas (1999) has also suggested that work development after illness onset is one of the major predictors of improvement in clinical symptoms, such as reduced negative symptoms, delusions, hallucinations, disorganization, and depression. These have highlighted the important role of vocational functioning as a treatment outcome after early psychosis.

The workplace is also an important setting for social interaction. There is some evidence that a person's social functioning before treatment is predictive of his or her outcome in psychosis. In a study investigating the relationship between level of social functioning prior to treatment and the severity of negative symptoms and social functioning after one year of treatment, a significant negative correlation was found (Meng et al., 2006). In that study, the Strauss and Carpenter Prognostic Scale (SCS) (Moller, Scharl, & von Zerssen, 1984) was used to assess social functioning. The SCS includes items such as the number and quality of social relations, and fulfilment in life during the previous year. Among these items, a major dimension is the quantity and quality of useful work or schooling. In other words, engagement in useful work is predictive of less severe negative symptoms in the early phase of psychosis.

Challenges in the workplace during recovery

While having a vocational role is an important part of recovery, for a person mid-treatment for early psychosis, the workplace can also pose difficulties.

In the Hong Kong working environment a person with early psychosis often cannot disclose the condition to his/her colleagues or employer. It may be challenging for him or her to take medications during the day, which can result in poor compliance and thus disease control. Some people may have difficulties getting sick leave, and may have to skip follow-up consultations. On the other hand, in many parts of Asia where stigmatization is rampant and the enforcement of anti-discrimination laws are less rigorous, patients may try every effort to hide his or her condition from employers and colleagues when applying for a new job in order to avoid any discrimination that may jeopardize the chance of securing the job. Many people are faced with the dilemma of risking being discovered later at work or not getting a job at all.

Attempts at hiding their condition at work can also cause much anxiety. The daily risk of being discovered raises stress levels for patients recovering from their disease. Such worries, fears, and guilt associated with the stress of having a "secret", which they are forced to hide in the workplace because of stigma and discrimination, might in turn impact negatively on patients' treatment outcomes. These difficulties pertaining to the workplace may partly explain why some patients experience a relapse soon after they resume work.

Suggestions for Employers and Colleagues of People with Psychosis

Given the impacts of a psychotic illness on a person, special accommodation may be needed in the workplace for the patient to be fully engaged. This does not, however, undermine the fact that many individuals with psychosis are gifted and talented in many ways. To bring the best out of a person with psychosis, as is true with other people, interaction in the workplace should focus on the person's relevant capabilities, rather than on the illness he or she faces.

Tragically, a common misconception is that a person at any stage of psychosis is unfit for work, and that he or she should be taken out of the workplace for treatment indefinitely, or until full recovery can be proven. For many, being in a supportive work environment is by itself therapeutic; for others, being able to return to work represents an important milestone in recovery.

As discussed above, individuals with psychosis face many barriers in job-seeking, remaining in a job position, interacting with workmates and business partners. They also have other difficulties specific to the workplace. However, any vocational role is an integral part of the holistic therapeutic process for people suffering from psychosis. Likewise, the workplace has a crucial role in early detection, development, and recovery of early psychosis. As with any person, individuals with early psychosis should not be deprived of the privilege to contribute in the workplace. Employers and healthcare professionals alike should offer the best possible support to people with a psychotic illness in the workplace, by encouraging active participation where appropriate and discouraging any form of discrimination during recruitment and daily interaction.

References

Fraser, R., Berger, G., Killackey, E., & McGorry, P. (2006). Emerging psychosis in young people, Part 3: Key issues for prolonged recovery. *Australian Family Physician, 35*(5), 329–333.

Meng, H., Schimmelmann, B. G., Mohler, B., Lambert, M., Branik, E., Koch, E., et al. (2006). Pretreatment social functioning predicts 1-year outcome in early onset psychosis. *Acta Psychiatrica Scandanavica, 114*(4), 249–256. doi: ACP773 [pii]10.1111/j.1600-0447.2006.00773.x

Moller, H. J., Scharl, W., & von Zerssen, D. (1984). [The Strauss-Carpenter Scale: Evaluation of its prognostic value for the 5-year outcome of schizophrenic patients]. *European Archives of Psychiatry in Neurological Science, 234*(2), 112–117.

Salokangas, R. K. (1999). [Prevention of the first-episode psychosis: A rational basis for the second large progress step in psychiatry]. *Duodecim, 115*(10), 1077–1078.

9
Enhancing Psychosis Detection through Gatekeepers

Chi-wing Law

One of the most significant challenges in running an early assessment and intervention programme for psychosis is how readily people with untreated psychosis can get in touch with services. According to the annual statistics of the Early Assessment and Services for Young People with Psychosis (EASY) in Hong Kong, schools and youth services social workers and counsellors contributed to more than 10% of all referrals, with the vast majority of cases assessed and managed on an outpatient basis. Looking into details of the pathway to care, more than 20% of all clients had had contact with social workers at some point of time before they were first seen by EASY. This shows that social workers and counsellors are important frontline gatekeepers, with whom early psychosis services need to collaborate closely to ensure a comprehensive coverage of referrals of potential clients suffering from psychosis.

Important Roles of Counsellors and Social Workers

Clients in their prodromal or initial phase of psychotic illness may be experiencing rather non-specific symptoms such as mood and personality changes, with resultant influences on their academic or work performance, as well as their relationships with family members and friends. These could easily be mistaken to be part of the schooling problems, adolescent crises, or family turmoil. Family and school social workers are most likely to be the first contact in this phase of the pathway to care.

Social workers have a wide network of contacts with those who are most deprived and in need. These include, for example, young people with a substance abuse problem and unengaged youth at home. These two groups are at higher risk for psychotic disorders, and yet are difficult for ordinary psychiatric services to reach. The more extensive social networks and in-depth outreach services known to social workers allow these potential clients to be reached more easily.

With the rapport and trust developed with their clients, counsellors and social workers are well placed to assist engagement of the client with an early psychosis service. In the subsequent course of treatment and rehabilitation, counsellors and social workers could also help in monitoring the person's condition in settings outside the clinic, such as at school and in the community. This connection would provide medical professionals with a more thorough understanding of any state of remission and recovery.

Potential Challenges in Collaborations with Frontline Gatekeepers

As with any kind of collaboration where multidisciplinary parties are involved, a number of potential challenges need to be tackled.

Increasing awareness in identification of psychosis among youngsters with various social or psychological problems

Training courses

Understandably, counsellors and social workers need to handle a huge variety of problems in young people and psychosis is only one of the many health issues they have to address. Frequent updates on clinical care and awareness building activities need to be offered repeatedly through different channels to keep the staff ready and able to respond effectively to any presenting psychosis. Specific education and publicity programmes are essential and may include in-depth discussions on case scenarios, or workshops on practical skills for handling people with psychosis. Education on psychotic disorders may also become core training for social workers and counsellors.

Quick references and accessories

Materials in the form of brief information booklets, CD-ROMs, etc., would be helpful for quick reference in case of need. More in-depth information could be provided through well-designed and preferably interactive web pages. Small souvenirs such as ball pens, bookmarks, and paper files with the web address and telephone number for assessment service printed on them can serve as easy reminders for target frontline workers.

Easily accessible services

The most important factor of all for enhancing frontline gatekeepers' support of early identification would be the availability of a simple, efficient referral channel for flexible and user-friendly service provision. This step would be useful in overcoming any perceived hurdles in referrals to medical specialists, a long-held concept for many people. Early psychosis services aim at providing flexible arrangements for clinical assessments of suspected cases of psychosis as promptly as possible. In cases where the potential client shows strong resistance to assessments in clinical settings, attempts can be made to collaborate with NGOs (see Chapter 22, "Working with Non-Governmental Organizations in Early Psychosis"), so that the first assessment can be done in a relatively less threatening and stigmatizing environment.

Referring out

Commonly, many cases screened via a telephone enquiry system or clinical triage are not psychotic. Simple tips and advice in handling these non-psychotic problems, as well as useful information to refer the person to other psychiatric services if needed, should be available for workers as far as possible. Non-rejecting attitudes should be maintained by staff. Better liaison with other psychiatric teams may help smooth inter-agency referrals and thus, attract future referrals to early psychosis services if frontline workers find the processes user-friendly.

Improving sensitivity of referrals from frontline gatekeepers

Improvement of "sensitivity" of referrals (number of true cases out of the total number of referrals) from frontline gatekeepers is an important issue that needs to be kept in reasonable balance. The preferred balance between referrals to early psychosis service which are inclusive and sensitive enough to detect cases with very early or even prodromal phase of psychosis, during when the symptoms are not always prominent, and over-referrals of non-psychotic cases, which could overload the services, is a delicate achievement that is often elusive in practice. Much of this balance is a by-product of educational content that emphasizes clear-cut symptoms such as hallucinations, delusions, and thought disorders, and less specific or more ambiguous features such as prodromal signs. Such well-prepared training can lead to a significant difference in the number and nature of referrals to the early psychosis service. This balance needs to be carefully adjusted with time, according to the service capacity and staff experience.

FAQs Raised by Frontline Gatekeepers in the Referral Process

The following questions often arise in the minds of frontline gatekeepers when referring potential clients to an early psychosis service. Careful handling of these enquiries would minimize unnecessary obstacles in service delivery.

Q: *How to motivate a young person with psychotic symptoms to receive assessment and treatment from the early psychosis service?*

A: Initially, some exploration of the client's resistance would be helpful, for example, why is he or she rejecting proper assessment or care from an early psychosis service? Issues of stigmatization, misconception, as well as fear about psychiatric services, need to be discussed (see Chapter 17, "Experience of Stigma in Early Psychosis Patients and Caregivers"). Young people are often worried about friends' and peers' perspectives of the illness. The possible consequences of a psychiatric label for future study or employment would also concern them. They may also worry about disclosing their problems to their parents or other family members, as they may be uncertain about family reactions towards this illness.

Frontline gatekeepers are advised to convey the following points to their clients:

1. During the initial contact, emphasize that only screening services will be provided for the time being. Visiting an early psychosis clinic for assessment does not necessarily mean being a psychiatric client.
2. Depending on the level of acceptance of the individual, the reason for seeking a psychiatric assessment is often flexibly "tailor-made" by the carers. Some may be interested in receiving a "psychological assessment" or getting psychological support for their problems. On the contrary, others may prefer to have a "physical check-up" for their perceived health problems. Whatever the motives, they could be a gateway to an early assessment service.

3. The provision of flexible assessment time and/or place is preferable. Carrying out the first assessment session at the referring NGO office offers a pleasant experience for the client, with the advantage of being in a non-stigmatizing setting. Many clients could be engaged in subsequent consultation and treatment at early psychosis clinics after rapport is established in the initial assessment sessions.
4. Sustained efforts of repeated persuasion from social workers and counsellors have been proven to be effective in clients with initial resistance.
5. Examples of successful and encouraging stories of treatment could be given for reassurance.

Q: *How to distinguish between the prodromal or early phase of a psychotic illness from the normal "emotional turmoil" of adolescence?*

A: First, professionals are advised to acknowledge that this is a difficult situation even for experienced clinicians to discern. As mentioned previously, symptoms experienced in the initial phases of a psychotic illness could be vague and non-specific, and it is sometimes difficult to make a distinction between an adjustment reaction and other psychiatric conditions (see Chapter 12, "Handling At-Risk Mental State").

In general, any *unexplained* change or decline in social interactions and academic performance needs particular attention, especially if those changes are *persistent* and *progressive* despite termination of potential stressors. Affected young people often report problems in concentration while studying, which accounts for their deterioration in academic performance. They often also lack interest in other aspects of life, and withdrawal from social activities becomes a common feature.

At the initial phase of a psychotic illness, young people may be rather sensitive in general, and hold over-valued paranoid ideas towards others. Perceived adverse or rejecting reactions from other students and peers are often exaggerated and leads to progressive deterioration in social relationships. In turn, a vicious cycle forms and feeds back to the over-valued paranoid ideas. School social workers or counsellors, having the privilege of more thorough understanding of the school community in general, are in a suitable position to clarify and reassure.

Q: *How to overcome resistance from the relatives of potential clients in receiving psychiatric services?*

A: Possible contributing factors for the resistance need to be addressed first. Apart from the abovementioned common factors that could hinder potential clients from receiving an early assessment, family members may face additional problems, such as guilt-laden feelings towards their children (see Chapter 17, "Experience of Stigma in Early Psychosis Patients and Caregivers"). Many parents believe that the development of their children's illness is related to problems in their upbringing, such as physical punishment and neglect of developmental needs. Consequently, parents often blame themselves for some perceived faults, and feel ashamed to let relatives or friends know about their children's problems.

On the other hand, some parents perceive the children's abnormal behaviours as some kind of rebellious or repelling acts against them. In these cases, the possibility of their children having an underlying illness is often overlooked. Some parents then resort to the use of hostile approaches towards them. Others would avoid any confrontation with their children at all, worrying that even the suggestion of a psychiatric consultation would worsen their children's problem and jeopardize their relationship.

Proper education for family members of potential clients is important. The biological nature of the illness should be emphasized. Explaining the stress-vulnerability model, that is, a genetic vulnerability or predisposition that interacts with the environment and life events (stressors) to trigger behaviours or psychiatric disorders, may also help. This step helps to reduce parental guilt feelings and avoid misunderstandings that could defer and lengthen the referral process.

Q: *How to collaborate with schools in helping young people with psychosis?*

A: During each stage of the illness, the young person may face different problems at school. In the initial phase when young people start developing psychotic symptoms and possibly abnormal behaviours, proper handling emerges as the immediate challenge. High levels of uncertainties, fears, and doubts will present in the client as well as in classmates and teachers, particularly before psychiatric assessment and treatment has commenced. The school would be concerned particularly about issues of safety, and the possibilities of violence and self-harm (see Chapter 26, "Suicide and Self-Harm Behaviour in Early Psychosis"). Prompt referral for complete psychiatric assessment and treatment from an early psychosis service is most crucial at this stage and frequently, the person may need to be temporarily removed from the potentially stressful environment of the school until a suitable remission of symptoms is achieved with treatment.

Another challenge sets in when the client reaches the initial phase of recovery and starts reintegrating into school life. Certain clinical features may still be present and include residual attenuated psychotic symptoms such as reference ideas and oversensitivity towards others' reactions, subjective cognitive impairments, as well as negative symptoms such as lack of volition and social withdrawal.

One of the immediate issues that he or she may face after resuming school activities is the difficulty of reintegrating into their former circle of peers. Full psychoeducation of classmates would help ease concerns and dispel myths about the person, so as to avoid unnecessary misunderstanding and stigmatization. For the client, psychological preparation would be necessary before they start the new course of study after a period of absence. This preparation would include areas such as handling possible queries raised by classmates about his or her illness. Preparation and rehearsal of "model answers and responses" would help avoid unnecessary stress.

The client may also face other problems after they resume studies. They may be lagging behind with classwork due to a prolonged period of absence. Problems in sustaining attention and concentration in academic tasks also surface and could be related to multiple factors, including presence of residual cognitive impairments, possible side-effects from medications such as drowsiness and extra-pyramidal symptoms, as well as possible negative and depressive symptoms. Progressive, gradual improvement of these residual symptoms is likely, but over time. Continuous persuasion and support for clients are essential in preventing a loss of interest and confidence in continuing studies.

School social workers appear to be an important bridge in facilitating communication and understanding among different parties including the client, his or her family members, schoolteachers, other students, as well as clinicians and case managers, in formulating a progressive yet feasible plan of rehabilitation and reintegration into the usual path of studies. The need for continuous adjustment to the pace of progress and future goals would be required through discussions among different parties in the process.

Q: *Early psychosis and substance abuse are handled by two subspecialty teams in Hong Kong. For young people with problems of both psychosis and substance abuse, from which psychiatric subspecialty should they seek help?*

A: The development of psychotic disorders is not uncommonly associated with the problem of substance abuse or dependence. The relationship between the two is multifaceted and often complicated (see Chapter 27, "Comorbid Substance Abuse in Early Psychosis"). Social workers and counsellors may find it difficult to decide which subspecialty is most appropriate for clients with a combination of these problems.

As a general rule, the appropriate choice of referral depends largely on the client's essential needs and critical issues. For example, for clients suffering from substance dependence who have frequent intoxications and drug-induced psychotic episodes that remit quickly after cessation of substance use, with difficulty in getting rid of the substance, the most important issue would be achieving abstinence from substance use. The episodic psychotic symptoms would likely disappear spontaneously afterwards. A referral to a substance abuse subspecialty team is more appropriate in this case. On the other hand, for those who have recreational use of substances but experience more persistent psychotic symptoms, and suffer mainly from the disabling effects of these symptoms despite cessation of substance use, a referral to an early psychosis intervention programme would be the better choice. Of course, this is only a simple rule of thumb; discussions and discretion are recommended for individual cases with more complicated conditions.

Summary

Frontline gatekeepers are important collaborators in early intervention programmes for psychosis, throughout the entire period from initial engagement with the service to subsequent chapters along their journey of recovery. A communicative partnership with ample chances of opinions, ideas, and experience sharing would provide an important impetus for further improvement in both individual client care and the prospective success of the service programme.

10
Initial Screening and Assessment: A Phone-Based Two-Stage Screening

Sherry Kit-wa Chan, Dana Yuk-yee Chun, and Kin-sheung Wong

One of the core objectives of early psychosis intervention service is to encourage potential clients to seek medical help as soon as possible in order to reduce the duration of untreated psychosis (DUP) (Bertolote & McGorry, 2005). To achieve this, a fast and easy access point for potential clients and their relatives for information and possible referral at the same time becomes essential. The referring system of early psychosis intervention service should therefore be open, direct, simple, accessible, flexible, and user-friendly. In Hong Kong, the Early Assessment Service for Young People with Psychosis (EASY) adopts a two-staged assessment and referral system. This chapter outlines the screening process, sources of referrals, and key skills for initial screening and assessment.

The Screening Process

The two-stage assessment system in EASY sees that every referral is first assessed by a case manager in the first-stage assessment, who is usually a psychiatric nurse. Potential cases are booked for clinical appointments with a psychiatrist (second-stage assessment) (Figure 10.1).

During the first-stage assessment, the case manager collects relevant information directly from the clients and/or their relatives and referrers, such as other family members, school social workers, and school teachers, if possible. Gathering information about clients from different perspectives and settings is crucial for establishing a comprehensive understanding of their current difficulties and complaints.

Before going into detailed psychopathological assessment, several core areas need to be screened to establish the eligibility of the client for EASY. First, the main concerns or problems of the clients are obtained from the referrers with an open and free-flow approach. Open-ended questioning skills supplemented

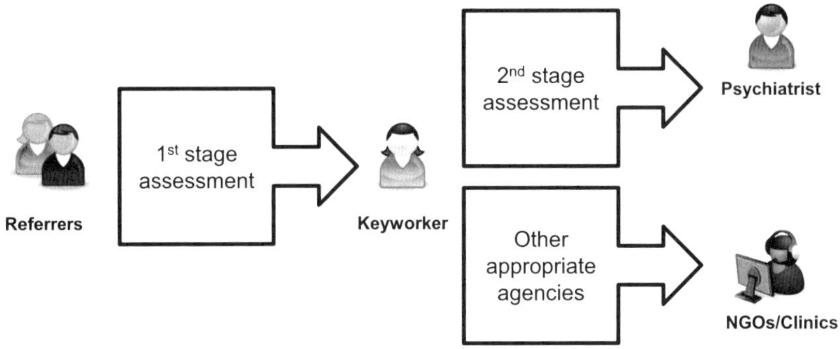

Figure 10.1

Workflow of the EASY referral system

with close-ended questioning skills are used to achieve maximum clarification of the main concerns.

This is then followed with detailed assessment of psychopathology. The standard assessment covers the following topics:

1. Presence of bizarre behaviours or change in behaviours, for example, self-muttering and giggling, preoccupation, and unwillingness to go out with someone who was previously active.
2. Change in perception including taste, feeling, smelling, hearing, and seeing such as hallucinations, illusions, or heightened sensation.
3. Odd beliefs suggestive of delusions, for example, the feeling that one's life is in danger or one is being monitored.
4. Idea of reference, for example, a feeling that one is being gossiped about.
5. Abnormal speech contents and flow.
6. Deterioration in work or studies performance, impairment in social functioning and self-care.
7. Change in affect, for example, emotional changes, such as becoming depressed, elated, or apathetic.

Before contacting the client, the case manager will ask the referrers to define the clients' perceptions of their problems. Such information is important for staff to decide what kind of strategies they can use in contacting the clients as the first contact is essential for successful engagement. For people who have poor insight into their problems and appear to be reluctant to receive services, the conversation can be started with topics that interest them or are relevant to their daily activities so as to establish trust and rapport. However, clients' capacity to explain their own problems and respond to conversations with mental health staff tends to vary as well. Therefore, a helpful, caring, and understanding staff attitude and flexible approach are crucial. A high level of patience across several assessment sessions is often needed at this stage.

Clients who do not meet the intake criteria of EASY are directed to appropriate services if necessary. Exclusion criteria are in place to target clients so as not to overlap psychiatric services by other agencies. Some clients are referred out as they may benefit more from other services; for instance, people suffering from substance abuse are directed to substance abuse clinics; clients aged under 15 years old with conduct or behavioural problems are referred to child and adolescent psychiatric services.

Since early psychosis intervention services emphasize early detection and early treatment, clients without prominent positive symptoms and unexplained deterioration in functioning such as deterioration in work or academic performance, impaired personal hygiene, or sudden personality change are also assessed by psychiatrists for possible prodromal phrase of the illness (see Chapter 12, "Handling At-Risk Mental State").

Sources of Referrals

A substantial proportion of the EASY target clients are referred from the community. To increase public awareness of early psychosis and encourage referrals from target groups, a public awareness campaign and a series of education talks publicized EASY when it was first launched.

Referrals can be grouped into two main categories, external and internal. External referrals are those from the community while internal referrals are those within the healthcare system, that is, referrals directly from psychiatrists of other medical specialties within the mental health service. The referral system of EASY is summarized in Figure 10.2.

External Referrals

Telephone-based assessment system

Telephone screening is an integral part of the assessment service in EASY. The telephone-based assessment system operated by case managers was set

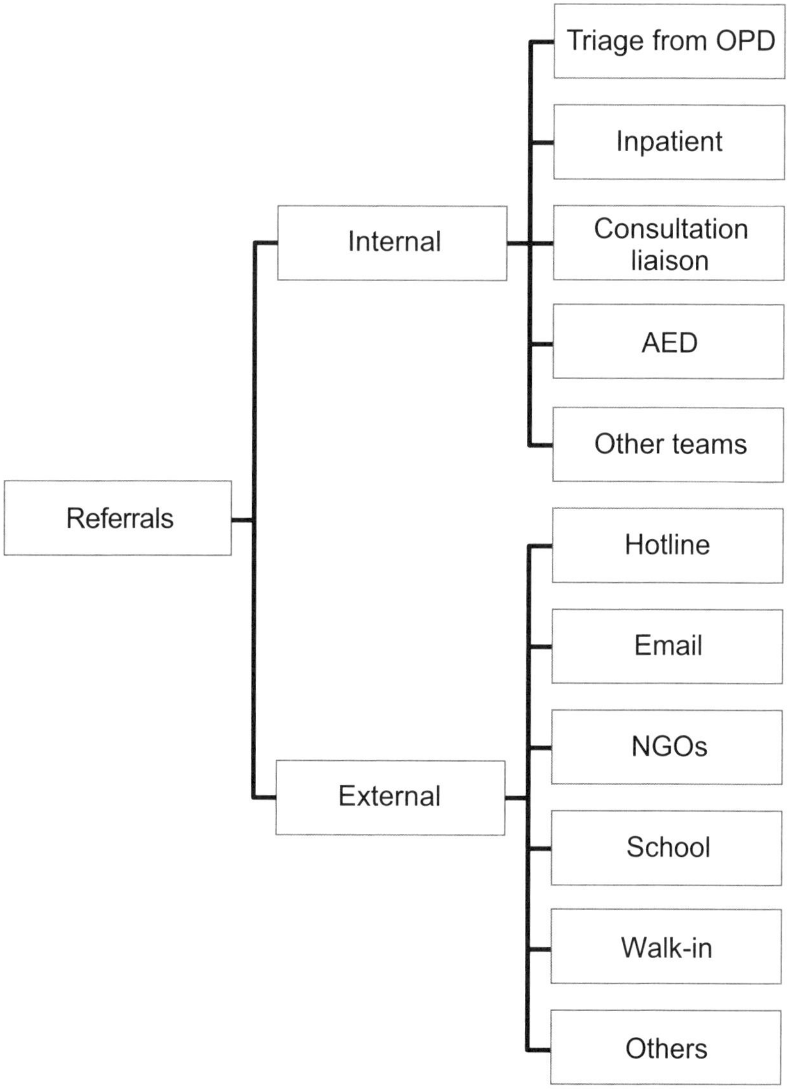

Figure 10.2

Referring system of EASY

up in 2001 after the official launch and provides a direct and easy access for services. The hotline is promoted via media such as road shows, public education, television and newspaper advertisements, radio interviews, press releases, and posters in public areas such as Mass Transit Railway stations and public housing estates.

This telephone-based assessment service operates during office hours and callers can leave a voicemail after office hours. Staff members in each centre will call back the next working day. Referrers or clients have direct telephone contact with an EASY case manager during office hours to obtain information about early psychosis and make referrals if necessary. To date, thousands of phone call referrals confirm this to be the main avenue of referrals.

Online referrals

An official website for EASY was established (www.ha.org.hk/easy/) to provide information about early psychosis and available services. The public can make referrals directly via the email form provided on the website. As the initial step, case managers of each team will respond to email referrals as soon as possible by contacting the referrer via phone or email.

Schools, NGOs and others

Teenagers in schools are one of the main target groups of EASY because epidemiological studies indicate that the peak onset age of psychosis is adolescence (Maurer & Riecher-R, 1993). Regular educational talks are arranged in schools so as to forge a close link and partnership between a particular EASY team and schools within its catchment area. This liaison will not only facilitate referrals and information sharing but also improve support for reintegration of clients back to school post recovery. The other advantage is that school social workers and teachers feel comfortable to make enquiries or referrals directly via phone calls to an EASY office when necessary.

NGOs provide a wide range of services to the public including teenagers. Information about EASY, including its referral mechanisms and knowledge of psychosis, is provided to NGOs on a regular basis to arouse their awareness about the illness. NGO workers are encouraged to make enquiries or referrals directly via phone calls to the EASY office (see Chapter 22, "Working with Non-Governmental Organizations in Early Psychosis").

Finally, without exception, EASY also welcomes enquiries and referrals from all other social agencies, private general practitioners, private psychiatrists and family service centres.

Internal Referrals

Triage from outpatient departments (OPD)

In Hong Kong, a common pathway of entering the public health system is via the OPD. Potential clients may be identified through the OPD triage system and referred to EASY for further assessment.

Accident and emergency departments (AED)

Some clients may go to AED to seek medical assistance. When doctors in AED meet a potential client for EASY, referrals can be made after attending to the person's immediate medical needs.

Consultation liaison team

Sometimes potential clients are admitted to a general ward, most commonly medical wards, for physical problems or organic work-up. Case doctors can also refer them to EASY for further assessment if appropriate.

Hospital inpatients

Inpatient services are another important source of referrals. Potential clients may be admitted to the hospital for acute problems or crises before their psychotic symptoms are identified. The case medical officer in the hospital can then refer them to EASY for further assessment and treatment if necessary.

Other teams or psychiatrists

EASY also welcomes referrals from other psychiatric teams, for example, the child psychiatric team and psychiatrists in other OPDs. Clinicians can make referrals directly if they have potential clients for early psychosis intervention service.

Skills in Initial Screening and Assessment

Listening skills

Screening via telephone is challenging as it is not possible to obtain non-verbal cues such as facial expressions, eye contact, gestures, and postures or movements on the phone. Listening for verbal cues is therefore of paramount importance. Case managers need to pay a lot of attention to verbal cues, especially when callers talk about odd experiences and emotional issues. Special attention is to be paid to any pausing, unwillingness to answer questions, stuttering, or changes in tone of voice or voice tension. Most potential clients, especially self-referrers, may have already experienced some distress from their psychotic symptoms. Paying special attention to these verbal cues can help to detect and identify psychotic symptoms. Explaining to them what these symptoms are, showing empathy, and relieving their stress and worries are an essential part of a telephone-based service. After gaining their trust via the telephone conversation, case managers may then advise them to seek help from psychiatrists.

Encouraging information giving

Some callers may hesitate before making the call to EASY as they may be unsure about the symptoms or unwilling to face the possibility that they or their loved ones may be suffering from psychosis. Showing concern and care for their worries and the impact of the problems on their life is important and will facilitate further disclosure of relevant information and sharing of sensitive issues.

In general, open questions are used to identify areas of concerns, while closed questions are used to narrow down essential information. Empathic understanding and support during the screening process to encourage callers to reveal more information about the illness is important. Rapport can be established by sharing feelings with the caller using empathic statements (e.g., "That must be difficult for you"), paying attention, listening patiently to what the caller is trying to convey (and jotting down all the information given while chatting), and most importantly considering issues from the caller's perspective.

Clarification of information

Naturally, there may be discrepancies between case managers' and the public's understanding of psychopathological terms. People interpret terms such as depression, auditory hallucination, and delusion to mean different behaviours. Thus, the screening process must clarify these mental states.

Since the start of using the new Chinese translation of "early psychosis" (思覺失調, *sijue shitiao*) in Hong Kong (see Chapter 17, "Experience of Stigma in Early Psychosis Patients and Caregivers"), numerous enquiries have been received from the public and professionals for clarification. Some wondered about the difference between psychosis and schizophrenia, while others would like to revise their diagnosis from schizophrenia, which was ascribed by psychiatrists more than 10 years ago, to early psychosis. Staff members need to clarify these issues and obtain concise information from callers before a second-stage assessment is arranged.

Guidelines in screening clients via a telephone-based assessment system

The following tips are helpful for screening clients via phone calls:

1. Respect callers and show concern with positive regard and non-judgemental attitude (i.e., allow callers to explain the psychotic symptoms in his or her own way rather than jumping to a conclusion prematurely).
2. Use active listening skills with a warm manner and be sensitive to the caller's needs.
3. Use simple and clear statements (avoid using jargons such as "hallucinations" and "ideas of reference").
4. Use open questions to identify areas of concern and closed questions to narrow down essential information; in either case, ask questions in a systematic way and jot down all information.
5. Be patient with less relevant content and allow ventilation of feelings.
6. Questions about sensitive issues such as sexual activities should be clear and reasonably direct.
7. End the call by summarizing and checking the information mentioned, making a clear concluding statement. Provide contact information for clients.

Summary

The EASY referral system aims to be open, direct, simple, accessible, flexible, and user-friendly. Therefore referrals are welcomed from diverse sources, both internal and external. External referrals include those from the telephone-based assessment system, emails, schools, family service centres, NGOs, walk-ins, and other agencies such as general practitioners.

Once a referral is received, a case manager will start the screening procedure. Screening is a complex process that requires skills, knowledge, and experiences of a trained professional. Areas of assessment and screening include psychotic experiences, speech, behaviour, affect, and thought processes. Apart from screening symptoms, allowing callers to freely express their concerns and problems is also crucial for initial screening. This allows better understanding of the clients' problems and their feelings, and also provides an opportunity for emotional ventilation.

Telephone-based initial screening is a challenging process of early psychosis intervention services. Since non-verbal cues and behaviours cannot be observed in a non-face-to-face interaction, hidden or underlying messages need to be detected with skill and experience. Case managers have to be sensitive to the callers' needs and be alert to any clues or hints, especially those who are suspicious with paranoid ideas. Despite these challenges in EASY, screening and first-stage assessment conducted by case managers are essential to ensure that clients receive the earliest and best initial psychiatric assessment to establish effective rapport and engagement.

References

Bertolote, J., & McGorry, P. (2005). Early intervention and recovery for young people with early psychosis: Consensus statement. *The British Journal of Psychiatry, 187*(48), s116–s119.

Maurer, K., & Riecher-R, A. (1993). The influence of age and sex on the onset and early course of schizophrenia. *The British Journal of Psychiatry, 162*(1), 80–86.

11
The Diagnostic Interview in Early Psychosis

Wing-chung Chang and Yip-chau Wong

Accurate diagnosis of psychosis in an early phase is important, as case formulation and management can be more confidently determined on this basis. Nevertheless, making a definitive psychiatric diagnosis during the initial interviews can be one of the most challenging aspects in early intervention services. The difficulties, to a certain extent, can be accounted for by the characteristics of young patients and the ambiguous and variable clinical pictures at this early phase. In this chapter, the challenges in ascertaining a definitive diagnosis of early psychosis are described. The approach to the patients presenting with a first-episode psychosis is also outlined.

Diagnostic Difficulties during Early Phase of Psychosis

With the development of the Early Assessment Service for Young People with Psychosis (EASY) in Hong Kong, patients with suspected first-episode psychosis can access psychiatric service earlier in the course of illness. Although the majority of patients presenting to EASY have clinical pictures conforming to the prototypical diagnostic entities defined by the current classification system, for instance, schizophrenia or bipolar affective disorder with psychotic features, it is not uncommon to see patients with subtle and non-specific symptoms that fail to fit into these discrete diagnostic categories in the early stage of illness and which may only evolve into a more definitive manifestation over time (McGorry, 1994). This matter is further complicated by the complex interplay between personality vulnerability, stressor, premorbid development, affective features, drug, as well as changing patterns of symptoms with age and phase of illness (McGorry, 1995). Growing evidence has shown that only a fraction of individuals who reported psychotic experience meet the criteria for a clinical disorder (Claridge et al., 1996; Johns et al., 2002; Peters, Joseph, & Garety, 1999; van Os et al., 2000).

Non-Specific Symptoms during Early Phase of Psychosis

The early course of schizophrenia is commonly divided into the premorbid phase, the prodromal phase, and the acute phase of psychosis (Beiser et al., 1993; Haas & Sweeney, 1992; Keshavan & Schooler, 1992; Loebel et al., 1992). The premorbid phase is the period before illness onset. The prodromal period is defined as the initial phase of disease process, though without any prominent psychotic symptoms (Malla & Norman, 1994). The acute psychotic phase is characterized by specific psychotic signs that fulfil the operational criteria of a diagnostic system.

High levels of non-specific or affective symptoms have been observed in individuals before their onset of psychosis (Owens et al., 2005). Depressed mood and attenuated negative symptoms such as social withdrawal are the most common symptoms identified with the prodromal phase of schizophrenia (an der Heiden & Hafner, 2000). Nonetheless, these symptoms are not specific to schizophrenia. It is also unclear whether these early features are, in fact, predictors, prodromal symptoms or an early manifestation of psychotic illness. To compound the problem, studies have repeatedly shown that only a proportion of individuals with these non-specific symptoms would experience full-blown psychosis in the future. In this regard, it is hard to clearly determine the case formulation and treatment plan for those individuals exhibiting these putatively prodromal, yet non-specific symptoms until the nature of these symptoms can be better elucidated.

Heterogeneity of Schizophrenic Symptomatology

The heterogeneity of schizophrenic symptomatology is well documented (Bleuler, 1950; Strauss, Carpenter, & Bartko, 1974; Crow, 1985; Andreasen, 1982). Research in recent decades has suggested classification of symptoms as either positive or negative (Crow, 1985; Andreasen & Olsen, 1982; Carpenter, Heinrichs, & Wagman, 1988). Depression is a common first presenting complaint in patients who later receive a revised diagnosis of schizophrenia. The finding that depressive symptoms are present in 75% of first-episode patients suggests that they may be a core part of schizophrenia, or a reaction to the experience of psychosis (Koreen et al., 1993). Chapman (1966) found intense anxiety to be almost invariable, and that perceptual disorders were common. In high-risk populations who later developed psychosis, a higher level of perceptual abnormalities was found (Owens et al., 2005). Given the high prevalence of atypical symptoms at the initial phase of psychosis, clinicians should take extra caution when excluding patient with non-specific symptoms from the diagnosis of psychosis.

Instability of Diagnosis

Many psychiatric diagnoses are subject to revision during a patient's lifetime, and this is particularly true for psychosis. Diagnostic stability is the degree to which a diagnosis remains unchanged at subsequent evaluations (Stanton & Joyce, 1993). Diagnostic change can be attributable to illness evolution and methodological artefacts such as information variance, unreliable assessment and inconsistent application of diagnostic criteria (Fennig et al., 1994). In recent years, a number of studies have been conducted to examine diagnostic stability in first-episode psychosis samples. The literature consistently shows that schizophrenia and bipolar affective disorder were the most stable diagnoses in functional psychosis (mostly above 90% and 80%, respectively) (Chang et al., 2009). Other non-affective psychoses such as delusional disorder and acute and transient psychoses were found to be diagnostically less stable with a significant proportion of patients having these diagnoses reclassified as schizophrenia over time (Chang et al., 2009).

Chang et al. (2009) conducted a five-year follow-up study investigating stability of diagnoses among Chinese young patients presenting with first-episode psychosis to EASY using systematic record review and consensus diagnostic assignment procedure. The study revealed that around 20% of patients had diagnostic revision at the end of the five-year follow-up period. Consistent with the literature, well-defined diagnostic entities i.e., schizophrenia and bipolar affective disorder were found to be diagnostically stable. The least stable baseline diagnoses were unspecified non-organic psychosis, acute and transient psychotic disorders and delusional disorder. The predominant pattern of diagnostic shift was towards schizophrenia. The results thus echoed the concept of differentiation, which hypothesized that the initial non-specific clinical picture of functional psychosis might become clearer over time and evolve into a typical syndrome such as schizophrenia (McGorry, 1994).

Given the fluidity of clinical presentation and the findings of frequent diagnostic change in the initial stage of psychotic illness, definitive diagnosis may not always be made after initial interview and assessment. Longitudinal validation with regular diagnostic reviews throughout the follow-up period should be emphasized.

Problem in Recognition or Expression of Symptoms

Although onset of psychosis can be acute, it was repeatedly shown that gradual onset is common (Beiser et al., 1993; Fenton & McGlashan, 1991). With slow changes, it is likely for patient's caregivers to have ignored the signs and symptoms and not being able to give an accurate account of the patient's progress. Owing to the nature of the negative symptoms (e.g., poverty of speech, anhedonia, and avolition), patients exhibiting prominent negative symptoms may have difficulty expressing their feelings clearly. And as the evolution of negative symptoms is mostly gradual with the manifestation being much less dramatic in comparison with positive psychotic symptoms, it is suggested that the presence of negative symptoms may be associated with treatment delay i.e., duration of untreated psychosis (Edwards et al., 1999; Larsen, McGlashan, & Moe, 1996).

Age-related factors

Schizophrenia and related psychotic disorders often set in during adolescence or early adulthood, with subsequent impact on psychosocial functioning (Hafner & Nowotny, 1995; Ritsner et al., 2003; Volkmar, 1996). Patients with earlier onset have been reported to show less differentiated presentation. Diagnosis is also less stable over time in adolescence-onset compared with adult-onset psychosis (Menezes & Milovan, 2000; Werry, McClellan, & Chard, 1991). Differences between these two groups are more quantitative than qualitative. Although the findings are not completely consistent, there is evidence that the younger-onset group has more affective symptoms (Joyce, 1984; Werry et al., 1991) and a higher frequency of behaviour problems and dysphoria (Menezes & Milovan, 2000; Werry et al., 1991). A higher level of negative symptoms has also been shown in adolescence-onset patients (Ballageer et al., 2005). The negative symptoms may not be easily differentiated from the emotional or behavioural manifestations that are commonly observed in this particular group of patients. In view of the above findings, additional difficulties may be encountered in diagnosing young patients with early psychosis.

Presence of other psychiatric disorders comorbidities

Clinical presentation of psychosis can be further compounded by comorbidities such as substance misuse and other psychiatric disorders in which patients may present with eccentric behaviours or odd verbal expression that cannot be easily differentiated from psychotic symptoms. Axis I diagnoses such as obsessive compulsive disorder and Asperger's syndrome, as well as axis II diagnoses such as mental retardation and personality disorder are some of the examples.

In Hong Kong, concern for substance misuse in adolescents is growing. An increasing trend of psychotropic substance use has been observed in the past decade, most significantly among young drug abusers who are aged below 21 years (Government Secretariat, 2008). Ketamine, ecstasy, methamphetamine, cannabis, and cocaine are the most prevalent illicit drugs misused in this age group. The harmful effects may range from attention deficits, cognitive impairment, depression, to full-blown psychosis. Furthermore, studies repeatedly found that slimming pills that contain sibutramine are also another cause of psychosis (e.g., see Khan et al, 1987; Carney, 1988). Psychotic experiences induced by these substances are thus increasingly seen in clinical settings. Clinically, it may not always be easy to differentiate between drug-induced and functional psychosis, especially when patients refuse to cooperate during interviews or decline urine screening for illicit drugs, or when a reliable history cannot be obtained from informants.

Obsessive symptoms may occur in the prodromal phase of schizophrenia (Rosen, 1957). In addition, schizophrenia patients with comorbid obsessive compulsive disorder have more emotional reactions and poorer executive function (Lysaker et al., 2000). Given these considerations, clinicians may need to be careful when assessing patients with obsessive symptoms, especially when atypical features are present.

Personality disorders that are found to be associated with liability to schizophrenia are schizotypal personality disorder (Baron et al., 1985; Battaglia et al., 1995; Battaglia et al., 1991; Kendler & Gruenberg, 1984; Kendler et al., 1993; Kendler et al., 1995), paranoid personality disorder (Baron et al., 1985; Kendler et al., 1993) and schizoid personality disorder (Kendler et al., 1993). Although these diagnoses tend to run a chronic course without definite onset and progression, the intensity of the symptoms may fluctuate intermittently and present as features that point to a diagnosis of psychosis.

Approach to Patients with First-Episode Psychosis

Although there is no single best approach applicable across patients and families, the assessment process can be facilitated by considering the nature of early psychosis and paying attention to the potential difficulties in making a diagnosis of psychosis. Clinicians may also wish to tailor the method of interview to suit the needs of patients with early psychosis and their informants.

Initial interview: Setting and approach

Preparation before the first interview may make the process of establishing therapeutic alliance easier. In EASY, after a case manager conducts first-stage screening, a multidisciplinary meeting will be held to determine the initial management plan. Before the first appointment, the case manager will normally brief the patient about the purpose of interview and its setting. For patients who refuse to come for assessment, family members may be interviewed, and feasible plan to contact the patient will be discussed. Initial interview is usually carried out in an EASY clinic to engage and gather information from patients and informants, such as family members, school social worker, teacher, friends, classmates, and church fellows.

Establishing trust and rapport is of paramount importance when assessing young patients with suspected psychosis. An empathic, calm, and friendly manner may encourage the patient to take part in the interview regardless of the setting. Therapeutic interaction, such as reflection and empathic listening, may ease anxiety in patients and help convince those who are sceptical about the interview. Understanding that youngsters need respect and privacy just as adults do, clinicians should have the opportunity to interview the patient in private. Sensitive issues, such as patient's view on their family, alcohol and substance misuse, sexual history, and forensic history should be handled with care. Confidentiality should not be breached unless fully justified. Their interaction with caregivers should also be tactfully handled. For instance, a caregiver's comments may be considered criticisms by the patient, especially when they are openly discussed in front of medical professionals. When a patient is reluctant to elaborate further about his or her experience or feedback on the caregiver's query, his or her feelings should be validated and emotional reaction should be timely addressed.

Support from and alliance with caregivers is of equal importance. Similarly, the emotion and reaction of caregivers should also be carefully assessed, as they are often in a phase of shock or grief in the initial illness stage. Sometimes they may displace their anger towards medical staff or the patient. Providing realistic expectations and an overview of the plan for subsequent assessment and management may minimize misunderstandings, disengagement, and negative emotional impact in caregivers. Caregivers should be educated early when there are difficulties in confirming a definitive diagnosis, emphasizing the risk of making diagnosis on inadequate grounds.

Look for changes in clarifying the phenomenon is essential. Regardless of how non-specific symptoms in early psychosis are conceptualized, some elements of change from a previous state, either objective or subjective, are integral to the concept of psychosis (Beiser et al., 1993; Keith & Matthews, 1991; Loebel et al., 1992; Yung & McGorry, 1996). Apart from systematic questioning, it is often useful to be sensitive and alert to factual cues, non-verbal as well as behavioural evidence, especially when assessing patients who are suggestible, guarded, or perplexed. Unexplained changes in lifestyle and social interaction may hint at probable underlying psychiatric problems. It is also common for young patients to display bizarre behaviours at the onset of psychotic illness (Ballageer et al., 2005). A similar approach can also be applied to patients who are cooperative but cannot clearly express their feelings, which may be caused by a cognitive impairment associated with the mental illness, immature verbal ability, borderline intelligence, or the non-specific nature of early symptoms in psychosis.

Differential diagnosis, work-up, and revision of diagnosis

After gathering information from patients and all informants, clinicians may have a list of differential diagnoses for guiding subsequent management such as further investigation, appropriate intervention, and setting of treatment. Sometimes, when the clinical presentation is atypical, differential diagnosis can only be made as the symptoms or signs unfold after several sessions.

On the basis of a sensible list of differential diagnoses, relevant and appropriate, the physical work-up should be determined at this phase. Medical or neurological causes should be excluded before confirming the diagnosis of functional psychosis, as organic conditions could be clinically similar to the classical presentations of schizophrenia (Davison & Bagley, 1969; Johnstone et al., 1986). Atypical features should be taken seriously, as they may point to possible organic causes. Background of family medical history, acute and rapid downhill course, as well as perceptual disturbance in visual, olfactory, or tactile modalities may be indicative of an organic nature of the psychosis. Common physical causes of psychotic phenomenon include metabolic disease, endocrine disease, intracranial pathology such as epilepsy or cerebral infection, poisoning, and side-effects of medication. Uncommon causes such as brain tumour or encephalopathy related to charcoal burning may run a subacute course. Thus, when presentation is atypical and treatment responses remain unsatisfactory after a reasonable period of time, clinicians should consider a further physical work-up and revision of diagnosis.

As mentioned above, clinicians should also be aware of the fact that comorbidities such as substance misuse are commonly seen in young people with early psychosis (see Chapter 27, "Comorbid Substance Abuse in Early Psychosis"). Covert drug-taking is not infrequently seen, and appropriate investigation should thus be done when substance abuse is suspected. Initial diagnosis of drug-induced psychosis needs to be followed up carefully, as a significant proportion of these patients will have a diagnosis shift towards schizophrenia. It should also be recognized that diagnoses of drug-induced psychosis and schizophrenia can coexist. Thus, underlying motives of substance misuse, such as self-medication to mask psychotic symptoms, to alleviate negative symptoms, or to mitigate side-effects of medication should be explored to minimize the risk of labelling the psychosis as purely drug-related.

All forms of psychosis should be considered when physical causes are excluded. Schizophrenia, affective psychosis, and drug-induced psychosis are amongst the most prevalent diagnoses in young patients. Less common diagnoses include acute and transient psychotic disorders, delusional disorder, and schizoaffective disorder. Depression can happen in the prodromal phase, or it can be a consequence of schizophrenia in the recovery phase. A diagnosis of unspecified psychosis is commonly given but also frequently revised, as it represents a group of patients who present with non-specific symptoms that could not fulfil the operationalized criteria of any specific type of psychotic disorder. Clinicians should be prepared to review the diagnosis when a change in clinical presentation becomes evident.

Conclusion

To ascertain a definitive diagnosis at the early phase of psychosis is one of the key challenges in early intervention services. Given that early symptoms can be non-specific and unstable, a definitive diagnosis should be determined with caution. Clearly, it is unwise to prematurely confirm a diagnosis of psychotic illness, as its consequence can be devastating for patients and their family. A longitudinal perspective should be taken into consideration in diagnostic assignment. A sensitive, pragmatic, and empathic approach may help engage patients and caregivers, even when a definitive diagnosis cannot be made in the initial interviews.

References

an der Heiden, W., & Hafner, H. (2000). The epidemiology of onset and course of schizophrenia. *European Archives of Psychiatry & Clinical Neuroscience, 250*(6), 292–303.

Andreasen, N. C. (1982). Negative symptoms in schizophrenia: Definition and reliability. *Archives of General Psychiatry, 39*(7), 784–788.

Andreasen, N. C., & Olsen, S. (1982). Negative v positive schizophrenia: Definition and validation. *Archives of General Psychiatry, 39*(7), 789–794.

Ballageer, T., Malla, A., Manchanda, R., Takhar, J., & Haricharan, R. (2005). Is adolescent-onset first-episode psychosis different from adult onset? *Journal of the American Academy of Child & Adolescence Psychiatry, 44*(8), 782–789. doi: S0890-8567(09)61739-1 pii]10.1097/01.chi.0000164591.55942.ea

Baron, M., Gruen, R., Rainer, J. D., Kane, J., Asnis, L., & Lord, S. (1985). A family study of schizophrenic and normal control probands: Implications for the spectrum concept of schizophrenia. *American Journal of Psychiatry, 142*(4), 447–455.

Battaglia, M., Bernardeschi, L., Franchini, L., Bellodi, L., & Smeraldi, E. (1995). A family study of schizotypal disorder. *Schizophrenia Bulletin, 21*(1), 33–45.

Battaglia, M., Gasperini, M., Sciuto, G., Scherillo, P., Diaferia, G., & Bellodi, L. (1991). Psychiatric disorders in the families of schizotypal subjects. *Schizophrenia Bulletin, 17*(4), 659–668.

Beiser, M., Erickson, D., Fleming, J. A., & Iacono, W. G. (1993). Establishing the onset of psychotic illness. *American Journal of Psychiatry, 150*(9), 1349–1354.

Bleuler, E. (1950). Dementia praecox or the group of schizophrenias. Oxford, England: International Universities Press.

Carney, M. W. (1988). Diethylpropion and psychosis. *British Journal of Psychiatry 152*, 146–147. doi: 10.1192/bjp.152.1.146.

Carpenter, W. T., Jr., Heinrichs, D. W., & Wagman, A. M. (1988). Deficit and nondeficit forms of schizophrenia: The concept. *American Journal of Psychiatry, 145*(5), 578–583.

Chang, W. C., Chan, S. S. M., Chung, D. W. S. (2009). Diagnostic stability of functional psychosis: A systematic review. *Hong Kong Journal of Psychiatry*, 19, 30–41.

Chang, W. C., Pang, S. L., Chung, D. W., & Chan, S. S. (2009). Five-year stability of ICD-10 diagnoses among Chinese patients presented with first-episode psychosis in Hong Kong. *Schizophrenia Research, 115*(2–3), 351–357. doi: 10.1016/j.schres.2009.09.037

Chapman, J. (1966). The early symptoms of schizophrenia. *British Journal of Psychiatry, 112*(484), 225–251.

Claridge, G., McCreery, C., Mason, O., Bentall, R., Boyle, G., Slade, P., et al. (1996). The factor structure of "schizotypal" traits: A large replication study. *British Journal of Clinical Psychology, 35 (Pt 1)*, 103–115.

Crow, T. J. (1985). The two-syndrome concept: Origins and current status. *Schizophrenia Bulletin, 11*(3), 471–486.

Davison, K., & Bagley, C. R. (1969). Schizophrenia-like psychoses associated with organic disorder of the central nervous system: A review of the liteature. In *Current Problems in Neuropsychiatry*, edited by R. N. Harrington, 113–184. Ashford, Kent: Headley.

Edwards, J., McGorry, P. D., Waddell, F. M., & Harrigan, S. M. (1999). Enduring negative symptoms in first-episode psychosis: Comparison of six methods using follow-up data. *Schizophrenia Research, 40*(2), 147–158. doi: S0920-9964(99)00043-2 [pii]

Fennig, S., Kovasznay, B., Rich, C., Ram, R., Pato, C., Miller, A., et al. (1994). Six-month stability of psychiatric diagnoses in first-admission patients with psychosis. [Research Support, U.S. Government, P.H.S.]. *The American Journal of Psychiatry, 151*(8), 1200–1208.

Fenton, W. S., & McGlashan, T. H. (1991). Natural history of schizophrenia subtypes. II. Positive and negative symptoms and long-term course. *Archives of General Psychiatry, 48*(11), 978–986.

Government Secretariat. (2008). *Central Registry of Drug Abuse: 1999–2008*. (58). Hong Kong Special Administrative Region.

Haas, G. L., & Sweeney, J. A. (1992). Premorbid and onset features of first-episode schizophrenia. *Schizophrenia Bulletin, 18*(3), 373–386.

Hafner, H., & Nowotny, B. (1995). Epidemiology of early-onset schizophrenia. *European Archives of Psychiatry and Clinical Neuroscience, 245*(2), 80–92.

Johns, L. C., Nazroo, J. Y., Bebbington, P., & Kuipers, E. (2002). Occurrence of hallucinatory experiences in a community sample and ethnic variations. *British Journal of Psychiatry, 180*, 174–178.

Johnstone, E. C., Crow, T. J., Johnson, A. L., & MacMillan, J. F. (1986). The Northwick Park Study of first episodes of schizophrenia. I. Presentation of the illness and problems relating to admission. *The British Journal of Psychiatry: The Journal of Mental Science, 148*, 115–120.

Joyce, P. R. (1984). Age of Onset in Bipolar Affective-Disorder and Mis-Diagnosis as Schizophrenia. *Psychological Medicine, 14*(1), 145–149.

Keith, S. J., & Matthews, S. M. (1991). The diagnosis of schizophrenia: A review of onset and duration issues. *Schizophrenia Bulletin, 17*(1), 51–67.

Kendler, K. S., & Gruenberg, A. M. (1984). An independent analysis of the Danish Adoption Study of Schizophrenia. VI. The relationship between psychiatric disorders as defined by DSM-III in the relatives and adoptees. *Archives of General Psychiatry, 41*(6), 555–564.

Kendler, K. S., McGuire, M., Gruenberg, A. M., O'Hare, A., Spellman, M., & Walsh, D. (1993). The Roscommon Family Study. III. Schizophrenia-related personality disorders in relatives. *Archives of General Psychiatry, 50*(10), 781–788.

Kendler, K. S., McGuire, M., Gruenberg, A. M., & Walsh, D. (1995). Schizotypal symptoms and signs in the Roscommon Family Study: Their factor structure and familial relationship with psychotic and affective disorders. *Archives of General Psychiatry, 52*(4), 296–303.

Keshavan, M. S., & Schooler, N. R. (1992). First-episode studies in schizophrenia: Criteria and characterization. *Schizophrenia Bulletin, 18*(3), 491–513.

Khan, S. A., Spiegel, D. A., & Jobe, P. C. (1987). Psychotomimetic effects of anorectic drugs. *American Family Physician, 36*(2), 107–112.

Koreen, A. R., Siris, S. G., Chakos, M., Alvir, J., Mayerhoff, D., & Lieberman, J. (1993). Depression in first-episode schizophrenia. *American Journal of Psychiatry, 150*(11), 1643–1648.

Larsen, T. K., McGlashan, T. H., & Moe, L. C. (1996). First-episode schizophrenia: I. Early course parameters. *Schizophrenia Bulletin, 22*(2), 241–256.

Loebel, A. D., Lieberman, J. A., Alvir, J. M., Mayerhoff, D. I., Geisler, S. H., & Szymanski, S. R. (1992). Duration of psychosis and outcome in first-episode schizophrenia. *American Journal of Psychiatry, 149*(9), 1183–1188.

Lysaker, P. H., Marks, K. A., Picone, J. B., Rollins, A. L., Fastenau, P. S., & Bond, G. R. (2000). Obsessive and compulsive symptoms in schizophrenia: Clinical and neurocognitive correlates. *Journal of Nervous and Mental Disorders, 188*(2), 78–83.

Malla, A. K., & Norman, R. M. (1994). Prodromal symptoms in schizophrenia. *British Journal of Psychiatry, 164*(4), 487–493.

McGorry, P. (1995). A treatment-relevant classification of psychotic disorders. *Australian and New Zealand Journal of Psychiatry, 29*(4), 555–558.

McGorry, P. D. (1994). The influence of illness duration on syndrome clarity and stability in functional psychosis: Does the diagnosis emerge and stabilise with time? [Review]. *The Australian and New Zealand Journal of Psychiatry, 28*(4), 607–619.

Menezes, N. M., & Milovan, E. (2000). First-episode psychosis: A comparative review of diagnostic evolution and predictive variables in adolescents versus adults. *Canadian Journal of Psychiatry, 45*(8), 710–716.

Owens, D. G., Miller, P., Lawrie, S. M., & Johnstone, E. C. (2005). Pathogenesis of schizophrenia: A psychopathological perspective. *British Journal of Psychiatry, 186*, 386–393. doi: 186/5/386 [pii]10.1192/bjp.186.5.386

Peters, E. R., Joseph, S. A., & Garety, P. A. (1999). Measurement of delusional ideation in the normal population: Introducing the PDI (Peters et al. Delusions Inventory). *Schizophrenia Bulletin, 25*(3), 553–576.

Ritsner, M., Kurs, R., Gibel, A., Hirschmann, S., Shinkarenko, E., & Ratner, Y. (2003). Predictors of quality of life in major psychoses: A naturalistic follow-up study. *Journal of Clinical Psychiatry, 64*(3), 308–315.

Rosen, I. (1957). The clinical significance of obsessions in schizophrenia. *Journal of Mental Sciences, 103*(433), 773–785.

Stanton, M. W., & Joyce, P. R. (1993). Stability of psychiatric diagnoses in New Zealand psychiatric hospitals. *The Australian and New Zealand Journal of Psychiatry, 27*(1), 2–8.

Strauss, J. S., Carpenter, W. T., Jr., & Bartko, J. J. (1974). The diagnosis and understanding of schizophrenia: Summary and conclusions. *Schizophrenia Bulletin* (11), 70–80.

van Os, J., Hanssen, M., Bijl, R. V., & Ravelli, A. (2000). Strauss (1969) revisited: A psychosis continuum in the general population? *Schizophrenia Research, 45*(1–2), 11–20. doi: S0920–9964(99)00224–8 [pii]

Volkmar, F. R. (1996). Childhood and adolescent psychosis: A review of the past 10 years. *Journal of the American Academy of Child & Adolescence Psychiatry, 35*(7), 843–851. doi: S0890–8567(09)62462-X [pii]10.1097/00004583–199607000–00009

Werry, J. S., McClellan, J. M., & Chard, L. (1991). Childhood and adolescent schizophrenic, bipolar, and schizoaffective disorders: A clinical and outcome study. *Journal of the American Academy of Child & Adolescence Psychiatry, 30*(3), 457–465. doi: S0890–8567(09)64566–4 [pii]10.1097/00004583–199105000–00017

Yung, A. R., & McGorry, P. D. (1996). The prodromal phase of first-episode psychosis: Past and current conceptualizations. *Schizophrenia Bulletin, 22*(2), 353–370.

12
Handling At-Risk Mental State

May Mei-ling Lam, Chi-chiu Lee, Wing-chung Chang, and Se-fong Hung

Various studies have demonstrated that schizophrenia is often preceded by a prodromal phase. It is suggested that the earlier the treatment begins, the faster the recovery and the better the overall outcome. The rationale for early intervention in psychosis has been extensively discussed in recent years (Corcoran, Malaspina, & Hercher, 2005; Larsen et al., 2001; Malla & Norman, 2002; McGorry et al., 2000; McGorry, Yung, & Phillips, 2001; Verdoux & Cougnard, 2003), and it is generally acknowledged that most psychosocial impairment develops in the prodromal and onset phase (Hafner et al., 1995).

Research on the prodrome has a long tradition in Germany, although most of the earlier studies have been retrospective in nature and mainly driven by psychopathological interests (Huber et al., 1980). More recently, prospective research in the emerging phase of psychotic disorders has aimed at building an evidence base to guide therapeutic intervention and clarify biological and psychosocial factors and mechanisms involved in the psychotic breakdown. The goal of this research is to prevent or at least ameliorate psychotic disorders.

This chapter will:

1. review the concept of prodrome and research approaches for identifying high-risk individuals;
2. review research findings on at-risk mental states and preventive studies in these individuals;
3. describe how high-risk cases are handled in early psychosis services in Hong Kong with reference to a local prodrome study; and
4. discuss obstacles and ethical issues concerning the intervention for high-risk individuals.

The Concept of Prodrome in Psychotic Disorders

The period prior to the clear-cut diagnosis of a psychotic disorder such as schizophrenia, has traditionally been referred to as the "pre-onset phase". The term covers two phases, the "premorbid phase" and the "prodromal phase". The premorbid phase is the period during childhood, and usually at least part of adolescence, in which emotional, cognitive, and behavioural functioning is not impaired. The prodromal phase is usually characterized by a sustained and clinically impaired deviation from the premorbid level of experience and behaviour.

Various studies have demonstrated that the prodromal period is characterized by non-specific symptoms, such as depressed mood and anxiety, attenuated negative symptoms, as well as subthreshold psychotic symptoms, and is associated with substantial levels of psychosocial impairment and disability (Hafner et al., 1999; Larsen, McGlashan, & Moe, 1996; Yung & McGorry, 1996). The subtle, subjectively experienced cognitive, vegetative, and perceptual disturbances, the so-called "basic symptoms", have also been described (Gross, 1989, 1997; Gross, Huber, & Klosterkotter, 1992). This prodromal period is often prolonged, lasting from two to five years (Beiser et al., 1993), and associated with substantial levels of psychosocial impairment and disability. Researchers and clinicians view the prodromal period as potentially important for early intervention and possible prevention of the development of psychotic disorders.

Up until now, reliable criteria for identifying impending psychosis are not yet available. The *Diagnostic and Statistical Manual of Mental Disorders*, third edition, revised (DSM-III-R), provided a list of nine criteria, mainly observable behaviours but also subjectively experienced changes, for identifying schizophrenia prodrome. But McGorry et al. (2000) challenged the non-specificity of these prodromal symptoms and, in addition, concerns such as whether these items give a valid description of the initial prodromal period have led to this list of criteria being dropped in the DSM-IV (Corcoran, First, & Cornblatt, 2010). The *International Classification of Diseases*, Tenth Revision (ICD-10) acknowledges prodrome as part of schizophrenic disorders; however, prodromal symptoms are not included in the ICD-10 description of schizophrenia because of their poor reliability for measurement and low specificity. Several research approaches can be used to address this issue.

Retrospective Studies

Initial efforts to chart the pre-psychotic pathway have followed a retrospective research strategy, that is, a reconstruction of prodrome by the patient or informants after the onset of psychotic illness. Hafner et al. (1992) developed the Interview for the Retrospective Assessment of the Onset of Schizophrenia (IRAOS) to predict onset of illness retrospectively by studying a population-based sample of 232 first-episode schizophrenia cases. A total of 73% of subjects showed a prodrome averaging five years in length. This phase characteristically began with negative symptoms. In 57% of the cases, social impairment began within two to four years before illness onset (Hafner et al., 1999). Positive symptoms were not included in the ten most frequent symptoms of schizophrenia prodrome. Other retrospective qualitative analyses revealed that prodromal symptoms were non-specific with subthreshold psychotic symptoms reported in up to 70% of patients.

Although informative, retrospective studies are subject to recall and selective bias. Factors that can affect accuracy of recall include family guilt, patient's mental state at the time of interview, and the degree of sealing over in either the patient or their family. In other words, the coping style of both patients and informants can affect the retrospective description of the prodrome.

Population Screening, Longitudinal Birth Cohort and Genetic High-Risk Studies

Large population screening would be costly and possibly impractical given the low annual incidence rate of schizophrenia (about 10 to 15 per 100,000) and other psychoses.

Longitudinal birth cohort studies are long-term projects that follow individuals from childhood or early adolescence through adulthood, covering the period of the highest risk of onset of schizophrenia. Follow-up assessments are performed at one- to five-year intervals, and outcome measures include the development of schizophrenia and schizophrenia spectrum disorders, as well as other psychotic disorders. Examples of such studies include the British 1946 birth cohort and Dunedin birth cohort in 1972.

In genetic high-risk studies, a group with presumably increased genetic risk, that is, offspring or other family members of a patient with schizophrenia, is identified. Additional risk factors that make transition to a frank psychotic disorder more likely can thus be examined. Such studies include the Copenhagen High Risk Project in 1962, the New York High Risk Project in 1971 and 1977, and the Edinburgh High Risk Study.

These longitudinal birth cohort and genetic high-risk studies have the advantage of guiding risk factors identification and providing clues about causality, thereby highlighting the premorbid deficits that treatment should target at. However, these are large-scale projects that require long-term commitment from research staff, and researchers acknowledge that a high transition rate to a psychotic disorder is unlikely. Findings from these studies are also not generalizable beyond the genetically defined high-risk group, while most people with schizophrenia do not have family members with the disorder. Patients with one schizophrenic parent constitute only 10% of the total population of schizophrenia. Only 19 new cases of schizophrenia would be identified by screening 10,000 first-degree relatives per year. The estimated annual yield of new cases is thus quite low for the purpose of accruing a sample of patients for research.

Prospective Follow-Up of Individuals with Subthreshold Symptoms

The Buckingham Study in 1992 was a pioneer study attempting to intervene in the pre-psychotic phase (Falloon, 1992). Kwapil et al. developed the Wisconsin Manual of rating psychotic-like symptoms on a continuum of deviancy from normal to grossly psychotic, defining symptoms that may indicate "psychosis proneness" (Kwapil, Chapman, & Chapman, 1999). They screened large numbers of college students in the United States to identify individuals who scored high on scales to detect attenuated and isolated psychotic symptoms. A control group of low scorers was also identified. Subjects were re-contacted 10 to 15 years later for follow-up and outcome measures of the development of psychotic disorders, schizotypal symptoms, and psychotic-like experiences were assessed. High scorers on one of the scales significantly exceeded controls on all of the above measures at follow-up, suggesting the predictive power of this approach. However, generalization of the findings is limited, as this sample was drawn from college students only.

Klosterkotter and colleagues (2001) assessed a cohort of patients with personality and neurotic disorders for the presence of "basic symptoms", which were subtle subjective experiences of cognitive, vegetative, and perceptual disturbance prior to the onset of psychosis, as described by Gross and Huber using the Bonn Scale for the Assessment of Basic Symptoms (BSABS). After an average follow-up period of 9.6 years, 79 of 160 subjects developed schizophrenia. Presence of certain basic symptoms, including thought interference, thought blockage, pressure of thought, visual disturbances, and disturbed reception of language, was found to be highly predictive of psychosis.

Another approach is in-depth observation of a small number of patients during the development of psychosis. This method has the advantage of being prospective, allowing observation and recording of changes in the individual as they develop. However, as it is not possible to predict with any reasonable degree of accuracy as to who will develop psychosis, it is difficult to know which individuals to study prospectively.

At-Risk Mental State and Preventive Studies

Since prodrome is a retrospective concept that is confirmed only after the development of full-blown psychotic illness, Yung and colleagues (2003) in Melbourne introduced the term "at-risk mental state" (ARMS), implying that a subthreshold syndrome can be regarded as a risk factor for subsequent development of psychosis. However, the onset of psychosis is not inevitable. The Melbourne group conducted studies in the Personal Assistance and Crisis Evaluation (PACE) clinic, which focuses on identifying precursors that occur just prior to psychosis onset; that is, to identify individuals who run a high risk of becoming psychotic in the short term in the absence of treatment. The operationalized ARMS criteria (or ultra high-risk criteria, UHR criteria) include three subgroups: (1) genetic risk in combination of functioning decline; (2) attenuated positive psychotic symptoms; and (3) transient psychotic episodes. Individuals with ARMS are followed up prospectively with monthly ratings of psychopathology. Initial data from the PACE clinic yielded a conversion rate of 30% to 50%.

Several other prospective studies have been initiated worldwide in the past few years using ARMS criteria similar to those adopted in PACE. Some of these include the Preventive through Risk Identification, Management and Education (PRIME) study, the Early Treatment of Psychosis Project (TOPP) in Norway and the Detection of Early Psychosis (DEEP) project in Finland. The conversion rates to psychosis reported for the early phases of these studies are between 30% and 60%. The Hillside Study of Risk and Early Detection of Schizophrenia (HSREDS) included a naturalistic study of 22 adolescents who were "clinically at risk", defined strictly on the basis of clinical characteristics and attenuated negative and disorganized symptoms, and attenuated positive and transient psychotic symptoms, which are similar to the ARMS. Recruited subjects were treated with symptomatic and psychosocial approach. Six months after initial assessment, only 14% of the putatively prodrome patients had developed psychotic symptoms (Correll et al., 2005).

The major challenge for an early detection and preventive approach based on the clinical high-risk strategy is to prospectively differentiate true from false-positive prodromal cases. However, thus far, no robust predictors of transition to psychosis have been identified and the sensitivity of this clinical high-risk approach remained low. Literature shows that psychosis transition rate of at-risk subjects identified by these UHR criteria ranged from 14% to 41% within the first 12 months (Cannon et al., 2008; Ruhrmann et al., 2010; Yung et al., 2003; Yung et al., 2007). A recent systematic review (Simon et al., 2011) found that, on average 76% of at-risk subjects remained non-psychotic during 6 to 40 months of follow-up. Alternatively, emerging evidence has suggested significant functional impairments in at-risk individuals when compared with non-psychiatric controls, irrespective of whether they developed psychosis or not at follow-up (Addington et al., 2011), thereby highlighting the treatment needs for this clinical high-risk group.

Handling High-Risk Cases in Early Intervention Services in Hong Kong

A significant proportion of young people who were assessed by the Early Assessment Service for Young People with Psychosis Programme (EASY) in Hong Kong are non-psychotic but markedly distressed. These "non-psychotic cases" would be referred to other appropriate psychiatric services such as child and adolescent psychiatric service or general adult psychiatric service for management of the identified psychiatric disorders, such as emotional conduct disorder, depressive or anxiety disorders, eating disorder, and hyperkinetic disorder, if any. Some of these individuals would be referred to other non-psychiatric services such as substance abuse counselling services and youth counselling services.

Among the EASY referrals, there are some distressed youths who are not floridly psychotic but have subthreshold psychotic symptoms, or significant functional decline. After being assessed as having a high risk for psychosis by a psychiatrist, they will be monitored regularly at the EASY outpatient clinic or in community settings where appropriate. At present, high-risk cases in EASY are defined based on individual psychiatrist's clinical assessment; since operationalized inclusion criteria for high-risk cases are yet to be adopted.

From the EASY data, there were 5,069 referrals from 2001 to 2005, of whom 4,102 (80.9%) received psychiatric assessment. Among these cases, 2,450 (59.7%) were psychotic and received intensive comprehensive treatment accordingly. With the remaining 1,652 "non-cases", 890 (53.9%) were assessed to be high-risk cases and were monitored regularly by the EASY team for a period of no more than 24 months.

Case Illustration of a High-Risk Individual Monitored by the EASY Team

John was an 18-year-old secondary school student. His elder brother had an onset of schizophrenia at age 13. His mother approached EASY via the telephone-based assessment system in view of John's concentration difficulties and poor motivation, in addition to falling behind drastically at school. At initial presentation, John reported a sense of uncertainty, that he felt something was not quite right with the world. He felt that his face and head looked somewhat different, and that he was not able to think clearly and follow through conversation with others. He reported that the change started after his head was hit by volleyball in the school playground 18 months ago. He became very sensitive and distressed whenever others came close to him, as he worried that others would touch his head and damage his brain. However, John was not always convinced in these unusual beliefs; at times, he retained insight and felt his worries were excessive and irrational. Feeling that his friends had changed somehow, John felt uneasy being around with others for a long period of time and he preferred to be alone.

John's mother reported that he was increasingly suspicious. John was noted to be very sensitive whenever his personal particulars got mentioned in the public as he worried that others would spread his particulars. John was also noted by his mother to have impaired will power and was not motivated to attend school.

At the initial assessment, John did not meet diagnostic criteria for psychosis but he was assessed by his clinician to be a high-risk case. John was monitored by the EASY team on a regular basis by psychiatrists and case managers. He received symptomatic treatment with benzodiazepine for his anxiety and sleep difficulties. John also had brief sessions with a clinical psychologist for stress management and relaxation skills training. Rapport with John increased over time. He was able to relax and even joke with his clinician and case manager. John's attenuated symptoms fluctuated in frequency and severity in the first nine months. Despite falling behind at school, he was still attending school regularly.

In the tenth month of treatment, John presented for several appointments in a row with increasing frequency and intensity of his paranoid beliefs. He was convinced that his brain was shaking inside after a drop of rain fell on his head. He had persistent unshakable belief that people unknown to him on the street were gossiping and following him. He developed a fleeting auditory hallucination of tapping noises. He subsequently received intensive comprehensive treatment for his psychotic illness.

A Prodrome Study in Hong Kong

A naturalistic prospective study was conducted in 2002 at Kwai Chung Hospital Clinic (one of the EASY centres) with the aim of assessing the rate of transition to psychosis in a group of Chinese youths, and comparing the groups who did with the one who did not become psychotic over a six-month follow-up period, specifically on variables such psychopathology and functional decline (Lam, Hung, & Chen, 2006). All participants met one or more of the three operationalized criteria defined in the 2002 version of the Comprehensive Assessment of At-Risk Mental State (CAARMS):

1. *Vulnerable Group:* Combination of trait risk factors, that are, a family history of psychosis in the first degree and a significant deterioration as measured by a 30% drop in Global Assessment of Functioning (GAF) score.
2. *Attenuated Symptom Group:* Symptoms that deviate from the normal phenomena but are not yet frankly psychotic, that is, of subthreshold intensity.

3. *Brief Limited Intermittent Psychotic Symptom Group:* Symptoms that are of psychotic intensity but infrequent, or which have a total duration of less than seven days before spontaneously remitting.

Subjects with a known history of psychotic episodes, previous or current treatment with antipsychotic or mood stabilizing medications were excluded from the study. The main outcome measure of this study was the development of psychosis. The point of onset was defined as a specific severity and frequency score on the subscales for disorders of thought content, perceptual abnormalities, or disorganized speech in the CAARMS.

Between June 2002 and April 2003, there were a total of 256 referrals made to the clinic, among which 153 were psychotic and treated accordingly. With the remaining 103 subjects, 67 met the operationalized intake criteria of the study, and 62 consented to participate in the project. They were not on antipsychotics or mood stabilizers at intake. They all received supportive counselling, and had access to symptomatic treatment with antidepressant and anxiolytic medications when needed. Over the six-month follow-up period, 18 subjects (29%) met the criteria for a psychotic disorder (Lam et al., 2006). In addition, significant differences were found in the intake Positive and Negative Syndrome Scale (PANSS), CAARMS, and GAF scores between the group that ultimately became psychotic and the group that did not. At one-year follow-up, 41.5% of the cohort made transition to a psychotic disorder. At two-year follow-up, 53% of the group made transition to psychosis (Lam et al., 2006).

The study results indicate that it is possible to identify a sub-sample of the Hong Kong population with a high rate of transition to psychosis (29%) within six months and 53% of the identified high-risk subjects developed psychosis within two years. The identified high-risk subjects had moderate levels of functional decline and psychopathology at the study intake. A lengthy delay was found between the onset of symptoms and the study intake from 11 days to 6.6 years.

Obstacles and Ethical Issues in Pre-Psychotic Intervention

With the vast and growing enthusiasm worldwide in pre-psychotic identification and intervention over the past few years, professionals working in this field need to be aware of the obstacles and ethical issues in this area. Many of these arise from the genuine problems associated with defining the onset of psychiatric disorders. The lack of a clear boundary between normality and psychotic disorders is especially relevant during onset, as syndromes emerge and progress from origins, which are indistinguishable from normal experiences.

The problems with false positives should be noted. Misunderstanding the implications of a false positive diagnostic test can lead to negative outcomes, including inappropriate stigmatization, discrimination in employment, and difficulties in obtaining life insurance. Communicating one's risk status to others can deprive him or her of social and occupational opportunities in several ways including overt discrimination. Self-stigma presents another potential hazard to subjects' psychological and social development, and is related to low self-esteem, diminished self-efficacy, and abandonment of developmental challenges and occupational goals. There are also growing concerns regarding specific risks associated with the use of antipsychotic medications in adolescents. There are too few data concerning the long-term and short-term consequences of exposing a developing brain to these drugs. The problems of false negatives are less frequently mentioned; however, being wrongly reassured may also undermine early detection.

References

Addington, J., Cornblatt, B. A., Cadenhead, K. S., Cannon, T. D., McGlashan, T. H., Perkins, D. O., et al. (2011). At clinical high risk for psychosis: Outcome for nonconverters. [Comparative Study Research Support, N.I.H., Extramural Research Support, Non-U.S. Government]. *The American Journal of Psychiatry, 168*(8), 800–805. doi: 10.1176/appi.ajp.2011.10081191

Beiser, M., Erickson, D., Fleming, J. A., & Iacono, W. G. (1993). Establishing the onset of psychotic illness. *The American Journal of Psychiatry, 150*(9), 1349–1354.

Cannon, T. D., Cadenhead, K., Cornblatt, B., Woods, S. W., Addington, J., Walker, E., et al. (2008). Prediction of psychosis in youth at high clinical risk: A multisite longitudinal study in North America. [Multicenter Study Research Support, N.I.H., Extramural Research Support, Non-U.S. Government]. *Archives of General Psychiatry, 65*(1), 28–37. doi: 10.1001/archgenpsychiatry.2007.3

Corcoran, C., Malaspina, D., & Hercher, L. (2005). Prodromal interventions for schizophrenia vulnerability: The risks of being "at risk". *Schizophrenia Research, 73*(2–3), 173–184. doi: S0920-9964(04)00218-X [pii] 10.1016/j.schres.2004.05.021

Corcoran, C. M., First, M. B., & Cornblatt, B. (2010). The psychosis risk syndrome and its proposed inclusion in the DSM-V: A risk-benefit analysis. [Research Support, N.I.H., Extramural Research Support, Non-U.S. Government]. *Schizophrenia Research, 120*(1–3), 16–22. doi: 10.1016/j.schres.2010.03.018

Correll, C. U., Lencz, T., Smith, C. W., Auther, A. M., Nakayama, E. Y., Hovey, L., et al. (2005). Prospective study of adolescents with subsyndromal psychosis: Characteristics and outcome. [Research Support, N.I.H., Extramural Research Support, U.S. Government, P.H.S.]. *Journal of Child and Adolescent Psychopharmacology, 15*(3), 418–433. doi: 10.1089/cap.2005.15.418

Falloon, I. R. (1992). Early intervention for first episodes of schizophrenia: A preliminary exploration. *Psychiatry, 55*(1), 4–15.

Gross, G. (1989). The 'basic' symptoms of schizophrenia. *British Journal of Psychiatry. Supplement* (7), 21–25; discussion 37–40.

Gross, G. (1997). The onset of schizophrenia. *Schizophrenia Research, 28*(2–3), 187–198.

Gross, G., Huber, G., & Klosterkotter, J. (1992). Early Diagnosis of Schizophrenia. *Neurology Psychiatry and Brain Research, 1*(1), 17–22.

Hafner, H., Loffler, W., Maurer, K., Hambrecht, M., & an der Heiden, W. (1999). Depression, negative symptoms, social stagnation and social decline in the early course of schizophrenia. *Acta Psychiatrica Scandinavica,100*(2), 105–118.

Hafner, H., Nowotny, B., Loffler, W., an der Heiden, W., & Maurer, K. (1995). When and how does schizophrenia produce social deficits? *European Archives of Psychiatry& Clinical Neuroscience, 246*(1), 17–28.

Hafner, H., Riecher-Rossler, A., Hambrecht, M., Maurer, K., Meissner, S., Schmidtke, A., et al. (1992). IRAOS: An instrument for the assessment of onset and early course of schizophrenia. *Schizophrenia Research, 6*(3), 209–223.

Huber, G., Gross, G., Schuttler, R., & Linz, M. (1980). Longitudinal studies of schizophrenic patients. *Schizophrenia Bulletin, 6*(4), 592–605.

Klosterkotter, J., Hellmich, M., Steinmeyer, E. M., & Schultze-Lutter, F. (2001). Diagnosing schizophrenia in the initial prodromal phase. [Comparative Study Research Support, Non-U.S. Government]. *Archives of General Psychiatry, 58*(2), 158–164.

Kwapil, T. R., Chapman, L. J., & Chapman, J. (1999). Validity and usefulness of the Wisconsin Manual for Assessing Psychotic-like Experiences. *Schizophrenia Bulletin, 25*(2), 363–375.

Lam, M. M., Hung, S. F., & Chen, E. Y. (2006). Transition to psychosis: 6-month follow-up of a Chinese high-risk group in Hong Kong. *The Australian and New Zealand Journal of Psychiatry, 40*(5), 414–420. doi: 10.1111/j.1440–1614.2006.01817.x

Larsen, T. K., Friis, S., Haahr, U., Joa, I., Johannessen, J. O., Melle, I., et al. (2001). Early detection and intervention in first-episode schizophrenia: A critical review. *Acta Psychiatrica Scandinavica, 103*(5), 323–334. doi: acp131 [pii]

Larsen, T. K., McGlashan, T. H., & Moe, L. C. (1996). First-episode schizophrenia: I. Early course parameters. *Schizophrenia Bulletin, 22*(2), 241–256.

Malla, A. K., & Norman, R. M. G. (2002). Early intervention in schizophrenia and related disorders: Advantages and pitfalls. *Current Opinion in Psychiatry, 15*(1), 17–23.

McGorry, P. D., McKenzie, D., Jackson, H. J., Waddell, F., & Curry, C. (2000). Can we improve the diagnostic efficiency and predictive power of prodromal symptoms for schizophrenia? *Schizophrenia Research, 42*(2), 91–100. doi: S0920–9964(99)00125–5 [pii]

McGorry, P. D., Yung, A., & Phillips, L. (2001). Ethics and early intervention in psychosis: Keeping up the pace and staying in step. *Schizophrenia Research, 51*(1), 17–29. doi: S0920–9964(01)00235–3 [pii]

Ruhrmann, S., Schultze-Lutter, F., Salokangas, R. K., Heinimaa, M., Linszen, D., Dingemans, P., et al. (2010). Prediction of psychosis in adolescents and young adults at high risk: Results from the prospective European prediction of psychosis study. [Comparative Study Multicenter Study Research Support, Non-U.S. Government]. *Archives of General Psychiatry, 67*(3), 241–251. doi: 10.1001/archgenpsychiatry.2009.206

Simon, A. E., Velthorst, E., Nieman, D. H., Linszen, D., Umbricht, D., & de Haan, L. (2011). Ultra high-risk state for psychosis and non-transition: A systematic review. [Review]. *Schizophrenia Research, 132*(1), 8–17. doi: 10.1016/j.schres.2011.07.002

Verdoux, H., & Cougnard, A. (2003). The early detection and treatment controversy in schizophrenia research. *Current Opinion in Psychiatry, 16*(2), 175–179. doi: 10.1097/01.yco.0000058616.61505.ec

Yung, A. R., & McGorry, P. D. (1996). The prodromal phase of first-episode psychosis: Past and current conceptualizations. *Schizophrenia Bulletin, 22*(2), 353–370.

Yung, A. R., Phillips, L. J., Yuen, H. P., Francey, S. M., McFarlane, C. A., Hallgren, M., et al. (2003). Psychosis prediction: 12-month follow up of a high-risk ("prodromal") group. [Comparative Study Research Support, Non-U.S. Government]. *Schizophrenia Research, 60*(1), 21–32.

Yung, A. R., Yuen, H. P., Berger, G., Francey, S., Hung, T. C., Nelson, B., et al. (2007). Declining transition rate in ultra high risk (prodromal) services: Dilution or reduction of risk? *Schizophrenia Bulletin, 33*(3), 673–681. doi: 10.1093/schbul/sbm015

Part III

Culturally Relevant Psychosocial Case Intervention

13 Implementing Psychological Intervention Programmes in Early Psychosis (PIPE)

Suzanne Ho-wai So

Over the past five decades or so, antipsychotic treatment has been and remains the mainstay of treatment for psychosis (Kapur & Mamo, 2003). Abundant evidence supports its efficacy in reducing the severity of psychotic symptoms such as hallucinations and delusions (see reviews by Miyamoto et al., 2005; Miyamoto et al., 2003). However, approximately 20%–50% of patients demonstrate persistent symptoms despite active antipsychotic treatment (Craig et al., 2004; Kane, 1996; Lieberman et al., 2005; Marder, 1996; Kane, 1999).

In the past two decades, there has been a surge of psychological interventions targeting psychotic symptoms and functional deterioration. Examples include cognitive-behavioural therapy for psychosis, family interventions, mindfulness-based treatment, social skills training, cognitive remediation, etc. (see reviews by Pilling et al., 2002; Tai & Turkington, 2009; Tarrier & Wykes, 2004; Wykes et al., 2011; Zimmermann et al., 2005). Psychological treatment approaches to psychosis flourish against a background where early detection and intervention for psychosis is promoted (spearheaded by clinicians in Australia, the US and the UK) and community treatment of psychiatric patients is advocated. The National Institute for Health and Clinical Excellence (NICE) in the UK has established treatment guidelines that recommend cognitive-behavioural therapy (CBT) and family interventions for psychosis (National Institute for Health and Clinical Excellence, 2009).

Background of PIPE

In 2001, when the Early Assessment Service for Young People with Psychosis (EASY) was launched in Hong Kong, this step was taken against a background that treatment of early psychosis called for timely and comprehensive psychosocial intervention in order to facilitate more enduring recovery. Psychological Intervention Programmes for Early Psychosis (PIPE) were developed by a group of clinical psychologists in Hong Kong who had extensive experience of providing psychological service to individuals with psychotic and other psychiatric illnesses (So, Wong, & Chong, 2002). The basic structure of the PIPE protocol was established in 2001, and has since been constantly updated with feedback and comments from case managers and service users, and to keep abreast with the growing literature. In order to sustain the effectiveness of the PIPE programme, clinicians of EASY constantly receive local and overseas training and supervision.

The acronym "PIPE" denotes "connection", "thoroughfare", and "outlet". The Chinese concept of *qudao* (渠道) also signifies "a way out", "a means to an end", and instils a sense of hope that is pivotal to recovering from first-episode psychosis. The content of the PIPE protocol was largely based on research findings in studies of psychological models of psychosis and associated interventions (mainly from Western countries), with adaptations made to take into account local Chinese cultural perspectives. This was especially important for PIPE-I (i.e. enhancing psychological adjustment to early psychosis) because cultural values are embedded in the way an individual and the family explain and deal with the psychotic experience. The PIPE protocol will likely serve as: (i) a guideline for clinicians of EASY when considering appropriate and evidence-based psychological intervention for individual service users; and (ii) a tool book for case managers about psychoeducation for psychosis. While this chapter gives an outline of the PIPE modules, the actual protocol consists of a set of handbooks, which are available from the author or EASY.

Structure of PIPE

In order to promote more lasting recovery from the psychotic episode, facilitate psychological adjustment, and prevent relapse, PIPE comprises three main modules of intervention for young adults with early psychosis, as well as their families. The three conceptual modules of the PIPE are:

- PIPE-I: Enhancing psychological adjustment to early psychosis
- PIPE-II: Intervention for secondary morbidity
- PIPE-III: CBT for drug-resistant psychotic symptoms

The structure and procedural delivery of the PIPE intervention modules for patients and their families are shown in Figure 13.1. PIPE is an integral component of the EASY service, which includes medical and other psychosocial interventions provided by a multidisciplinary team. Treatment needs for each service user are regularly reviewed by this team. In Figure 13.1, the PIPE modules are indicated in boxes with thick frames. The dotted arrows point to service modules that only select patients and families with specific treatment needs receive, whereas the other boxes carry core service modules that all patients and families are presented. While PIPE-I is conducted by case managers to every service user of EASY, other modules (PIPE-IA,-II, and -III) are provided based on referrals to a clinical psychologist by the treating psychiatrist. Therefore, the PIPE module(s) received differ between individuals,

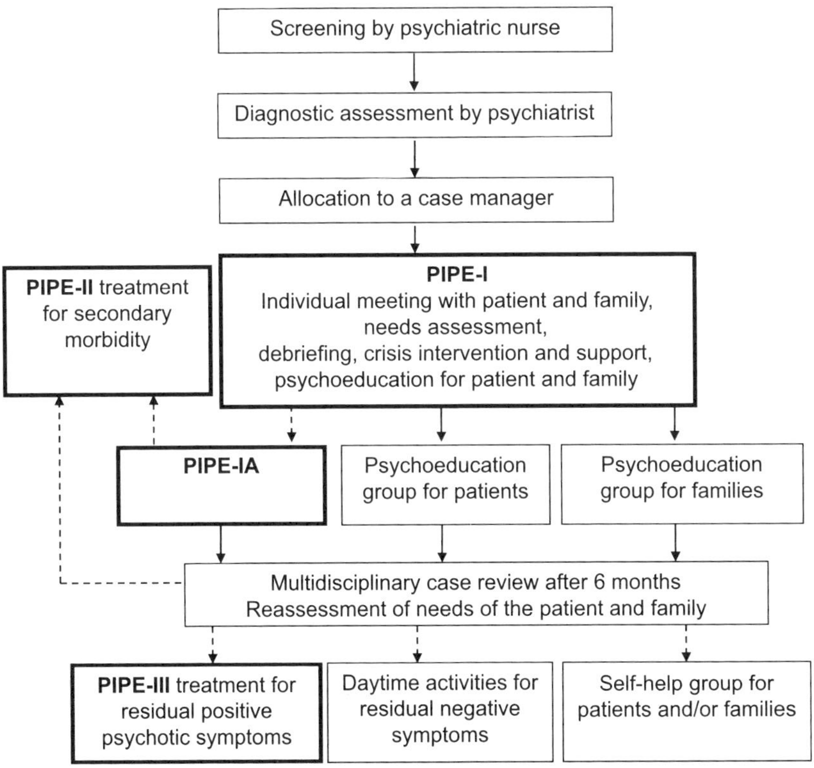

Figure 13.1

Psychosocial intervention for first-episode psychosis

according to specific therapeutic goals identified through a comprehensive needs assessment.

Assessment of Treatment Goals and Suitability

Recovery takes different forms in different individuals. In a 10-year longitudinal follow-up study of first-episode schizophrenia, Srivastava, Thakar, Shah, and Stitt (2008) found that clinical recovery was achieved in 61% of patients on a clinical global impression scale, 25% on multiple clinical criteria, and 26% on social recovery criteria; only 23% of patients showed both clinical and social recovery. About half of the patients who remitted symptomatically or clinically did not experience functional recovery, and 5% to 7% of patients who experienced functional recovery did not show remission of symptoms. Therefore, clinical recovery is not equivalent to social recovery, and it is important to identify treatment goals individually.

Driven by the traditional "medical model", patients and clinicians alike have held the common view that recovery equates with complete symptom remission, cessation of medications, and the resumption of normal psychosocial functioning (Harding et al., 1987; Hopper, Harrison, & Wanderling, 2007; Ng et al., 2011; Robinson et al., 2004). However, a newer "social recovery" model maintains that, rather than "becoming normal", being in recovery is a process of gaining and regaining lost targets in life and discovering new ones, through coming to terms with the illness experience (Deegan, 1996). Therefore, it is emphasized that PIPE clinicians have open and continuous discussions with each individual patient, understanding their unique illness model (i.e., what they think has happened to them during the illness and why), and identify treatment needs individually.

PIPE-I: Enhancing Psychological Adjustment to Early Psychosis

Psychological reactions to first-episode psychosis

First-episode psychosis can be a confusing and traumatic experience for patients and their families. Patients often report feeling confused and dread when they first encounter the unusual experiences during the psychotic episode, which are novel to them and which they cannot name. After an initial feeling of shock and anger, they commonly react to the experiences with denial and avoidance. Frightened by the symptoms, some patients may attempt to control or reduce them, without much benefit. So and Wong (2008) found that most people with hallucinations reported unpleasant voices and tried to cope with them using various strategies, which they found to be only moderately effective. Some patients complied with commands given by the voices, shouted back at them, or tried to resist their influence by sleeping all day; these efforts added to the distress and disrupted their lifestyle even further.

Patients with delusions also often acted on their symptoms through safety behaviours such as avoidance, which in turn lead to persistent delusions (Freeman et al., 2007). Therefore, one of the aims in PIPE-I (and PIPE-IA) is to provide systematic psychoeducation of the illness and help patients develop more effective ways of dealing with psychotic symptoms.

Case Vignette 1

Ambrose was brought to the early intervention clinic because of sudden emergence of visual hallucinations and disorganized behaviours. The psychotic symptoms were quickly controlled by antipsychotic medications. However, Ambrose decided to withdraw from medical treatment as he believed that the abnormal experiences were related to some religious rituals that he had been through. Both Ambrose and his mother planned to go through some rites in order to break the spell and expel the spirits.

Few patients obtain insight into their illness the first time they experience it. Not knowing what the experience is about, patients typically attribute the events to stress or something external to the self, such as possession by evil spirits. Some patients, like Ambrose, explain the psychotic experience by cult beliefs. Instead of seeking timely treatment from mental health professionals, they resort to spiritual or superstitious means. Others may believe that the abnormal experience is a form of punishment from the Divine, which they deserve in return for something bad they have done. Therefore, they tend to passively tolerate it or try to "make up for it" by engaging in good deeds. These myths and misunderstandings of psychosis inevitably delay effective treatment.

A well-established fact, that individuals with psychosis have different recovery styles (see also Chapter 30, "Concepts of Recovery in Early Psychosis"). According to McGlashan, Levy, and Carpenter (1975), this fact is borne out by patients who "seal over" to avoid thinking about their symptoms or engaging in treatment and services, thus generating poorer long-term outcomes. Jackson, Knott, Skeate, and Birchwood (2004) suggested that sealing over might be a psychological defence against the trauma of early psychosis. McGorry (1992) observes, in his clinical practice, that it often takes several episodes and many years for patients to adjust to the potentially relapsing illness while maintaining a secure identity and self-esteem. It is the clinicians' task, during PIPE-I and PIPE-IA, to help patients to come to terms with the illness in an objective yet empathic and non-confrontational manner.

Alongside insight, the social stigma attached to mental illness is another factor that affects patients' and families' reaction to the diagnosis of early psychosis. Local surveys found that patients in Hong Kong experience marked stigma associated with their mental illnesses and tend to conceal their illnesses (Chung & Wong, 2004; Lee, Lee, Chiu, & Kleinman, 2005; see Chapter 17, "Experience of Stigma in Early Psychosis Patients and Caregivers"). A common scene in clinical practice is for patients and families to seek alternative medicines, traditional herbal drugs, mind-body-spiritual exercises, nutritional supplements, or even rests and holidays instead of engaging in psychiatric treatments.

Another aim of PIPE-I (and PIPE-IA), therefore, is to correct patients' and carers' myths and misunderstandings about psychosis and its treatment, so as to promote more adaptive help-seeking behaviours and stronger treatment adherence. EASY, as a whole, is also devoted to enhancing public awareness and acceptance of mental illness through public education.

Treatment components of PIPE-I

As shown in Figure 13.1, PIPE-I is intended for all young persons with first-episode psychosis entering EASY and aims at allaying misguided fears and anxieties through psychoeducational procedures about mental illness. Thus helping to engage patients, foster treatment compliance, and build up the psychological attributes that are essential for coping and recovery, and enhance a congenial therapeutic environment at home and in the community where rehabilitation takes place. The case manager will provide the full set of psychoeducation for the patient and his or her family.

In all practicality, the core ingredients of PIPE-I reel into action as soon as the patient is engaged in EASY. All patients and their families receive core treatment components of PIPE-I by their case managers. Information is carefully tailored to each individual case, and there is a need to be selective. Depending on the individual needs of the patients and the collaborative decision between the patients and the case managers, PIPE-I typically consists of eight to ten 30-minute sessions. Core elements of PIPE-I are as follows:

1. engagement;
2. correction of myths about mental illness;
3. psychoeducational information concerning the illness and treatment;
4. treatment compliance;
5. appraisal of remaining strengths, assets and controls;
6. coping and stress management; and
7. relapse prevention.

The procedures and skills required for conducting PIPE-I are detailed in the set of three PIPE-I protocol handbooks. The first handbook is entitled *Psychosis and Treatment* includes information about the nature of psychosis as an illness of the brain, common myths and misconceptions about psychosis and treatment, risk and protective factors affecting illness development, and evidence-based treatment domains. The illness model of psychosis is conceptualized in accordance with vulnerability-stress models (Strauss & Carpenter, 1981; Zubin & Spring, 1977). Case Managers, guided by the handbook, are encouraged to explore any attempt that the patient may have taken to try and cope with the psychotic experience, and whether these methods are helpful or not, gradually establish insight and facilitate compliance to evidence-based treatment. Handouts on stages of psychosis, aetiological factors, and treatment options (in Chinese) are included in the handbook, to be printed out for the service users to keep for reference.

Engaging psychotic patients into services can be challenging, and may be limited by factors such as poor insight, social anxiety or oversensitivity, sense of threat or danger, and self-stigmatization (see Chapter 16, "Engagement and Outreach in Early Psychosis Management"). They may also have been rejected or criticized by others for "talking nonsense", subsequently becoming less willing to discuss the strange experiences. Therefore, the second handbook,

Engagement and Assessment, focuses on therapeutic skills that are conducive to effective engagement and development of therapeutic alliance with service users, e.g. empathic listening, reflection of feelings, collaborative goal setting, etc. Numerous examples are given in Chinese to illustrate some of the patients' common responses during engagement, and useful engagement strategies. Table 13.1 includes do's and don'ts of engagement suggested in the handbook. This handbook also includes a symptom checklist, an intake interview record form, and a treatment goal form to facilitate needs assessment and instil insight. The short form of the Depression Anxiety Stress Scale (Lovibond & Lovibond, 1995) is included in the handbook as a quick screening for emotional problems and referral for more specialized treatment.

The third handbook, entitled *Recovery and Relapse Prevention*, emphasizes the importance of identifying risk factors for relapse and learning to cope with stress and residual symptoms, so as to enhance patients' confidence in controlling the illness in the longer term. The content of this handbook draws substantially on Birchwood and colleagues' work on relapse prevention (Hewitt & Birchwood, 2002), and includes exercises such as a onset/relapse timeline, early sign detection, and an action plan, which have been adopted from Birchwood's 'Back in the Saddle' package with permission. This handbook also includes a

Table 13.1
Engagement with psychotic patients

Dos	Don'ts
• Be genuine and respectful • Listen rather than confront • Adopt a reassuring tone • Validate the patient's feelings • Explain the purpose before you ask sensitive questions • Talk to, not about, the patient • Be prepared to answer questions • Engage in a conversation with the patient rather than going through the symptom checklist • Try to understand the underlying emotions of the patient's words/acts • Beware of your body language • Be flexible about pacing, duration, frequency, and locality of contact	• Do not joke about the patient or his/her symptoms • Keep from confronting the symptoms until therapeutic alliance is readily established • Do not breach confidentiality • Do not be defensive • Do not judge or label • Do not be elusive about the diagnosis or treatment goals • Avoid collusion on the delusions — agree to differ • Do not assume the patient's feelings when you are not sure • Do not give false hope too soon about recovery

section on supporting carers and families. As a large proportion of the young EASY patients live with their families, it is important to educate the relatives as well as the patients about the illness and to suggest ways of creating a low-stress family environment. Emphasis is given to alleviating self-blame and stigma in the family, and promoting a more positive communication style. All in all, knowledge acquisition in PIPE-I directs towards positive changes in the sense of meaning, mastery, and help-seeking behaviours. The illness is considered potentially controllable and for which the patients must take some responsibility, such as in preventing relapses.

Despite having received the PIPE-I module, some patients or their significant others may still hold strong attitudes or beliefs that are not conducive to adaptive adjustment to the illness and treatment. Others may resist psychiatric service and have poor medication adherence. In cases like these, patients and families are referred to a clinical psychologist for more goal-directed and individualized PIPE-IA intervention, which is a more specialized version of PIPE-I. Apart from PIPE-I and PIPE-IA, psychoeducation for patients and families under early psychosis service may also take the form of group intervention. Both groups focus on knowledge about psychosis, coping and stress management, and relapse prevention. Psychological services for the carers of psychotic patients are especially important in patients' recovery in Hong Kong, since most of the patients are young and likely to be living with their families. In view of the fact that most carers of patients in EASY are working parents, the groups are designed to be brief (i.e., four sessions for patients and six sessions for carers). Despite its relatively short duration, initial data found that the caregiver group improves participants' knowledge about psychosis and coping of caregiving burden (So et al., 2006).

Readers are encouraged to look up the treatment manuals for detailed procedures of conducting essential elements of PIPE-I and PIPE-IA: Turkington, Kingdon, and Turner's (2002) insight-oriented cognitive-behavioural therapy; Kemp, David, and Hayward's (1996) compliance therapy; Hogarty et al.'s (1997) personal therapy; Hewitt and Birchwood's (2002) relapse prevention techniques; and McFarlane et al.'s (1995) multifamily group therapy. Some useful instruments for assessment are: Coping Style Questionnaire (Drayton, Birchwood, & Trower, 1998); Personal Beliefs about Illness Questionnaire (PBIQ; Birchwood et al., 1993); Insight Scale (Birchwood et al., 1994); and Depression Anxiety Stress Scale (Lovibond & Lovibond, 1995).

PIPE-II: Intervention for Secondary Morbidity

Secondary morbidity

Patients with first-episode psychosis often present with more than one psychiatric diagnosis. Other forms of morbidity such as depression, anxiety and post-traumatic stress disorder before, during, and after the psychotic episode are well documented (Birchwood, 2003; Chisholm, Freeman, & Cooke, 2006; McGorry et al., 1991; see Section "Managing Complications and Comorbidities of Psychosis"). Emotion is clearly implicated in the ontogeny of psychosis. Studies have shown that neuroticism (namely depression, anxiety, and in particular social anxiety) is among the strongest risk factor for psychosis (Freeman & Garety, 2003; Garety et al., 2005; Krabbendam et al., 2005; Owens et al., 2005).

Case Vignette 2

Bridget, a Hong Kong-born Chinese, was studying in a prominent university in America when her psychotic illness developed. She was suspended from the university and was hospitalized in Hong Kong. For months after the onset of her illness, Bridget suffered from flashbacks and nightmares about her bizarre behaviours during the psychotic episode. She could not forget how she behaved under the delusions of persecution and grandiosity; and she wondered how others would think about her. She could not enjoy one single meal without recalling how the voices had commented on her weight and body shape. She cut off contact from everyone she knew and lost confidence in applying for even the least demanding jobs. She was admitted to the hospital again as she was found to have gestures of deliberate self-harm.

In view of the disturbing nature of psychotic symptoms and the resultant functional impairment, it is understandable that emotional morbidity arises from the psychotic experience and one's appraisal of it. Like Bridget, some patients are traumatized by the unusual experiences and their abnormal reactions to them. Sometimes they describe themselves as having "awakened from the nightmare", not knowing what they have done and why. Apart from the experience of the symptoms itself, subsequent interpretation of the symptoms also causes the associated distress and disability (Birchwood & Chadwick, 1997; Garety et al., 2001). It has been shown that prior emotional distress influences the content of delusions and that delusion content in turn influences level of emotional distress (Chisholm et al., 2006; Freeman, Garety, & Kuipers, 2001; Green et al., 2006). Many patients with first-episode psychosis have had bizarre behaviours at school or work, making their subsequent social environment even less congenial. Following the negative and often uncontrollable events in the psychotic episode, patients may develop a depressive mood together with negative implications about themselves, the future, and the world. It has been consistently shown in studies that an increased insight into psychosis is associated with levels of depression (Jackson et al., 1998; McGlashan & Carpenter, 1976; Schwartz, 1994).

Depression amongst people with psychosis may be akin to the process of grieving (Appelo et al., 1993; Lafond, 1998). Grief in this sense refers to reactions to the reality of the loss of one's health, personal capacities to function, as well as key roles and status. This formulation highlights the similarities between the emotional reactions of people with psychosis and those with other longer-term physical disabilities, such as heart disease and diabetes. Similarly, the way in which patients make sense of the diagnosis per se may also provide the main causal pathway to post-psychotic depression (Iqbal et al., 2000).

Apart from emotional morbidity, other problems may also warrant psychiatric attention. Some patients, like Bridget, develop eating disorders as their psychotic symptoms are closely related to their body images. Other patients may try to cope with their anomalous experiences or negative emotions by taking psychotropic drugs, hence becoming substance dependent (see Chapter 27, "Comorbid Substance Abuse in Early Psychosis").

Treatment components of PIPE-II

PIPE-II is intended for patients with a secondary morbidity that stems from primary psychotic disorders. Careful screening is required before a patient is referred to a clinical psychologist for the PIPE-II intervention. In treating specific secondary conditions, clinicians may resort to intervention protocols with established efficacy for that particular disorder in its primary state, for example, depression in the non-psychosis domain. However, caution is given to the unique and complex interaction between psychosis and other psychiatric disorders. Examples of some relevant treatment manuals are as follows:

motivational interviewing for addictive behaviour (Miller & Rollnick, 1991) and CBT for mood disorders (Beck, 1976; Salkovskis, 1996). Recent studies on treatment for psychotic patients with comorbidity also provide important references for the PIPE-II intervention (e.g., Birchwood et al., 2000; Hall & Tarrier, 2003; Iqbal et al., 2000; Myin-Germeys, Delespaul, & van Os, 2005).

PIPE-III: CBT for Drug-Resistant Psychotic symptoms

Drug-resistant psychotic symptoms

In spite of advances in antipsychotics over the past half-century, medicines are not a perfect cure for psychosis. A substantial group of patients (25%–60%) experience persistent psychotic symptoms even when treatment adherence is not an issue (Curson et al., 1988; Kane, 1996). Each psychotic episode is associated with an increase in residual positive symptoms (Wiersma et al., 1998) and the experience of positive symptoms is one of the strongest predictors of rehospitalization (Tarrier et al., 1991). Mizrahi and colleagues (2005) reported that, from the patient's perspective, antipsychotics work by making them feel more detached from the psychotic symptoms, rather than eradicating the symptoms completely. Kapur, Agid, Mizrahi, and Li (2006) argued that antipsychotics are effective in dampening the sense of aberrant salience (where everything seems novel and important to the patient), but psychological treatment is required to help the patient "work through" and re-appraise the psychotic experience.

Case Vignette 3

Carl was described by his treating psychiatrist as "treatment-resistant". He tried to stay hopeful every time he was prescribed a new antipsychotic medicine. Despite multiple attempts, however, he began to convince himself that he might have to live with the remaining psychotic symptoms. He continued to hear voices whenever he was bored or angry. He no longer felt being followed as before, but he remained rather suspicious. He enjoyed no privacy as he felt that his every act was being broadcasted in real time on a "true-man show". He considered medical treatment "partially helpful" (e.g. in helping him sleep and stay calm), but his residual psychotic symptoms were still rather debilitating.

Like Carl in Case Vignette 3, some patients are disturbed by drug-resistant psychotic symptoms such as suspiciousness and hallucinations. While they may be aware that these perceptions are not real, these experiences remain distressing and impairing. Realizing that the symptoms are not totally removed by medications, some patients may lose hope in controlling the illness and even in longer-term relapse prevention.

Treatment components of PIPE-III

In recent decades, there has been fast and dynamic development in the theoretical and clinical approaches of CBT for psychosis. Examples of these include coping skills approach (Tarrier, 2001), normalizing approach (Kingdon & Turkington, 1991), and the newer mindfulness-based approach (Bach & Hayes, 2002; Gaudiano & Herbert, 2006), among many others. More than 20 clinical trials have evaluated different forms of CBT deployed to reduce positive psychotic symptoms as an adjunct to standard psychiatric care (see reviews by Gould et al., 2001; Pfammatter, Junghan, & Brenner, 2006; Pilling et al., 2002; Tarrier, 2005; Tarrier & Wykes, 2004; Turkington, Kingdon, & Weiden, 2006; Zimmermann et al., 2005). Reviews and meta-analyses all conclude that there is good evidence that CBT is effective in reducing positive symptoms. Effect sizes are generally small to medium and are most consistent for persistent positive symptoms (see review by Garety et al., 2008). Based on current research evidence, CBT is recommended for treatment of schizophrenia by the UK National Institute for Clinical Excellence (2009). However, other treatment approaches (e.g., supportive approaches) may also have beneficial effects, but there is yet little empirical support to demonstrate the superiority of any one CBT theoretical approach over the others.

PIPE-III of EASY is intended for patients who, despite pharmacological treatment, still exhibit persistent positive psychotic symptoms. Key references for PIPE-III are drawn from Fowler, Garety, and Kuipers (1995) and Chadwick, Birchwood, and Trower (1996). These CBT protocols are grounded in cognitive models of psychotic symptoms (Birchwood & Iqbal, 1998; Chadwick & Birchwood, 1994; Close & Garety, 1998; Freeman & Garety, 1999; Garety & Freeman, 1999) and firmly supported with replicated efficacy studies among medication-resistant psychotic patients (Garety et al., 2008; Kuipers et al., 1998; Kuipers et al., 1997). Data have shown that the significant benefits in terms of symptom reduction as a result of this form of CBT are sustained at follow-up at 18 months (Kuipers et al., 1998). The effects are not only apparent in positive symptoms, as Garety et al. (1994) and Garety et al. (2008) also found reductions in depression scores.

The broad aims of cognitive-behavioural therapy for people with medication-resistant psychosis are threefold (Fowler et al., 1995): (1) to reduce the distress and disability caused by psychotic symptoms; (2) to reduce emotional disturbance; and (3) to help the individual arrive at an understanding of psychosis that promotes his or her active participation in reducing the risk of relapse and levels of social disability. The stages of CBT for psychosis are as follows (Garety, Fowler, & Kuipers, 2000):

1. engagement and assessment;
2. cognitive-behavioural coping strategies;
3. developing an understanding of the experience of psychosis;
4. working on delusions and hallucinations;
5. addressing negative mood and self-evaluations;
6. managing the risk of relapse and social disability.

For details of each therapeutic phase and the required skills, readers are advised to refer to Fowler et al.'s (1995) treatment manual.

Summary

This chapter introduces the psychological intervention programme for patients and families of EASY in Hong Kong–PIPE, which consists of various treatment modules targeting different aspects of psychological recovery from psychosis. It is theoretically driven, suitable for the early stage of psychosis, and incorporates the cultural characteristics of the population. The combination of basic treatment modules (for all service users) and specific treatment modules for selected individuals with special needs allows for flexible, cost-effective and individually tailored service delivery, which is particularly essential for early intervention services with limited resources. Due to space constraints, relative emphasis has been given to PIPE-I, because the structure of the PIPE-I components was specifically designed for EASY and detailed handbooks are available. The theoretical background and treatment manuals that serve as the bases of PIPE-II and -III have been extensively published elsewhere; readers are directed to the citations with the hope that the PIPE programme may serve as a reference to similar services in other regions.

References

Appelo, M. T., Slooff, C. J., Woonings, F. M. J., Carson, J., & Louwerens, J. W. (1993). Grief: Its significance for rehabilitation in schizophrenia. *Clinical Psychology and Psychotherapy, 1*(1), 53–59.

Bach, P., & Hayes, S. C. (2002). The use of acceptance and commitment therapy to prevent the rehospitalization of psychotic patients: A randomized controlled trial. [Clinical Trial Randomized Controlled Trial Research Support, Non-U.S. Government Research Support, U.S. Government, P.H.S.]. *Journal of Consulting and Clinical Psychology, 70*(5), 1129–1139.

Beck, A. T. (1976). *Cognitive Therapy and the Emotional Disorders*. New York: Penguin Books.

Birchwood, M. (2003). Pathways to emotional dysfunction in first-episode psychosis. [Editorial]. *The British Journal of Psychiatry: TheJjournal of Mental Science, 182*, 373–375.

Birchwood, M., & Chadwick, P. (1997). The omnipotence of voices: Testing the validity of a cognitive model. *Psychological Medicine, 27*(6), 1345–1353.

Birchwood, M., Iqbal, Z., Chadwick, P., & Trower, P. (2000). Cognitive approach to depression and suicidal thinking in psychosis. 1. Ontogeny of post-psychotic depression. [Research Support, Non-U.S. Government]. *The British Journal of Psychiatry: The Journal of Mental Science, 177*, 516–521.

Birchwood, M., Mason, R., MacMillan, F., & Healy, J. (1993). Depression, demoralization and control over psychotic illness: A comparison of depressed and non-depressed patients with a chronic psychosis. *Psychological Medicine, 23*(2), 387–395.

Birchwood, M., Smith, J., Drury, V., Healy, J., Macmillan, F., & Slade, M. (1994). A self-report Insight Scale for psychosis: Reliability, validity and sensitivity to change. *Acta Psychiatrica Scandinavica, 89*(1), 62–67.

Birchwood, M. J., & Iqbal, Z. (1998). Depression and suicidal thinking in psychosis: A cognitive approach. In *Outcomes and Innovation in Psychological Management of Schizophrenia*, edited by T. Wykes, N. Tarrier and S. Lewis, 81–100. Chichester: John Wiley & Sons.

Chadwick, P., & Birchwood, M. (1994). The omnipotence of voices. A cognitive approach to auditory hallucinations. [Case Reports]. *The British Journal of Psychiatry: The Journal of Mental Science, 164*(2), 190–201.

Chadwick, P., Birchwood, M. J., & Trower, P. (1996). *Cognitive Therapy for Delusions, Voices and Paranoia*. Chichester and New York: Wiley.

Chisholm, B., Freeman, D., & Cooke, A. (2006). Identifying potential predictors of traumatic reactions to psychotic episodes. [Research Support, Non-U.S. Government]. *The British Journal of Clinical Psychology/The British Psychological Society, 45*(Pt 4), 545–559. doi: 10.1348/014466505X90136

Chung, K. F., & Wong, M. C. (2004). Experience of stigma among Chinese mental health patients in Hong Kong. *The Psychiatrist, 28*(12), 451–454.

Close, H., & Garety, P. (1998). Cognitive assessment of voices: Further developments in understanding the emotional impact of voices. *The British Journal of Clinical Psychology/The British Psychological Society, 37 (Pt 2)*, 173–188.

Craig, T. K. J., Garety, P., Power, P., Rahaman, N., Colbert, S., Fornells-Ambrojo, M., Dunn, G. (2004). The Lambeth Early Onset (LEO) Team: Randomised controlled trial of the effectiveness of specialised care for early psychosis. *British Medical Journal 329*, 1067. doi: 10.1136/bmj.38246.594873.7C

Curson, D. A., Patel, M., Liddle, P. F., & Barnes, T. R. (1988). Psychiatric morbidity of a long stay hospital population with chronic schizophrenia and implications for future community care. *British Medical Journal, 297*(6652), 819–822.

Deegan, P. (1996). Recovery as a journey of the heart. *Psychiatric Rehabilitation Journal, 19*(3), 91–97.

Drayton, M., Birchwood, M., & Trower, P. (1998). Early attachment experience and recovery from psychosis. *The British Journal of Clinical Psychology/The British Psychological Society, 37 (Pt 3)*, 269–284.

Fowler, D. R., Garety, P. A., & Kuipers, L. (1995). *Cognitive Behaviour Therapy for Psychosis: Theory and Practice*. Chichester: Wiley.

Freeman, D., & Garety, P. A. (1999). Worry, worry processes and dimensions of delusions: An exploratory investigation of a role for anxiety processes in the maintenance of delusional distress. *Behavioural and Cognitive Psychotherapy, 27*(1), 47–62.

Freeman, D., & Garety, P. A. (2003). Connecting neurosis and psychosis: The direct influence of emotion on delusions and hallucinations. [Review]. *Behaviour Research and Therapy, 41*(8), 923–947.

Freeman, D., Garety, P. A., & Kuipers, E. (2001). Persecutory delusions: Developing the understanding of belief maintenance and emotional distress. *Psychological Medicine, 31*(7), 1293–1306.

Freeman, D., Garety, P. A., Kuipers, E., Fowler, D., Bebbington, P. E., & Dunn, G. (2007). Acting on persecutory delusions: The importance of safety seeking. [Multicenter Study Research Support, Non-U.S. Government]. *Behaviour Research and Therapy, 45*(1), 89–99. doi: 10.1016/j.brat.2006.01.014

Garety, P. A., Fowler, D., & Kuipers, E. (2000). Cognitive-behavioral therapy for medication-resistant symptoms. [Review]. *Schizophrenia Bulletin, 26*(1), 73–86.

Garety, P. A., Fowler, D. G., Freeman, D., Bebbington, P., Dunn, G., & Kuipers, E. (2008). Cognitive-behavioural therapy and family intervention for relapse prevention and symptom reduction in psychosis: Randomised controlled trial. [Multicenter Study Randomized Controlled Trial Research Support, Non-U.S. Government]. *The British Journal of Psychiatry: The Journal of Mental Science, 192*(6), 412–423. doi: 10.1192/bjp.bp.107.043570

Garety, P. A., & Freeman, D. (1999). Cognitive approaches to delusions: A critical review of theories and evidence. [Review]. *The British Journal of Clinical Psychology/The British Psychological Society, 38 (Pt 2)*, 113–154.

Garety, P. A., Freeman, D., Jolley, S., Dunn, G., Bebbington, P. E., Fowler, D. G., . . . Dudley, R. (2005). Reasoning, emotions, and delusional conviction in psychosis. [Multicenter Study Randomized Controlled Trial Research Support, Non-U.S. Government]. *Journal of Abnormal Psychology, 114*(3), 373–384. doi: 10.1037/0021–843X.114.3.373

Garety, P. A., Kuipers, E., Fowler, D., Freeman, D., & Bebbington, P. E. (2001). A cognitive model of the positive symptoms of psychosis. *Psychological Medicine, 31*(2), 189–195.

Garety, P. A., Kuipers, L., Fowler, D., Chamberlain, F., & Dunn, G. (1994). Cognitive behavioural therapy for drug-resistant psychosis. [Clinical Trial Controlled Clinical Trial Research Support, Non-U.S. Government]. *The British Journal of Medical Psychology, 67 (Pt 3)*, 259–271.

Gaudiano, B. A., & Herbert, J. D. (2006). Acute treatment of inpatients with psychotic symptoms using Acceptance and Commitment Therapy: Pilot results. [Randomized Controlled Trial]. *Behaviour Research and Therapy, 44*(3), 415–437. doi: 10.1016/j.brat.2005.02.007

Gould, R. A., Mueser, K. T., Bolton, E., Mays, V., & Goff, D. (2001). Cognitive therapy for psychosis in schizophrenia: An effect size analysis. [Meta-Analysis Research Support, Non-U.S. Government]. *Schizophrenia Research, 48*(2–3), 335–342.

Green, C., Garety, P. A., Freeman, D., Fowler, D., Bebbington, P., Dunn, G., & Kuipers, E. (2006). Content and affect in persecutory delusions. [Research Support, Non-U.S. Government]. *The British Journal of Clinical Psychology/The British Psychological Society, 45*(Pt 4), 561–577. doi: 10.1348/014466506X98768

Hall, P. L., & Tarrier, N. (2003). The cognitive-behavioural treatment of low self-esteem in psychotic patients: A pilot study. [Clinical Trial Randomized Controlled Trial]. *Behaviour Research and Therapy, 41*(3), 317–332.

Harding, C. M., Brooks, G. W., Ashikaga, T., Strauss, J. S., & Breier, A. (1987). The Vermont longitudinal study of persons with severe mental illness, II: Long-term outcome of subjects who retrospectively met DSM-III criteria for schizophrenia. [Comparative Study Research Support, U.S. Government, P.H.S.]. *The American Journal of Psychiatry, 144*(6), 727–735.

Hewitt, L., & Birchwood, M. (2002). Preventing relapse of psychotic illness: Role of self-monitoring of prodromal symptoms. *Disease Management & Health Outcome, 10*, 395–407.

Hogarty, G. E., Greenwald, D., Ulrich, R. F., Kornblith, S. J., DiBarry, A. L., Cooley, S., et al. (1997). Three-year trials of personal therapy among schizophrenic patients living with or independent of family, II: Effects on adjustment of patients. [Clinical Trial Randomized Controlled Trial Research Support, U.S. Government, P.H.S.]. *The American Journal of Psychiatry, 154*(11), 1514–1524.

Hopper, K., Harrison, G., & Wanderling, A. (2007). An overview of the course and outcome in ISoS. In *Recovery from Schizophrenia: An International Perspective. A Report from the WHO Collaborative Project, the International Study of*

Schizophrenia, edited by K. Hopper, A. Harrison, A. Janca and N. Sartorius. New York: Oxford University Press.

Iqbal, Z., Birchwood, M., Chadwick, P., & Trower, P. (2000). Cognitive approach to depression and suicidal thinking in psychosis. 2. Testing the validity of a social ranking model. [Research Support, Non-U.S. Government Validation Studies]. *The British Journal of Psychiatry: The Journal of Mental Science, 177*, 522–528.

Jackson, C., Knott, C., Skeate, A., & Birchwood, M. (2004). The trauma of first episode psychosis: The role of cognitive mediation. *The Australian and New Zealand Journal of Psychiatry, 38*(5), 327–333. doi: 10.1111/j.1440–1614.2004.01359.x

Jackson, H., McGorry, P., Edwards, J., Hulbert, C., Henry, L., Francey, S., et al. (1998). Cognitively-oriented psychotherapy for early psychosis (COPE). Preliminary results. [Clinical Trial Research Support, Non-U.S. Government]. *The British Journal of Psychiatry. Supplement, 172*(33), 93–100.

Kane, J. M. (1996). Treatment-resistant schizophrenic patients. [Review]. *The Journal of Clinical Psychiatry, 57 Suppl 9*, 35–40.

Kane, J. M. (1999). Pharmacologic treatment of schizophrenia. [Research Support, U.S. Government, P.H.S. Review]. *Biological Psychiatry, 46*(10), 1396–1408.

Kapur, S., Agid, O., Mizrahi, R., & Li, M. (2006). How antipsychotics work-from receptors to reality. [Research Support, Non-U.S. Government Review]. *NeuroRx: The Journal of the American Society for Experimental NeuroTherapeutics, 3*(1), 10–21. doi: 10.1016/j.nurx.2005.12.003

Kapur, S., & Mamo, D. (2003). Half a century of antipsychotics and still a central role for dopamine D2 receptors. [Historical Article Research Support, Non-U.S. Government Review]. *Progress in Neuro-psychopharmacology & Biological Psychiatry, 27*(7), 1081–1090. doi: 10.1016/j.pnpbp.2003.09.004

Kemp, R., Hayward, P., Applewhaite, G., Everitt, B., & David, A. (1996). Compliance therapy in psychotic patients: Randomised controlled trial. [Clinical Trial Randomized Controlled Trial Research Support, Non-U.S. Government]. *British Medical Journal, 312*(7027), 345–349.

Kingdon, D. G., & Turkington, D. (1991). The use of cognitive behavior therapy with a normalizing rationale in schizophrenia. Preliminary report. [Case Reports]. *The Journal of Nervous and Mental Disease, 179*(4), 207–211.

Krabbendam, L., Myin-Germeys, I., Hanssen, M., de Graaf, R., Vollebergh, W., Bak, M., & van Os, J. (2005). Development of depressed mood predicts onset of psychotic disorder in individuals who report hallucinatory experiences. *The British Journal of Clinical Psychology/The British Psychological Society, 44*(Pt 1), 113–125. doi: 10.1348/014466504X19767

Kuipers, E., Fowler, D., Garety, P., Chisholm, D., Freeman, D., Dunn, G., et al. (1998). London-east Anglia randomised controlled trial of cognitive-behavioural therapy for psychosis. III: Follow-up and economic evaluation at 18 months. [Clinical Trial Randomized Controlled Trial Research Support, Non-U.S. Government]. *The British Journal of Psychiatry: The Journal of Mental Science, 173*, 61–68.

Kuipers, E., Garety, P., Fowler, D., Dunn, G., Bebbington, P., Freeman, D., & Hadley, C. (1997). London-East Anglia randomised controlled trial of cognitive-behavioural therapy for psychosis. I: effects of the treatment phase. [Clinical Trial Multicenter Study Randomized Controlled Trial Research Support, Non-U.S. Government]. *The British Journal of Psychiatry: The Journal of Mental Science, 171*, 319–327.

Lafond, V. (1998). The grief of mental illness: Context for the cognitive therapy of schizophrenia. In *Cognitive Psychotherapy of Psychotic and Personality Disorders*, edited by C. Perris and P. D. McGorry. New York: John Wiley & Sons.

Lee, S., Lee, M. T., Chiu, M. Y., & Kleinman, A. (2005). Experience of social stigma by people with schizophrenia in Hong Kong. [Comparative Study Research Support, Non-U.S. Government]. *The British Journal of Psychiatry: The Journal of Mental Science, 186*, 153–157. doi: 10.1192/bjp.186.2.153

Lieberman, J. A., Stroup, T. S., McEvoy, J. P., Swartz, M. S., Rosenheck, R. A., Perkins, D. O., Keefe, R. S., Davis, S. M., Davis, C. E., Lebowitz, B. D., Severe, J., Hsiao, J. K. (2005). Effectiveness of antipsychotic drugs in patients with chronic schizophrenia. *The New England Journal of Medicine, 353*(12), 1209–1223. 10.1056/NEJMoa051688

Lovibond, P. F., & Lovibond, S. H. (1995). The structure of negative emotional states: Comparison of the Depression Anxiety Stress Scales (DASS) with the Beck Depression and Anxiety Inventories. *Behaviour Research and Therapy, 33*(3), 335–343. doi: 0005-7967(94)00075-U [pii]

Marder, S. R. (1996). Pharmacolgoical treatment strategies in acute schizophrenia. *International Clinical Psychopharmacology, 11*(Suppl. 2), 29–34.

McFarlane, W. R., Lukens, E., Link, B., Dushay, R., Deakins, S. A., Newmark, M., et al. (1995). Multiple-family groups and psychoeducation in the treatment of schizophrenia. [Clinical Trial Comparative Study Randomized Controlled Trial Research Support, Non-U.S. Government]. *Archives of General Psychiatry, 52*(8), 679–687.

McGlashan, T. H., & Carpenter, W. T., Jr. (1976). Postpsychotic depression in schizophrenia. [Review]. *Archives of General Psychiatry, 33*(2), 231–239.

McGlashan, T. H., Levy, S. T., & Carpenter, W. T., Jr. (1975). Integration and sealing over: Clinically distinct recovery styles from schizophrenia. *Archives of General Psychiatry, 32*(10), 1269–1272.

McGorry, P. D. (1992). The concept of recovery and secondary prevention in psychotic disorders. *Australian and New Zealand Journal of Psychiatry, 26*(1), 3–17.

McGorry, P. D., Chanen, A., McCarthy, E., Van Riel, R., McKenzie, D., & Singh, B. S. (1991). Posttraumatic stress disorder following recent-onset psychosis: An unrecognized postpsychotic syndrome. *The Journal of Nervous and Mental Disease, 179*(5), 253–258.

Miller, W. R., & Rollnick, S. (1991). *Motivational Interviewing: Preparing People to Change Addictive Behavior*. New York: Guilford Press.

Miyamoto, S., Duncan, G. E., Marx, C. E., & Lieberman, J. A. (2005). Treatments for schizophrenia: A critical review of pharmacology and mechanisms of action of antipsychotic drugs. [Research Support, Non-U.S. Government Research Support,

U.S. Government, P.H.S. Review]. *Molecular Psychiatry, 10*(1), 79–104. doi: 10.1038/sj.mp.4001556

Miyamoto, S., Lieberman, J. A., Fleischhacker, W. W., Aoba, A., & Marder, S. R. (2003). Antipsychotic drugs. In *Psychiatry*, 2nd edition, edited by A. Tasman, J. Kay and J. A. Lieberman, 1928–1964. Chichester John Wiley & Sons, Ltd.

Mizrahi, R., Bagby, R. M., Zipursky, R. B., & Kapur, S. (2005). How antipsychotics work: The patients' perspective. [Clinical Trial]. *Progress in Neuro-psychopharmacology & Biological Psychiatry, 29*(5), 859–864. doi: 10.1016/j.pnpbp.2005.03.001

Myin-Germeys, I., Delespaul, P., & van Os, J. (2005). Behavioural sensitization to daily life stress in psychosis. [Research Support, Non-U.S. Government]. *Psychological Medicine, 35*(5), 733–741.

National Institute for Health and Clinical Excellence (Ed.). (2009). *Schizophrenia. NICE Clinical Guideline 82*. London: National Institute for Health and Clinical Excellence.

Ng, R. M., Pearson, V., Chen, E. E., & Law, C. W. (2011). What does recovery from schizophrenia mean? Perceptions of medical students and trainee psychiatrists. *The International Journal of Social Psychiatry, 57*(3), 248–262. doi: 10.1177/0020764009354833

Owens, D. G., Miller, P., Lawrie, S. M., & Johnstone, E. C. (2005). Pathogenesis of schizophrenia: A psychopathological perspective. [Comparative Study Research Support, Non-U.S. Government]. *The British Journal of Psychiatry: The Journal of Mental Science, 186*, 386–393. doi: 10.1192/bjp.186.5.386

Pfammatter, M., Junghan, U. M., & Brenner, H. D. (2006). Efficacy of psychological therapy in schizophrenia: Conclusions from meta-analyses. [Meta-Analysis]. *Schizophrenia Bulletin, 32 Suppl 1*, S64–80. doi: 10.1093/schbul/sbl030

Pilling, S., Bebbington, P., Kuipers, E., Garety, P., Geddes, J., Orbach, G., & Morgan, C. (2002). Psychological treatments in schizophrenia: I. Meta-analysis of family intervention and cognitive behaviour therapy. [Comparative Study Meta-Analysis]. *Psychological Medicine, 32*(5), 763–782.

Robinson, D. G., Woerner, M. G., McMeniman, M., Mendelowitz, A., & Bilder, R. M. (2004). Symptomatic and functional recovery from a first episode of schizophrenia or schizoaffective disorder. [Research Support, U.S. Government, P.H.S.]. *The American Journal of Psychiatry, 161*(3), 473–479.

Salkovskis, P. M. (Ed.). (1996). *Trends in Cognitive and Behavioural Therapies*. Chichester: W J Wiley & Sons.

Schwartz, C. E. (1994). Insight in psychosis: State or trait? [Comment Letter]. *The American Journal of Psychiatry, 151*(5), 788–789.

So, S., Wong, C. W., & Chong, H. C. (eds.). (2002). *Psychological Intervention Programme for Early Psychosis (PIPE) Handbook for EASY Service*. Hong Kong: Early Assessment Service for Young People with Psychosis.

So, S. H. W., & Wong, C. W. (2008). Experience and coping with auditory hallucinations in first-episode psychosis: Relationship with stress coping. *Hong Kong Journal of Psychiatry, 18*(3), 115–121.

Srivastava, A., Thakar, M., Shah, N., & Stitt, L. (2008). Outcome in schizophrenia: How good is "good outcome" schizophrenia in long-term in developing countries? Paper presented at the XIV World Congress of Psychiatry, Prague, Czech Republic.

Strauss, J. S., & Carpenter, W. T., Jr. (eds.). (1981). *Schizophrenia*. New York: Plenum Press.

Tai, S., & Turkington, D. (2009). The evolution of cognitive behavior therapy for schizophrenia: Current practice and recent developments. [Review]. *Schizophrenia Bulletin, 35*(5), 865–873. doi: 10.1093/schbul/sbp080

Tarrier, N. (2001). The use of coping strategies and self-regulation in the treatment of psychosis. In *A Casebook of Cognitive Therapy for Psychosis*, edited by A. Morrison, 79–107. Cambridge, UK: Cambridge University Press.

Tarrier, N. (2005). Cognitive behaviour therapy for schizophrenia: A review of development, evidence and implementation. [Review]. *Psychotherapy and Psychosomatics, 74*(3), 136–144. doi: 10.1159/000083998

Tarrier, N., Barrowclough, C., & Bamrah, J. S. (1991). Prodromal signs of relapse in schizophrenia. *Social Psychiatry and Psychiatric Epidemiology, 26*(4), 157–161.

Tarrier, N., & Wykes, T. (2004). Is there evidence that cognitive behaviour therapy is an effective treatment for schizophrenia? A cautious or cautionary tale? [Meta-Analysis]. *Behaviour Research and Therapy, 42*(12), 1377–1401. doi: 10.1016/j.brat.2004.06.020

Turkington, D., Kingdon, D., & Turner, T. (2002). Effectiveness of a brief cognitive-behavioural therapy intervention in the treatment of schizophrenia. [Clinical Trial Multicenter Study Randomized Controlled Trial Research Support, Non-U.S. Government]. *The British Journal of Psychiatry: The Journal of Mental Science, 180*, 523–527.

Turkington, D., Kingdon, D., & Weiden, P. J. (2006). Cognitive behavior therapy for schizophrenia. [Review]. *The American Journal of Psychiatry, 163*(3), 365–373. doi: 10.1176/appi.ajp.163.3.365

Wiersma, D., Nienhuis, F. J., Slooff, C. J., & Giel, R. (1998). Natural course of schizophrenic disorders: A 15-year followup of a Dutch incidence cohort. [Research Support, Non-U.S. Government]. *Schizophrenia Bulletin, 24*(1), 75–85.

Wykes, T., Huddy, V., Cellard, C., McGurk, S. R., & Czobor, P. (2011). A meta-analysis of cognitive remediation for schizophrenia: Methodology and effect sizes. [Meta-Analysis Research Support, Non-U.S. Government]. *The American Journal of Psychiatry, 168*(5), 472–485. doi: 10.1176/appi.ajp.2010.10060855

Zimmermann, G., Favrod, J., Trieu, V. H., & Pomini, V. (2005). The effect of cognitive behavioral treatment on the positive symptoms of schizophrenia spectrum disorders: A meta-analysis. [Comparative Study Meta-Analysis]. *Schizophrenia Research, 77*(1), 1–9. doi: 10.1016/j.schres.2005.02.018

Zubin, J., & Spring, B. (1977). Vulnerability: A new view of schizophrenia. [Research Support, U.S. Government, Non-P.H.S.]. *Journal of Abnormal Psychology, 86*(2), 103–126.

14
The PASTE that Binds: Culturally Relevant Psychological Interventions for First-Episode Psychosis Individuals in Singapore

Eugene Puay Chong Tay and Lyn Chua

Introduction

Unlike people with other disorders, individuals who are afflicted with psychosis are most likely to experience disturbances in their perception and cognition. Compounded with the psychotic experiences and the presence of symptoms, their ability to engage in fruitful social interactions and usual role functioning are often impaired. Moreover, individuals may experience comorbid conditions and must be closely monitored for related emotional reactions of social anxiety, depression and suicidality, hostility or trauma, so as to incorporate interventions that help them function optimally.

Besides the use of antipsychotic medication, which is the mainstay of treatment, psychological interventions have been identified as the other arm that bears paramount importance in an individual's recovery from the illness. Amongst the various biopsychosocial interventions covered in this book (for group-based psychosocial programmes, see Chapter 19, "Community Psychosocial Intervention in Early Psychosis"), psychotherapy has consistently been demonstrated to be useful, if not the most useful form of intervention. The evidence-base for psychotherapy as a treatment for psychosis is demonstrated extensively in the literature (Garety, Fowler, & Kuipers, 2000; Haddock et al., 1998; Rector & Beck, 2001; Turkington, Kingdon, & Chadwick, 2003).

Many psychotherapeutic approaches have placed emphasis symptom remission through cognitive behavioural therapy (CBT) (Garety et al., 2000), social support, relapse prevention, and recovery through psychoeducation, active listening, empathy, crisis management, reinforcement of health-seeking behaviours, and advocacy, also known as supportive therapy (Pinto et al., 1999). These methods validate the distress of the psychotic experiences and the stigma attached to the illness, and develop a collaborative explanation of symptoms and experiences, with a theoretical mechanism of effectiveness to increase control and decrease distress related to residual positive symptoms (Marlowe, 2003).

This chapter does not purport to provide an exhaustive coverage of the application of these therapeutic approaches but will provide a brief overview of a unique therapeutic modality that is culturally relevant and sensitive, known as the Personal and Strategic Coping Therapy for Early Psychosis (PASTE; Chua, Choo, & Chan, 2004). PASTE was developed specifically for patients in Singapore's Early Psychosis Intervention Programme (EPIP). The case illustrations describe the applications of PASTE across different phases of the illness ranging from acute, stabilization, to the maintenance phase.

Stages of Schizophrenia Recovery

The acute phase of psychosis is a period when the individual is affected by intense psychotic symptoms such as hallucinations, delusions, paranoia, and disordered thinking. During this period, individuals are usually hospitalized and treated with medications to control the positive symptoms. Studies have shown that early engagement at this stage forges a strong therapeutic alliance, enabling the individual to feel supported and understood, helping them to make better recovery in functioning, and pre-empting or alleviating secondary morbidities (Jackson et al., 1998; Jackson et al., 2001).

Stabilization is a period when the psychotic symptoms are gradually coming under control. Individuals may still have attenuated symptoms that continue to affect their daily lives. They are also particularly vulnerable to relapses. This is also a period when some can be helped to gain insight but faced with the stigma of the illness some individuals may develop comorbid conditions.

In the maintenance phase, emphasis is placed upon ensuring long-term recovery whereby individuals seek to sustain symptom remission and reduce risks of relapse and hospitalization. To ensure this, individuals need to continue with medications and be engaged in psychosocial interventions, such as supportive therapy, psychoeducation for patients and caregivers, cognitive remediation, and vocational and social rehabilitation.

Personal and Strategic Coping Therapy for Early Psychosis (PASTE)

Individuals may be referred for psychotherapy at different stages of their recovery. Consequently, the psychological approach needs to be customized according to their needs, strengths, as well as stage of recovery.

Bearing this in mind, PASTE was developed as a holistic, sensitive, and culturally relevant psychotherapeutic approach to address an individual's needs and distress from the start of the psychotic episode through to the stabilization phase. This approach enables the individual to explore personal beliefs about the causes of the symptoms to gain insight, support and validation of their experiences, and sense of control over the illness. PASTE also incorporates elements of CBT and psychoeducation. Strategic coping therapy enables a stabilized patient to deal with the trauma, grief, fear, and any losses and comorbid conditions that may arise (Table 14.1).

Table 14.1
Components of PASTE

• Supportive therapy
• Personal therapy
• Cognitive-behavioural therapy
• Psychoeducation
• Strategic coping therapy

As psychotic episodes can be frightening, especially during the acute phase, much focus is placed upon the supportive component, which involves developing rapport, forming therapeutic alliance with the individual by providing an active listening ear, as well as validating the personal distress.

Supportive Therapy: Therapeutic Alliance

Uniquely, PASTE is highly cognizant of and places great emphasis on the cultural and religious background of the individual, which is important for understanding the origin of the individual's explanatory model. This insight contributes to a sound therapeutic alliance and helps the individual feel understood, supported, and validated.

Therapeutic alliance is the working relationship between the patient and therapist in developing a bond and having mutually agreed goals and targets for treatment. It has its roots in both psychodynamic theory (in relation to the concept of transference) and Rogers' work on client-centred therapy. Some of the core elements include active listening, being empathic and warm, genuineness, and unconditional regard (Rogers, 1957); complemented with providing assurance, reinforcing correct perceptions, being open to and non-judgemental or dismissive of the individual's experience, and being mindful of any trauma.

Case Example 1 is an excerpt of an interaction with a patient who was brought into the inpatient ward. The patient was initially guarded and refused to divulge any information at the start of his admission. The non-judgemental and unchallenging approach of the therapist encouraged the patient to share further about his psychotic symptoms that involved a long-standing paranoid delusion towards his neighbours.

Case Example 1

Pang is a 39-year-old man with 10 years' duration of untreated psychosis. He lives with his elder sister. He had been shouting out from his bedroom window and playing his TV at loud volume throughout the day and night for years. The neighbours made repeated police reports and he was eventually brought to service when he went up to one of the neighbour's home with a stick to create a scene.

(Introductions made to the patient; T: therapist, P: Pang)

T: Tell me a little more about what brought you here?

P: I don't know, I was just resting at home watching TV in my room when the police came knocking on my door. Next thing I know I was brought to the ward. Must be the neighbours. They just want to have me locked up.

T: Sounds like you feel rather displeased with being brought to the hospital and feel it is unwarranted.

P: *(in a loud agitated tone)* Yes, I did not do anything.

T: I see, what do you think may be the reason for the police to come over?

P: *(still speaking angrily)* The stupid neighbours. It must be them. I am sure they want to harm me. I hear them talking all the time. I hear them talking at night, outside the window along the corridor. They keep saying that they want me to die and I am good for nothing. All I did was increase the volume and shout for them to stop.

T: Seems like you feel harassed by them yet you have been trying to avoid confrontation by doing various things, like increasing the sound volume.

P: *(less agitated, engaged in brief eye contact)* You are absolutely right! I never bothered them but they keep disturbing me.

T: You mentioned hearing "them" talk. Who might "them" be referring to?

P: Don't know, them . . . You may laugh when I tell you, but sometimes I hear my neighbour on the 15th floor talking *(patient stays on the 8th floor)* and they throw lizards into my house to spy on me.

T: Tell me more . . .

Personal Therapy: Explanatory Model

Often individuals' assertions about their symptoms may sound bizarre and implausible. Usually, at the time of service entry, they may not be amenable to the medical model presented to them, as each individual may have his or her own explanation for their psychotic experience. The dissonance between personal explanations and those of the professionals' is likely to affect help-seeking behaviour, adherence to medication (Foulks, Persons, & Merkel, 1986), and satisfaction (Callan & Littlewood, 1998). Arthur Kleinman (1980) suggests that explanatory models of illness should encompass the *what*, *why*, *how*, and *who* questions so as to better understand patients and their families.

Consequently, the personal therapy component of PASTE seeks to accede to this by understanding the individual's perception about the nature of his or her problem(s), its cause(s), prognosis, and treatment preferences. By adopting an inquisitive approach to the exploration of their problems, the therapeutic relationship is enhanced, so that the individual feels safe and secure in expressing any explanations for the cause of their problems and "illness".

The explanatory model is personal to the individual and is based on their own beliefs, which are often influenced by their cultural and/or religious background and earlier life experiences (see Case Example 2). When their mental state becomes more stable, the individual may be amenable to psychoeducation and CBT, to re-examine and modify these beliefs, and to resolve cognitive distortions.

Case Example 2

Cynthia was a 16-year-old student who lived with her parents. She was referred for therapy as she had presented with ideas of reference and paranoid ideas. Earlier in school, she had become violent towards some of her classmates and had threatened to beat them if they continued to stare at her. In public places, she constantly felt that strangers were talking about her and had this foreboding sense that they wanted to harm her. Cynthia also shared about feeling increasingly annoyed seeing people frown. She attributed all of this to her classmates. She believed that her classmates might have blogged or written negatively about her on Facebook. She was referred for therapy as the school had considered expelling her due to the danger she posed to her classmates and also her poor grades. Cynthia had also met with the school counsellor but felt that adult was in cahoots with her classmates. Her parents also reported her poor sleep patterns and increasing defiant behaviours when she stayed up late at night.

Presenting concerns:
- Psychotic symptoms
- Sleep problems
- Impending suspension from school due to poor grades, impulsive and aggressive behaviours (e.g., threatening to hit people, using vulgarities)
- Relationship problems with peers, teachers, and family

Aim of therapy:
- To help address anger issues and the consequences of her behaviours (e.g., beating up people, using vulgarities, defying instructions from authoritative figures)

- Addressing her explanatory model
- Learning to challenge and modify her beliefs

The initial sessions sought to develop the therapeutic alliance and also to make a risk assessment of her ongoing defiant behaviours. The therapeutic alliance was of paramount importance as Cynthia came from a school with a culture of bullying and gang activities. She also had difficulty in trusting people. The supportive therapy component of PASTE sought to validate her experiences in an empathic manner. She was also disappointed with the school counsellor, whom she felt was reporting to the principal, teachers, as well as her classmates. Socratic questioning was used to explore Cynthia's interpretation of the situation and her defiant behaviour in school where she would hurl vulgarities and threaten to inflict injury on others. To help understand her aggressive actions and behaviours, the therapist encouraged Cynthia to share her explanatory model of her "illness"—what, why, how, and who she believed caused her current problems.

Explanatory model

Cynthia revealed that she had become involved with gangs when she was 13 years old (in Secondary Form 1) to protect herself from the constant bullying in school. Since then, she had been involved in multiple fights as well as harassing people. Some weeks prior to her illness onset, she claimed to have seen a member of the rival gang whom she had extorted money from at a shopping mall conversing with her classmate. Shortly after when she started to become unwell, Cynthia chanced upon her classmate's photos on Facebook and learnt that these two individuals were indeed friends. She believed that her classmate might have learnt something about her past and might have "bad-mouthed" her. In her search online, she had also seen some class excursion photos and saw pictures of the school counsellor posing with her classmates.

Cynthia's explanatory model was that the girl from the rival gang was spreading rumours about her because of their past altercation of money extortion. This explanatory model helped the therapist understand her initial ambivalence towards the school counsellor as she thought that the counsellor might have colluded with her classmate to disparage her.

Cynthia explained that by seeing the photo online, she was immediately certain that the counsellor was conspiring with her friends.

In therapy, her initial conviction about this delusional belief was assessed. As the session progressed, the therapeutic alliance strengthened and Cynthia was encouraged to consider alternative explanations. For homework, she was assigned to check her friends' photos online. Cynthia noticed that even her best friend in school had appeared in the excursion photo. Cynthia claimed that she trusted her best friend, who, incidentally had been the reason for her to leave the gangs. Her ability to question this dysfunctional assumption helped cast doubt over her delusion of a conspiracy (reality testing technique). To help Cynthia internalize this further, the therapist helped her evaluate the positive and negative consequences of holding onto this belief.

(T: therapist; C: Cynthia)

T: Cynthia, you had mentioned that those who were in the photos, including the counsellor and the classmate you saw at the shopping centre, were scheming with the rival gang member to harm you.

C: Uh-huh. The photo I saw on Facebook just confirms it.

T: Hmm . . . and previously you have rated 90% on your conviction to this feeling.

C: Yes, I still feel it though I am not so sure as my best friend was in the photo too. Funny thing is that I did not notice her previously.

T: Interesting, so your friend was also in the photos as well but you do not feel that she is part of the conspiracy?

C: Ya, and that is the confusing part for me.

T: Okay, let's examine the advantages and disadvantages to you holding the view that people who were in the photograph were going to harm you. *(Patient had put up a slight resistance but was assured that she could cease this exercise if she felt uncomfortable.)*

C: Well, the advantage of having that thought would be that I need to be careful with people around me. I need to be sure nobody can hurt me.

T: Hmm . . . so it serves as a protective barrier for you.

C: Yes, you can never be sure of whom you trust for they might just hurt me.

T: Any other advantages that you could think of?

C: *(pauses)* No . . . can't think of any.

T: Alright, if you come up with any, do let me know. What about the disadvantages?

C: Ok. Well, if it is not true then I look like a complete fool. My best friend would be so disappointed in me. *(sighed heavily)*

T: Sounds like you do not want to appear foolish in blaming people. Any other disadvantages if you hold the notion that they want to harm you?

C: Well, it also means that I will make fewer friends, people in school will think I am crazy as I am constantly telling them that I will beat them up.

T: What are the consequences to that?

C: I get really stressed out and cannot sleep at night as I am constantly checking online. Also, I will get expelled from school as I cannot focus in class and my grades keep dropping.

By having the patient examine the advantages and disadvantages of holding onto her beliefs, she came to realize that alternative interpretations existed. Similarly, by helping the client weigh through the advantages and disadvantages of discarding the belief helped her gain emotional commitment and focus upon more adaptive outcomes.

Stabilization Phase

As her psychotic symptoms gradually came under control, the sessions sought to reduce risk behaviours (i.e., threats to inflict physical pain onto others) and anger management (i.e., shouting expletives and throwing tantrums at family members). She learnt to express her feelings such as anger, appropriately, seeing other's perspectives, and appreciating the impact of their behaviour on others. As symptoms went into remission, she was taught social skills to improve her social relationships with classmates and family members.

Cognitive-Behavioural Therapy and Strategic Coping Therapy

In PASTE, the CBT component is modified to be less confrontational and challenging, and gentler and more persuasive than the usual CBT.

CBT focuses on positive symptoms and uses a systematic and structured approach of reality testing and belief modification, encouraging individuals to consider alternative explanations through guided discovery in an unchallenging manner. The aim of CBT is to help the individual develop new and rational beliefs for causes of symptoms and also learn more adaptive coping skills (Chadwick, Birchwood, & Trower, 1996).

When stabilized, individuals need help to integrate back to the community and to adjust to their new role. Such strategic coping therapy helps the individual move on. Usually, at this stage, the symptoms are in remission, but individuals still face a multitude of problems with stigma, skills deficits (e.g., social, communication or interpersonal skills), fear, anger, confusion, loss of confidence and losses due to the psychotic illness. At this stage, individuals would reflect on their illness and its impact on their lives. Psychoeducation and case management are complementary components that support the individual through recovery. Individuals are taught coping skills and encouraged to resume previous activities to reconnect in the various life domains. This is also an important stage to prevent secondary morbidities such as social anxiety, depression, and post-traumatic stress disorder.

Case Example 3

Peter was a 21-year-old man who had completed his National Service (NS) and about to enter tertiary education. He was referred for psychotherapy whilst he was still in NS where he had reported poor sleep and onset of auditory hallucinations and grandiose delusions. He believed that he was able to communicate with people from an alternate world telepathically. He further claimed to hear the voices of ex-classmates from college (whom he had never been close or in contact with since enlistment), camp mates, celebrities (Adam Lambert from *American Idol*), and even strangers in this alternate world. Peter became increasingly distressed as he believed that he had created "clones" of these individuals and somehow they were trapped in the alternate world. He also believed that he was causing these people to repeat their daily events (e.g., having Adam Lambert sing repeatedly until his throat was hoarse), resulting in their wrath. Peter shared that in the alternate world these individuals had threatened to harm his loved ones. He was worried that it might happen in real life and was increasingly concerned that new classmates he might meet at university would also be affected. According to his mother, Peter had always been a soft-spoken and shy boy in school.

Explanatory model

During the sessions, Peter shared that he had always been reticent in Junior College (JC) and did not have many friends. He was afraid that his classmates might laugh at him and consider him as being weird. Peter revealed that he distanced himself from his peers after entering JC. He had regretted his decision of selecting a different school to his secondary school friends'. In JC, he felt inadequate as most of his classmates were performing better academically. He had wanted to be seen as one of the "coolest kids". He tried to represent the school in sports events but, the repeated defeats made him feel even more dejected. He realized that he was not popular and avoided forging any social interactions with his classmates.

Moreover, he would come home after school and would carry out imaginary conversations in his head until late at night. When he started hearing voices, he was initially curious but became elated when the voices encouraged him. At times, he felt that he needed to depend upon them and would seek advice from the voices for approval. However, the voices became overwhelming when he noticed that they commented on almost everything he did. They made it difficult for him to concentrate. Peter was distressed and felt helpless as he believed that they wanted to torture him for he had incarcerated them within the alternate world. At times, he would raise his voice and shout at them.

Stabilization phase: Presence of symptoms

To help Peter feel less affected and "controlled" by the voices, efforts were made for him to consider an alternative to his explanatory model, and realize that the voices formed part of his illness. CBT was used to gradually shift his reactivity towards the voices. He was then taught to use strategic coping techniques to ignore them and proceed with life even though the voices might still be present (as in the case of a treatment-resistant situation). While he was still constantly being troubled by the voices, certain distraction techniques were employed.

In the sessions, Peter learnt to identify antecedents to the voices as well as his current coping mechanisms. Peter identified that he would usually yell but realized that this would cause the voices to remain and at times to even increase in volume disappear. One of the strategic coping techniques he learnt was that whenever he put on his earphones, the voices dissipated. Other alternative coping strategies were provided for Peter to practise outside the sessions.

Some coping strategies for voices:

- Listening to his iPod or mp3 player
- Calling a friend or family member
- Reading a book, magazines, or newspapers
- Engaging in activities (e.g., playing computer games with headphones on or physical exercise)
- Delay talking to the voices or seeking feedback from them
- Using the "coping response" card to handle the voices
- Considering the voices to be "little pests", "little children", "small-sized people like in *Gulliver's Travels*"

In Peter's case, he perceived the voices to be omniscient and was thus drawn towards them whenever he needed guidance and support. When the voices became ominous in nature, they frightened him. One of the strategies proposed to Peter was to have him perceive the voices differently. Peter felt better when he imagined the voices to be that of "little children" as they appeared to be less powerful and dangerous.

Maintenance phase: Developing social skills

As Peter had a rather small social network and few friends, he had turned inwards to seek solace in the voices. He acknowledged his social difficulties that stemmed from his lack of confidence in making social interactions with others and his negative beliefs that people would not want to form social connections with him. During therapy, Peter shared about his interests in computer games and table tennis. He was encouraged to identify camp friends with similar interests. Through role-plays and role-modelling within the sessions, Peter gradually gained confidence to initiate and sustain conversation. He eventually made friends with his camp mates as they shared a common interest in PS2 games.

(T: therapist; P: Peter)

T: So how has camp been?

P: Okay, I tried to talk to one of my colleagues (camp mate) about this game I was playing . . . Actually, he came over to ask me.

T: Sounds like your colleague was interested to learn more about the game.

P: Ya, I started sharing with him and he told me that he played PS2. We have been playing together. We exchanged some games. *(Peter was encouraged to continue conversing with his friend. In a subsequent session, he was asked on the experience.)*

T: So Peter, how are things with you and your PS2 friend in camp?

P: He invited me along with some of the other camp mates to go play LAN games. We went out a few times and I enjoyed the time with them. I am now like a popular person in camp (smiles nervously).

T: How did you become a "popular person"?

P: 'Cos of the PS2 game, many of them come to me for tips.

T: How does that make you feel?

P: Good, something different.

T: Seems like you enjoyed the company and time you spent with your friends.

P: Yes, but I am not sure how things will be when I go to university. I will not see my friends in camp anymore.

T: Sounds like you may miss their company and would want to maintain contact with them?

P: Ya, wish I could continue hanging out with them.

T: What are some of the things that you could do?

P: Perhaps I can call them up for outings or MSN them about school.

T: They sound like good ideas. How about we look at them together?

P: Yes, I would like that.

Conclusion

PASTE is a culturally sensitive psychotherapeutic intervention that provides supportive therapy throughout the psychotic episode and encourages the expression of the individual's explanatory model. Through reflective dialogue and good therapeutic relationships, individuals come to share their internal experiences and distress. With guided discovery, individuals are able to assess their beliefs, assumptions and cognitive distortions, and the negative consequences associated with them. Various techniques of appraisal and cognitive restructuring, such as generating alternative explanations, reality testing, behavioural experiments from CBT, are helpful in challenging and modifying their delusions. Adaptive strategies to cope with auditory hallucinations and residual symptoms are also useful to help individuals gain confidence towards their abilities to be in better control of their symptoms. As psychotic symptoms go into remission, there are other aspects of skills deficits that may require assistance, some of which include social skills deficits, cognitive deficits, self-esteem issues, trauma and concerns about grief and loss, as well as stigmatization. Learning to appraise their emotional reactions appropriately would also bring about improvements in their functioning and assist reintegration into the community.

Case conceptualization is one of the most important aspects of CBT as it helps to identify the individual's reasoning and core beliefs for interpreting events in a particular fashion and can also be used to formulate management plans. Detailed case conceptualization is outside the scope of this chapter; for more discussion about case management, see Chapter 18, "The Phase-Specific Progress Supervision Model for Case Managers".

References

Callan, A., & Littlewood, R. (1998). Patient satisfaction: Ethnic origin or explanatory model? *The International Journal of Social Psychiatry, 44*(1), 1–11.

Chadwick, P., Birchwood, M. J., & Trower, P. (1996). *Cognitive Therapy for Delusions, Voices and Paranoia*. Chichester and New York: Wiley.

Chua, L., Choo, L., & Chan, S. (2004). Psychotherapy for early psychosis in an Asian culture of exorcism and superstitions. *Schizophrenia Research, 70*(Suppl. 1), 128.

Foulks, E. F., Persons, J. B., & Merkel, R. L. (1986). The effect of patients' beliefs about their illnesses on compliance in psychotherapy. [Research Support, Non-U.S. Government]. *The American Journal of Psychiatry, 143*(3), 340–344.

Garety, P. A., Fowler, D., & Kuipers, E. (2000). Cognitive-behavioral therapy for medication-resistant symptoms. [Review]. *Schizophrenia Bulletin, 26*(1), 73–86.

Haddock, G., Tarrier, N., Spaulding, W., Yusupoff, L., Kinney, C., & McCarthy, E. (1998). Individual cognitive-behavior therapy in the treatment of hallucinations and delusions: A review. [Review]. *Clinical Psychology Review, 18*(7), 821–838.

Jackson, H., McGorry, P., Edwards, J., Hulbert, C., Henry, L., Francey, S., et al. (1998). Cognitively-oriented psychotherapy for early psychosis (COPE). Preliminary results. [Clinical Trial Research Support, Non-U.S. Government]. *The British Journal of Psychiatry. Supplement, 172*(33), 93–100.

Jackson, H., McGorry, P., Henry, L., Edwards, J., Hulbert, C., Harrigan, S., et al. (2001). Cognitively oriented psychotherapy for early psychosis (COPE): A 1-year follow-up. [Clinical Trial Research Support, Non-U.S. Government]. *The British Journal of Clinical Psychology/The British Psychological Society, 40*(Pt 1), 57–70.

Kleinman, A. (1980). Major conceptual and research issues for cultural (anthropological) psychiatry. [Comparative Study]. *Culture, Medicine and Psychiatry, 4*(1), 3–13.

Marlowe, K. (2003). Cognitive-behavioural therapy for psychosis. [Comment Letter]. *The British Journal of Psychiatry: The Journal of Mental Science, 183*, 262–263.

Pinto, A., La Pia, S., Mennella, R., Giorgio, D., & DeSimone, L. (1999). Cognitive-behavioral therapy and clozapine for clients with treatment-refractory schizophrenia. [Clinical Trial Randomized Controlled Trial]. *Psychiatric Services, 50*(7), 901–904.

Rector, N. A., & Beck, A. T. (2001). Cognitive behavioral therapy for schizophrenia: An empirical review. [Research Support, Non-U.S. Government Review]. *The Journal of Nervous and Mental Disease, 189*(5), 278–287.

Rogers, C. R. (1957). The necessary and sufficient conditions of therapeutic personality change. *Journal of Consulting Psychology, 21*(2), 95–103.

Turkington, D., Kingdon, D., & Chadwick, P. (2003). Cognitive-behavioural therapy for schizophrenia: Filling the therapeutic vacuum. [Editorial]. *The British Journal of Psychiatry: The Journal of Mental Science, 183*, 98–99.

15

Cultural Issues in Early Psychosis Management

K. Pushpa

Singapore is a multi-religious country due to its diverse ethnic mix of peoples from various origins. Most of the key religious denominations are represented in Singapore (see Figure 15.1) and the government promotes religious tolerance. In 2000, Singapore had a population of about 4 million. It is comprised mainly of Chinese (76.8%), the majority of whom are Buddhist or atheists; Malays (13.9%), who are generally Muslim; and Indians (7.9%), who are mostly Hindus; another 1.4% is of other ethnicities (Statistics Singapore, 2007).

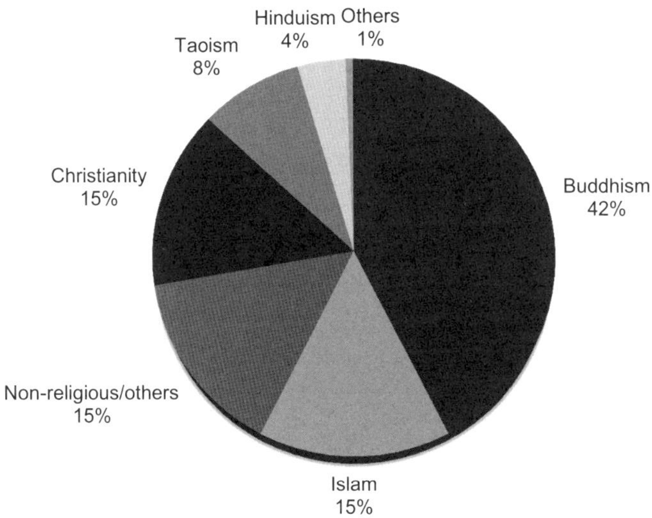

Figure 15.1

Religious distribution in Singapore

These statistics are relevant and of high importance in understanding the explanatory model of patients afflicted by mental disorders in Singapore. Understanding the cultural influence makes it easier for mental health professionals to work with clients. To patients, culture is a perspective, just like biological, psychological, and sociological perspectives, which explains the cause of mental illness. This chapter depicts several case examples to provide a better understanding for working with clients who present with strong cultural and traditional values.

Case Example 1

K was a 34-year-old lady brought to the emergency room by a student nurse. She had approached the student nurse for help when she felt confused and odd that she was hearing her religious leader's voice saying he no longer existed. However, on the contrary, K would see him in the mosque. K is Malay and proficient in that language. She had a firm Muslim upbringing. She was raised in Malaysia, married a Singaporean, and settled in Singapore.

K knew her experience was not normal and thus sought help. Upon service contact, she was clearly hallucinating and was also assessed to be depressed. As part of the usual practice, the Early Psychosis Intervention Programme (EPIP) team spoke to K's husband for corroborative history. It was an uphill task to make him understand K's distress. He strongly believed that K had been cast an evil spell by someone with malicious intent. The husband was consulting Malay healers while K was still in the ward.

K's explanatory model

K's husband allowed K to continue with treatment because she had come for help of her own accord. K would voluntarily request admission whenever she felt distressed at home. She relapsed and heard the voice of religious leaders every time she stopped her medications. K admitted feeling unheard by her husband and she had "no love for her husband". She felt much stressed from handling her four children, of whom one has autism. K was passively aggressive by being noncompliant and admitting herself to the hospital when her husband paid no attention to her unspoken request of wanting to be loved. K's explanation after gaining insight was that there was no evil spell but a strained marital relationship.

Husband's (main caregiver) explanatory model

K's husband continued to believe in the evil spell. He frequently asked healers to come to the house to cleanse it as he complained of the odour of dead corpses. He had videos of evil possessions and would sit all his children to watch and understand this spirit dimension. He attributed K's experience to his cousin, who had loved him many decades ago, who was jealous and pained about this marriage and therefore, had put a curse on K.

K avoided any intimacy with her husband and slept alone. K's husband, who slept in the living room, did not understand her non-feelings for him and claimed that the separation was to prevent "spirits" from disturbing the family. He felt a strong need to protect the family and the marriage. He tended to externalize problems to the spirit for everything that went wrong in his marriage. He even blamed the cousin's spirit when he lost his job. Asserting that the spirit had changed target from K to him, as his efforts to protect the family were an obstacle.

K's husband witnessed K's improvement whenever she had regular follow-ups, but still perceived that she improved due the strong occult practice of the healers. Although there was a mixture of religious and mystical beliefs, he encouraged K to come for any doctor follow-up after her many self-admissions. Her hospital stays had disrupted their family life since he would have to be absent from work to take care of the children whenever K was admitted. Once K had become stable, he thought that the spirit targeted him instead.

In this society, supernatural causes for illnesses are widely acknowledged and considered "real" especially within Islam. That said, in a Muslim community, people need to be educated to recognize mental illness as a legitimate medical condition that is distinct from illnesses of a supernatural nature. In this way, individuals learn to acknowledge or accept their mental illness and seek treatment and more community support along with less stigma that would be otherwise associated with their diagnoses.

Interventions

In this case, the difficulty with interventions was not with the patient but the main caregiver, as K had deep insight into her illness. Her stressors included handling an autistic child with special needs. We immediately engaged the special school's social workers for assistance.

A case conference with the social worker, K, and her husband updated the social worker about K's illness. Her child with special needs got a placement and subsidy for transport and school fees from the school, as those expenses were another source of family stress.

The husband played an active role in school affairs and K got some respite while the child attended school. As for their marital issues, she was not keen on couple counselling because of the husband's poor insight into their marital problems. Although it was hard for the husband to gain insight into K's illness, he did cooperate well with the treatment team whenever K relapsed. Delicate handling of the family's strong cultural beliefs by the case manager, and sensitive regard for their traditions helped K to continue with follow-ups and remain well.

Case Example 2

J was a 33-year-old Indian married lady with two children; one aged 12 and one aged 10. She was a homemaker for a few years before her first admission to hospital a diagnosis of schizophreniform disorder. She walked into the emergency room herself. J complained of two to three weeks of auditory hallucinations, which were derogatory and religious in content. She was increasingly religious and was observed to be frequently meditating. Her husband claimed that she had been withdrawn for a few years and neglected household chores. J was noted to look preoccupied and at times talking to herself prior to admission. Her symptoms abated in three weeks and she was discharged with medications and follow-up appointments.

J came for regular follow-ups alone and continued to be compliant. She soon found a job as a trainer in software programmes. During this period, her case manager conducted a home visit and found out that J had been sleeping separately from her husband. Her husband had never revealed much about their relationship but was observed to have minimal contact during her first admission in the hospital.

J relapsed after 18 months with similar symptoms and walked into the emergency room again by herself. She complained of hearing voices, was irritable but played down her symptoms whenever spoken to. She was observed to be meditating more during this admission. The only way to get her express her symptoms was to show interest and some awareness of her explanation, especially in the context of "karma" and in reverence to her Hindu guru.

After further exploration, J revealed that there had been marital strain for many years. She also finally shared that her husband was a Christian and that he had become more fervent just before her relapse. There were many issues in addition to their longstanding marital problems such as their disagreements about religious beliefs, and the children's confusions and struggles concerning choice of faith.

J's explanatory model

J always spoke in riddles. Clarifications were needed to understand her explanations. She attributed her psychotic experience to her bad karma, which had come from her past lives and the present, such as cooking non-vegetarian food for her family when she was a vegetarian, as well as her disloyalty to her guru whom she had ignored. She strongly felt that she should have continued with her practice in meditation and prayers as prescribed by her first guru so as to advance spiritually. She was further confounded by guilt for entering another school that taught meditation techniques. For her, all these steps had contributed to her bad karma and invoked the mental illness.

Her explanatory model of "karma" being the cause of mental illness enabled her to comply with medications and follow-up consultations. However, her explanation model coloured her judgement of the underlying cause of her relapses, which was in fact related to her longstanding marital strain. This denial inevitably had an effect on her treatment efficacy and speed of recovery.

Intervention

J had no insight to her illness and, given the marital discord, it was hard to achieve much improvement in her mental state. Although she complied with medication in the ward, she would relapse whenever she returned home because of the influence of her cultural beliefs and the strained relationship with her husband. In this case, it was hard to get passed the first stage of helping her understand some of her behaviours and thoughts. All her helpers' knowledge of the religious beliefs made more exploration possible. Otherwise, she refused to share as she felt misunderstood by and suspicious of and guarded with her treatment team.

Case Example 3

P was a 26-year-old Indian housewife who was not conversant in English. She was married with a 4-year-old daughter. She was referred to our department for acute psychosis. She and her family of origin understood her psychotic experience as a spiritual attack. She had been having erratic mood swings—intermittently irritable, sad, and then remorseful. Mood swings were not pervasive throughout the day. Her sleep and appetite were normal.

For the previous 12 months, her husband claimed that she had been "possessed by a spirit sent by his family". She repeatedly expressed guilt about her past extra-marital affair two years ago and she also accused her family of using black magic against her. The family brought her to a church so that the pastor could exorcise the evil spirits from her. They would then stay in the church for a few days for deliverance from the evil spirit.

Report by husband

P's husband reported that P would suddenly alternate between using a hoarse voice and her own soft voice, accusing her family members of being sinful for committing sexual sins. There was no history of delusions of passivity or ideas of reference. Her voice would suddenly change and she would display unusual movements, such as head swinging and movements like a snake. She would be shouting throughout these episodes, which would last for a few seconds. She claimed that she did not recollect these episodes and, in between episodes, she functioned normally. The team was also told that she had similar episodes of being "possessed" during a pregnancy that she eventually terminated.

Childhood and significant events

P was born and raised in a village in India. She has a brother who is seven years younger. Her paternal aunt played a major role in her strict upbringing alongside her biological parents. Nobody was allowed to visit the family and P was not encouraged to have friends. Nor was she encouraged to express her thoughts or feelings with family. She was often canned whenever she was seen to disrespect the adults. She lived in fear and dared not speak up. Her parents were initially Hindu but converted to Christian Pentecostal before P's birth. Hence, P was also Pentecostal from birth and disliked association with the Hindu religion. She had an arranged marriage in her late adolescent years and migrated to Singapore.

She was pregnant four times but the first three were all terminated (the first two were terminated because they were unprepared, and the third due to "spirit possession"). P revealed that due to a decrease in intimacy with her husband, she had an extra-marital affair with a colleague for a few months. She expressed to us that she was lonely and had "no dear friend". After some time, her parents and younger brother also moved to Singapore and resided with them upon her husband's invitation. P was upset about this arrangement, feeling a loss of privacy.

Psychological and social stressors

P was born and bred to a traditional family in India who had converted from Hinduism to Christianity. Although the concept of possession and exorcism exist in both faiths, they are spoken of in different ways. Her childhood was turbulent with much physical abuse and emotional neglect. Without question, the move from village life to a metropolitan society in Singapore, her three pregnancy terminations and the known extra-marital affair had a huge impact on her psychologically. Given the parent's background and her being raised according to a strict religious and strong cultural code, any perception of a good, moral daughter would exclude an extra-marital affair and abortions.

Clearly, the best hypothesis for this case is founded in her being extremely guilt stricken. In P's case, the guilt feelings that stem from doing wrong had escalated out of control and interfered with her healthy psychological function.

Culture and life events play a critical part in shaping all people, the product of upbringing, experiences, and choices. From a psychodynamic perspective, P's upbringing in a traditional family strung between two religious beliefs, combined with her own choices and poor coping mechanisms, may have contributed to the psychotic episodes. Studies have shown that guilt is a significant predictor of dissociative experiences and may have explained P's abnormal behavioural changes.

Explanatory model

P's husband and family were not keen on her going to follow-up consultations for treatment, and her experience was described as a "spiritual attack". It was more comforting for the family to buy in the beliefs of spirits and possession and engage the religious healers to exorcise than to believe that it was the behavioural manifestation of psychological stressors.

They reported that P had no further episodes and had resumed her duties as a homemaker with no functioning decline. The church played a significant role in supporting them emotionally. All of them were still upholding the explanation that she was possessed.

Intervention

The team was toiling with diagnosis before her discharge from the ward. With the given presentation she could be perceived to be unwell or experiencing a brief psychotic episode; however, if we take into consideration her upbringing, strong cultural values, migration stress and marital problems, she should be given the benefit of doubt that she is free from mental illness. The team decided to stop medication and observe her for the next 6 months. She was eventually discharged from our department due to absence of psychotic symptoms. It is possible that the manifestation can be explained from the perspective of culture. The question remains whether this was "the effects of culture on recovery from transient psychosis" (Castillo, 2006).

Case Example 4

LK was a 39-year-old Chinese married lady, with two children; both aged under 13 years. She is a homemaker with a diagnosis of schizophrenia. In the hospital ward, LK reported auditory and tactile hallucinations and insomnia. She was very psychotic upon admission. She walked backwards from the ward lobby to her room and had "trance-like" state frequently. She claimed that the "spirits" were doing this to her body.

Explanatory model

LK believed that she was possessed and she was the "chosen one". She did not buy into the medical model but agreed to take antipsychotic medication as it helped her sleep better. A few months later, when she returned as an outpatient in the clinic, her explanatory model shifted a little. She continued to believe that the experience was spiritual, but started to entertain that she might have a mental illness due to stress. She also began to question if she was genetically vulnerable because her mother had schizophrenia. Before she was discharged from our service after two years, her explanatory model shifted again. She was convinced that she had a mental illness and her earlier symptoms were not caused by spirit possession.

Intervention

In order to work with her, LK's case manager accepted and respected her cultural beliefs without pushing her too hard with the medical model. The case manager focused on other benefits of the medication, such as helping her calm her mood and induce better sleep even during times when she was non-compliant with medication. She was allowed to experience the difference between with and without medication.

The case manager continued to explore her psychosocial needs, which include growing up with a parent with mental illness and how her upbringing impacted her self-esteem and coping skills. Trust was built by being there when in times of crisis as she suffered from side-effects of medications. Psychoeducation was initially focused on how stress caused by the external environment and her own expectation of life could have an impact on her mental health. The biological model of psychosis was carefully introduced at her own pace. The case manager's patience and respect for her explanatory model paid off eventually.

Popular Beliefs about Mental Illness

Mental illness and its effects on individuals are often misunderstood and negatively construed in many communities and cultures across the world. It is often understood and explained in people's own familiar and popular beliefs. In Asian cultures, mental illness is commonly viewed as a punishment from God, a result of possession by evil spirits (Jinn), effects of evil eye, and effects of evil objects that are transferred to the individual (the evil spirit is put into an object by someone with malicious intent) (Pridmore & Pasha, 2004; Stein, 2000).

Islam

Islam views mental illness as a condition that results from an unbalanced lifestyle (diet, sleeping patterns, spiritual activities, and remembrance of God) or body (Rahman, 1998). It is important to note that supernatural causes to illnesses are widely acknowledged and are considered very real within Islam. Traditionally, Islams do not link all mental illnesses to supernatural causes (Rahman, 1998). Furthermore, one of the early Muslim scholars in psychiatric healthcare, Ibn Sina, rejected the popular notion that mental illnesses originated from evil spirits (Pridmore & Pasha, 2004).

Hinduism

Among Hindus, beliefs and health are intrinsically linked. The Hindus believe that physical, emotional, mental, and spiritual health are all inseparably linked and therefore must all be balanced to have good health, and that the entire universe is connected. Magnetic influences, planetary influences, spiritual influences, as well as personal actions, beliefs, thoughts, diet, and exercises, are all seen as having various effects on physical and mental health.

In Hindu medicine, the four elements of earth, fire, water, and air represent the four elements of mankind—physical, emotional, mental, and spiritual. If all four of these are in balance, there is a state of health. If any of these is out of balance to any degree, there is a state of illness. In the West, health is understood as freedom from disability, but in Hinduism, it is understood as soundness of the body and mind. Many Hindus consider illness simply as part of ordinary life experience and a test from God. Another commonly held belief among Hindus is that illness is instigated by bad karma.

Karma theory

Karma refers to action at three levels—physical (body), mental (mind), and speech. Action at any level has consequences. Uncomfortable actions reap uncomfortable consequences or situations, which are not limited to the current life; results could be outcomes of doings from previous lives.

Karma is accumulated through prior existences and it defines your character, tendencies, capacities, and caste. Hindus seek a high quality of life, as measured by one's longing for God instead of worldly things. The system of karma perpetuates transmigration that results from ethical or unethical consequences. In Hinduism, one's perpetual soul's future and the quality of one's rebirth and progress towards liberation depend on one's actions in life. The law of karma states that every event has a cause and effect, and every cause has a destiny. It signifies the interplay between fate and free will. Hindus are not fatalists who believe that humans have no freedom, are subject to preordained forces, and are puppets of fate.

Buddhism and Taoism

Buddhists and Taoists believe that people can be attacked by ghosts. Ghosts may attack human beings to prompt them to meet their needs, or at least to draw attention to the reason they are haunting a person, location, or object.

A spirit may be unhappy because it had a bad death, an improper burial, or had no descendants to perform proper rituals after its death for which it became a ghost (sometimes called a "hungry ghost", a term with Buddhist origins). The Ghost Festival is celebrated during the seventh month of the Chinese Lunar calendar. It also falls on a full moon day and coincides with the new season, the fall harvest, the peak of Buddhist monastic asceticism, the rebirth of ancestors, and the assembly of the local community. During this month, the gates of hell are opened and ghosts are free to roam on earth, where they seek food and entertainment. These ghosts are believed to be ancestors of those who have forgotten to pay tribute to them after they die, or those who never give a proper ritual for a send-off. Family members offer prayers to their deceased relatives, with food and drinks, and burn joss paper. Such paper items are only valid in the underworld, which is why they burn it as an offering to the ghosts that come from the gates of hell.

It is common to attribute the symptoms to possession by ghosts, especially when a person is afflicted by mental illness during this month. The sufferers may be seen as having offended the ghosts.

Christianity

In Christianity, the associations between mental illness and beliefs are the guilt of having sinned and spiritual attacks. Forgiveness of sins is a key characteristic of Christianity. Depression, anxiety, hostility, fear, tension, and in more serious cases, psychosis, are regarded as ailments of the conscience—symptoms that result from violating the principles and refusing to live honestly and responsibly. The only means of being cleansed from sins is through repentance and faith in Christ.

Christian patients and families often report difficulties in differentiating between demonic possession and schizophrenia. Mental illness is often explained as wrongdoings and evil actions, of which the patient may be the actor or victim of such actions of others. It takes time for Christian patients and families to accept that it is a medical problem and not a moral problem.

Demonic possession (the fallen angels) or spiritual attacks are often the term used to describe the control over a human form by the devil himself or one of his assigned advocates. Descriptions of demonic possessions often include erased memories or personalities, convulsions, and fits and fainting as if one is dying. The subject has no control over the possessing entity, which will persist until forced to leave the victim, usually through prayers in effort to cast out demons.

Conclusion

Spirit possession is a concept of paranormal, supernatural and/or superstitious belief in which spirits, gods, demons, animas, or other disincarnate entities may take control of a human body, resulting in noticeable changes in behaviour. Many cultures and religions contain some concept of demonic possession, but the details vary considerably. The concept of spiritual possession exists in all contemporary religions and can also be seen in the mythology and folklore of many cultures.

The case examples in this chapter narrate the impact of cultural and religious belief in individuals suffering from psychosis. In a society like Singapore with various ethnic groups from different cultural and religious background, not to mention the stigma of mental illness, it is important for mental healthcare professionals to take into account the sufferers' explanatory model, and avoid taking on a top-down approach when it comes to psychoeducation of mental illness. It does not only improve rapport, but also drives a holistic intervention approach, which can hopefully create a stronger positive impact on the lives of sufferers and their families.

References

Castillo, R. J. (2006). Effects of culture on recovery from transient psychosis. *Psychiatric Times, 23*(14), 46–48.

Pridmore, S., & Pasha, M. I. (2004). Psychiatry and Islam. *Australasian Psychiatry: Bulletin of Royal Australian and New Zealand College of Psychiatrists, 12*(4), 380–385. doi: 10.1111/j.1440-1665.2004.02131.x

Rahman, F. (1998). *Health and Medicine in the Islamic Tradition: Change and Identity.* Chicago, IL: ABC International Group. *Statistics Singapore.* (2007). Singapore.

Stein, D. (2000). Views of mental illness in Morocco: Western medicine meets the traditional symbolic. [Historical Article Research Support, Non-U.S. Government]. *CMAJ: Canadian Medical Association Journal (Journal de l'Association Medicale Canadienne), 163*(11), 1468–1470.

16
Engagement and Outreach in Early Psychosis Management

Kai-tai Chan and Gloria Hoi-kei Chan

According to the Oxford Advanced Learner's Dictionary, engagement means "locking together, fitting into; of part of a machine, etc." (Hornby, 2005). Yet, in psychology or psychiatry literature, there is little consensus on the definition and measurement of engagement or disengagement (see reviews by O'Brien, Fahmy, & Singh, 2009; Tetley et al., 2011) and this construct is often conflated with concepts related to the treatment progression or therapeutic alliance. Despite this, it is well recognized that therapeutic engagement is important for patients to receive appropriate help and achieve better outcomes.

Engagement is especially important in first-episode psychosis. First of all, failure in engaging patients may cause delays in treatment, which in turn affects patients' outcomes. Late presentation of first-episode psychosis has been shown to be associated with slower and less complete recovery (Harrigan, McGorry, & Krstev, 2003; Helgason, 1977, 1990; Loebel et al., 1992; McGorry et al., 1996) and earlier intervention demonstrated to improve subsequent levels of disability (McGorry, 1992). Secondly, successful engagement, which consists of a strong therapeutic alliance, is significantly related to maintenance of psychotherapy, medication compliance, better outcomes, and less medications among non-chronic schizophrenia patients (Frank & Gunderson, 1990). From the evidence available, a strong therapeutic alliance is apparently necessary to enable change (Hewitt & Coffey, 2005) and may maximize the therapeutic effects and benefits of intervention on patients' and their caregivers' well-being.

Therapeutic engagement is more than therapeutic alliance, however, according to Tetley et al. (2011). In evaluating whether an individual is "actively participating in the treatment on offer", he or she will show attendance in arranged treatment, completion of treatment, completion of between-session tasks, willingness to self-disclose, and supportive behaviours (in group sessions), in addition to a working alliance. Successful therapeutic engagement is not easy to attain and should never be taken for granted. Its success often depends on the various parties concerned, including the service provider, staff, service, patients, and caregivers.

Service Provider

A case management system has been adopted by the Early Assessment Service for Young People with Psychosis (EASY) in Hong Kong. The case manager serves as a key person to provide comprehensive care to patients and help them in different aspects of their life, with an aim of ensuring continuous and specialized care for patients.

In engaging patients in EASY, accessibility to services is also of paramount importance. Case managers in EASY can be readily contacted by telephone during office hours. Voice messages can be left after office hours, and case managers will respond to them the next working day and provide appropriate and timely management according to the urgency and nature of the presenting problems. With this high accessibility, patients appreciate the service provider more often and start to gain confidence in the service. This in turn enhances patients' willingness to seek help when they encounter further problems. In this way, patients are more eager to remain in service and the therapeutic alliance is further enhanced.

For patients who refuse to attend follow-up consultations—a situation that is often due to poor mental state or lack of insight—outreach services can be arranged. With this type of service, patients can be re-engaged in services with regular psychiatric reviews.

Moreover, in EASY, a multidisciplinary team composed of doctors, clinical psychologists, nurses, occupational therapists, and medical social workers working in close collaboration has proven to be important for engaging patients in services. This team holds regular and ad hoc meetings for patients' management to facilitate accurate information sharing and timely responses to patient's problems ranging from clinical management to school or occupational issues. With this collaborative effort, patients' problems can be more thoroughly handled with due consideration to many different aspects.

Staff

In managing patients' problems, the attitude of the staff when providing care is often influential. It has a special impact on patients' willingness to disclose their feelings and thoughts. Disclosure of information and problems is important as further deterioration in mental well-being can be prevented when problems are handled at an early stage.

In order to foster information disclosure, staff members take an empathetic, proactive, and collaborative approach, which encourages patients and their caregivers to seek help in times of difficulty. This step maximizes therapeutic effect.

Services

Early psychosis intervention service emphasizes psychoeducation, support, social integration of patients and their caregivers, and liaison with service partners in the community. Regular psychoeducational talks, in collaboration with schools and non-governmental organizations, can be held to enable patients and their caregivers to gain more knowledge about mental illness, and hence better understand their problems (see Chapter 22, "Working with Non-Governmental Organizations in Early Psychosis"). Patients and their caregivers are referred to community partners for social support and social activities. Regular liaison with community partners is held to review the collaborative programmes and share information about patients to ensure that patients and their caregivers receive the services they need. Outreach service by nurses and doctors to facilitate effective community assessment and treatment is another important area in this early psychosis intervention service.

Patients

Denial and resistance are common psychological reactions in people with early psychosis. Patients in their first episode of psychosis may have symptoms of persecutory ideas and suspiciousness, which prevent them from interacting with others, even the ones whom they originally trusted. During such an active state of psychosis, social withdrawal is not uncommon among patients.

A key factor that hampers engagement in treatment, and even help-seeking, is lack of insight. In the National Comorbidity Survey (Von Korff et al., 1985), a large-scale community-based survey conducted in the United States found that over half of the individuals with serious mental illness never sought help because they did not believe they had a problem that required treatment. Some believed that the problem would get better by itself, or that they wanted to solve it by themselves because treatment would be unlikely to help. Indeed, lack of insight, which involves undermining the severity and impact of the illness, is correlated with service disengagement (Tait, Birchwood, & Trower, 2003). This factor must be appropriately addressed and handled with sensitivity when delivering intervention and psychoeducation especially during the initial period of treatment.

Additionally, comorbidities such as depression and substance abuse will render patients unwilling to receive and be engaged in services (see Chapter 27, "Comorbid Substance Abuse in Early Psychosis"). Fear of stigma is another challenge when establishing therapeutic and treatment engagement, but can be reduced by public education, and probably through sharing of experiences by other patients (see Chapter 17, "Experience of Stigma in Early Psychosis Patients and Caregivers" and Chapter 7, "Public Awareness Approaches in Early Psychosis"). At an individual level, psychoeducation with an emphasis on the need for and importance of early intervention can help instil hope and relieve fear in patients and their caregivers.

Caregivers

Caregivers play an important role in the process of treatment, especially in the establishment of a therapeutic alliance since most young people with early psychosis in Hong Kong live with their family (see Chapter 2, "Early Psychosis Services in an Asian Urban Setting: EASY and Other Services in Hong Kong"). Frequently, family members find it difficult to accept the fact that someone in the family has a mental illness, and may resist seeking help (see Chapter 17, "Experience of Stigma in Early Psychosis Patients and Caregivers"). Chinese people in particular may think that the person is disturbed by spirits and they may seek help from religious agencies rather than medical assistance. These cultural beliefs should always be respected when engaging patients and their family members in the service, but an alternative explanation should be offered from a psychiatric point of view at the same time so that psychiatric management can commence promptly (see Case Vignette 1).

Case Vignette 1

Jane was a 20-year-old single unemployed lady newly referred to a mental health service and living with her mother and siblings. She was distressed by an unsatisfactory interpersonal relationship and stress in her new job. Jane quit her job and felt guilty for making her family rely on social welfare. She presented with one week of low and anxious mood, poor sleep and appetite, mild loss of energy and interest, passivity, symptoms of being controlled by two selves, auditory hallucination (one voice asking her to do good things and another asking her to do bad things), persecutory ideas, and vague thought-broadcasting.

At first, the family sought help from a spiritualist. On the day of admission, the patient said she was controlled by a "self" which tried to make her harm herself. Her mother was worried and sought help from the early psychosis intervention service through the telephone-based assessment system. As the patient also had problem of decreased oral intake, a referral to the outreach doctor and nurse was made promptly. Through discussion and persuasion, the family began to accept that Jane's problem was psychiatric in nature. Jane was then admitted voluntarily to a psychiatric hospital and maintained regular follow-up visits thereafter. At the same time, the family also sought help from spiritualists to perform rituals even during her hospital stay. Jane remained in remission after discharge. With the advice from the spiritualist, she also changed her first name to change her "bad luck".

Discussion

In this scenario, although the family and the patient held a religious and cultural interpretation of the psychotic experience, they nevertheless accepted psychiatric management for the problems. Any intervention and psychoeduation, therefore, had to respect the patients' and caregivers' perspective so as to facilitate effective treatment and therapeutic engagement. Further psychoeducation and insight instillation, necessary for further engagement of the patients and their family in treatment, was then activated.

In summary, engagement is a prerequisite for effective psychiatric treatment for early psychosis, and can be achieved with a proactive, multidisciplinary, user-friendly, culture-sensitive, flexible, and collaborative approach. Engagement requires an empathic and non-confrontational attitude by early intervention staff, as well as self-efficacy in patients. In this way, the "locking together" of patients, caregivers, and service enables the "machine" of psychiatric management to run at full efficiency.

Outreach Services

Outreach services are an important element of community-based psychiatry, in which psychiatric services are extended to the community in a flexible, client-centred, and assertive manner. Outreach usually involves psychiatrists, nurses, and other disciplines when necessary. The venue may be the patient's school, workplace, or social centre. In early psychosis, outreach intervention services are of particular importance for the following reasons:

Timely Assessment: A patient may be unwilling to attend a diagnostic interview at the early stage of the illness for several reasons. First of all, new clients may still be in a stage of denial about their mental problems such that he or she refuses to accept any explanation that the changes in mental state and/or behaviour are due to psychiatric factors. They may therefore be ambivalent about receiving mental health services. Secondly, some patients may fear being stigmatized if they receive mental health services. In addition, some clients may harbour paranoid ideas against people around them or experience abnormal perceptions about the reality, especially during the active phase of psychosis, thus rendering any communication difficult or making them reluctant to share with others properly. Under these circumstances, potential clients referred to service may not receive a timely assessment and intervention because they are not willing to come to an outpatient department. Outreach services in the community provided by doctors and nurses the clients is an appropriate alternative for these cases who need immediate intervention, especially for those whose mental condition may be endangering their safety or others' well-being. Outreach services can assess risks and patients' mental conditions for further psychiatric management in a timely way.

Restore Treatment Continuity: Some existing patients stop attending their psychiatric appointments after a series of follow-up consultations. Reasons for disengagement include lack of insight, bad experience with treatment, deterioration of mental state, prominent negative symptoms, side-effects of medications, difficulty in social reintegration, or even caregivers' rejecting attitude. Outreach staff can perform formal psychiatric assessment, understand of patients' problems, and engage with patients and caregivers with the aim of restoring regular psychiatric treatment.

Case Vignette 2

Susan was a 24-year-old single, unemployed lady living with family and was newly referred to the mental health service. Her mother suffered from depression. She was distressed by repeated job-hunting failures, parental conflicts, her father's extra-marital affairs, and isolation from friends. She developed delusions of reference, grandiosity, misidentification and persecution, auditory hallucination, mood fluctuation, social withdrawal, and used irrelevant speech for three weeks. She broke an umbrella and tried to climb out of a window, saying that she wanted to drive Satan out of her father. She even attempted to strangle her mother, because she misidentified her as her father's mistress. She had on-and-off poor feeding. Outreach services were arranged in view of the potential risks to herself and the family. Susan was finally admitted to hospital under compulsory status.

Discussion

In this case, the patient refused psychiatric admission by covering herself up with a blanket in bed when the outreach team arrived. After discussion, her mother remained ambivalent about the need for admission so the doctor and nurse had to wait until her father returned to Hong Kong from China late in the evening to conclude the discussion. Being a Chinese herbalist, her father initially showed resistance towards psychiatric admission and thought that Susan's problems were not that severe and could be cured by Chinese medicine. After further explanation emphasizing the seriousness of her psychiatric problems, the effectiveness of psychiatric treatment, and the risk of poor feeding, her father finally approved his daughter's compulsory admission. This is a good example showing the need for and advantages of outreach services, for timely risk management and relevant psychoeducation.

Streamlining Regular Services

Outreach is an effective way of streamlining regular psychiatric service. In early psychosis intervention services, outreach enables doctors and nurses to gain deeper appreciation of patients' living environment, especially for socially withdrawn patients, including meetings with the patient's family, schoolteachers, social workers, and community partners. Such liaisons might not be possible in an outpatient setting. Sometimes, intervention (e.g., injection of depot medication) can be given in outreach settings, and unnecessary psychiatric admissions can be avoided. An outreach service is particularly important in first-episode psychosis, as it is desirable to avoid admissions to prevent further traumatic experiences in young patients.

Special Considerations in Outreach Service

Staff safety: Safety of the visiting staff during outreach is of utmost importance, and risks should be ascertained before each visit. In order to ensure contact with the patient, liaison with his or her caregivers is necessary to make sure that the patient can be met in a comfortable atmosphere at the meeting point, and be accompanied if needed. In case of emergency, for example, when the patient needs compulsory psychiatric admission and immediate control, help from ambulance staff and police should be arranged. However, such decisions should be the last resort to avoid the likelihood that neighbours, especially in crowded living environments, will witness the patient being escorted away from home. If neighbours view such events, the patient may find it difficult to face them after discharge. Explanation of the purpose of outreach at the beginning of the visit will avoid unnecessary fear and paranoia on the part of the patient.

An empathetic attitude: An empathetic, open, and flexible attitude is always desirable to allay the patient's anxiety and fear. Understanding and managing the patients' problems according to their developmental stage is also important for adolescent patients. Appreciation of their environment and the caregivers' attitudes towards them can deepen understanding about the patients. Therapeutic options should be offered whenever possible, as therapeutic alliance and engagement is a prerequisite for successful treatment outcomes in the long run. After the outreach, clear documentation is necessary to enable further information sharing and case management. In most cases, the aim of the outreach should be to restore continuity of regular psychiatric service instead of replacing it.

In summary, outreach service is an important component of effective community early psychosis service. It also serves as a timely and client-centred intervention supplementing and streamlining the regular service. It is of particular importance in early psychosis intervention service that a "low-threshold principle" be adopted in arranging outreach service for potential and existing patients, so that their difficulties and problems can be handled in a user-friendly and prompt way. Engagement and therapeutic alliance can thus be improved, enhancing patients' and caregivers' well-being in the long term.

References

Frank, A. F., & Gunderson, J. G. (1990). The role of the therapeutic alliance in the treatment of schizophrenia: Relationship to course and outcome. [Clinical Trial Randomized Controlled Trial Research Support, Non-U.S. Government Research Support, U.S. Government, P.H.S.]. *Archives of General Psychiatry, 47*(3), 228–236.

Harrigan, S. M., McGorry, P. D., & Krstev, H. (2003). Does treatment delay in first-episode psychosis really matter? *Psychological Medicine, 33*(1), 97–110.

Helgason, L. (1977). Psychiatric services and mental illness in Iceland: Incidence study (1966–1967) with 6–7 year follow-up. *Acta Psychiatr Scand Supplement*(268), 1–140.

Helgason, L. (1990). Twenty years' follow-up of first psychiatric presentation for schizophrenia: What could have been prevented? *Acta Psychiatrica Scandinavica, 81*(3), 231–235.

Hewitt, J., & Coffey, M. (2005). Therapeutic working relationships with people with schizophrenia: Literature review. [Review]. *Journal of Advanced Nursing, 52*(5), 561–570. doi: 10.1111/j.1365-2648.2005.03623.x

Hornby, A. S. (2005). *Oxford Advanced Learner's Dictionary of Current English* (7th ed.). Oxford, UK: Oxford University Press.

Loebel, A. D., Lieberman, J. A., Alvir, J. M., Mayerhoff, D. I., Geisler, S. H., & Szymanski, S. R. (1992). Duration of psychosis and outcome in first-episode schizophrenia. *American Journal of Psychiatry, 149*(9), 1183–1188.

McGorry, P. D. (1992). The concept of recovery and secondary prevention in psychotic disorders. *Australian and New Zealand Journal of Psychiatry, 26*(1), 3–17.

McGorry, P. D., Edwards, J., Mihalopoulos, C., Harrigan, S. M., & Jackson, H. J. (1996). EPPIC: An evolving system of early detection and optimal management. *Schizophrenia Bulletin, 22*(2), 305–326.

O'Brien, A., Fahmy, R., & Singh, S. P. (2009). Disengagement from mental health services. A literature review. [Review]. *Social Psychiatry and Psychiatric Epidemiology, 44*(7), 558–568. doi: 10.1007/s00127-008-0476-0

Tait, L., Birchwood, M., & Trower, P. (2003). Predicting engagement with services for psychosis: Insight, symptoms and recovery style. *British Journal of Psychiatry, 182*, 123–128.

Tetley, A., Jinks, M., Huband, N., & Howells, K. (2011). A systematic review of measures of therapeutic engagement in psychosocial and psychological treatment. [Review]. *Journal of Clinical Psychology, 67*(9), 927–941. doi: 10.1002/jclp.20811

Von Korff, M., Nestadt, G., Romanoski, A., Anthony, J., Eaton, W., Merchant, A., et al. (1985). Prevalence of treated and untreated DSM-III schizophrenia: Results of a two-stage community survey. *The Journal of Nervous and Mental Disease, 173*(10), 577–581.

17
Experience of Stigma in Early Psychosis Patients and Caregivers

Desiree Yan Wong, Dicky Wai-sau Chung, and May Mei-ling Lam

Psychotic disorders often emerge in late adolescence and young adulthood with a prolonged delay between onset of symptoms and the first effective treatment. Such delays affect symptom severity, treatment response, relapses, and quality of life. The stigma associated with psychosis may be one of the major factors associated with delays in seeking medical help. For diagnosed patients and their family members, the negative stigma attached to psychotic disorders also often cause psychosocial repercussions. This chapter discusses some concepts of stigma in psychosis, with reference to the subjective experience of stigma and reactions to the diagnosis among patients and caregivers in Hong Kong.

Public Stigma of Psychosis

Social stigma attached to mental illness is universal regardless of culture and ethnic group. In a broad and non-judgemental sense, any feature that marks a person out as different from others can be considered a stigma. However, more often, stigma is a mark of shame or discredit: it emerges through the social processes of labelling, stereotyping, and discrimination (Link & Phelan, 2001). By labelling, people are distinguished as different, and seen as "them" and "not us". These people are then linked to undesirable characteristics that form stereotypes. Stereotypes of mental illness held by the public have four common components (Hayward & Bright, 1997): (1) the mentally ill are dangerous; (2) they are unpredictable and unable to follow accepted social roles; (3) they are responsible for their behaviours and conditions; and (4) mental illness is chronic, difficult to treat with poor prognosis. The labelled people are subsequently discriminated against, leading to status loss, unfair treatment, and unequal outcomes.

Many factors contribute to the stereotyping and discrimination of psychosis. Media reports of violence or crime can lead to reactions of fear and anger in society. Anger can be further exacerbated if the mentally ill offenders get lenient sentences due to their unwell mental state. Fear easily leads to an increase in social distance from the neighbourhood, and hence marginalization (Tsang et al., 2003). Many people also despise the mentally ill, not only because of the attribution to their personality and responsibility for their own behaviour, but also the high prevalence of coexisting substance abuse in that population (see Chapter 27, "Comorbid Substance Abuse in Early Psychosis"). People's pessimistic view of mental illness being irreversible and untreatable, in addition to not being able to arouse sympathy, can heighten despair and neglect.

Internalization of Public Stigma and Concealment

Stigmatization has two interrelated aspects: public stigma on the mentally ill, and the stigma perceived by patients and their relatives. These two influence each other, forming a vicious cycle. The internalization of others' negative valuation gives rise to low self-esteem and a sense of incompetence in patients. This further jeopardizes their social skills and limits the social circles. The difficulty in reintegrating into society is a self-driven marginalization (Mueller et al., 2006). Patients may also pessimistically perceive themselves as suffering from a devastating illness.

Recent research has emphasized the adverse effects of stigma on patients who have suffered from psychosis. In particular, the social stigma associated with the illness is debilitating to patients, and their family who also suffer the brunt of the social reaction. A study on people with schizophrenia in China (Phillips et al., 2002) shows an association between perceived stigma in family members and higher expressed emotion, with the latter increasing the chance of relapse, resulting in poorer treatment outcomes. Both parties have a tendency to conceal the psychosis due to the fear of being stigmatized and discriminated against. Concealment of mental illness may delay medical treatment and thus lead to poorer outcomes.

Either for the hereditary or upbringing factor attributed to having caused the mental illness, parents are blamed when they have a mentally ill child either because of hereditary factors or style of upbringing, that give raise to the disgrace for having mental illness in the family. The relatives readily handle this situation with defence mechanisms of suppression or denial (e.g., attribution to supernatural forces or trivialization of the problem). In Japan, even psychiatrists were reluctant to tell patients with schizophrenia the exact diagnosis (Ono et al., 1999). A study in Hong Kong found that concealment of having a mentally ill family member was common (Lee et al., 2005). More than half of the family members of patients with schizophrenia wanted to conceal from others the presence of a psychiatric patient in their family, as compared with only 3.9% in patients with diabetes. Such reaction from the family is much more hurtful than that from the public. In India, concealment of mental illness in a daughter by the family serves another purpose. As over 90% of marriages are still arranged by parents, mental illness infers "damaged goods" and hence, this diagnosis cannot be revealed (Thara & Srinivasan, 2000).

Besides family members, mental health workers are also found to be stigmatized. In a Singaporean study, others laughed at 60% of mental health workers for having joined that profession (Lai, Hong, & Chee, 2001). In fact, some subtle discrimination stems from the psychiatric profession itself. In Hong Kong and some European countries, psychiatric nurses are awarded a higher salary than their counterpart professionals because they have to work with mentally ill patients, who might be allegedly more violent. This decision contributes to "iatrogenic stigmatization" (Sartorius, 2002).

Patients' and Caregivers' Experiences

In Hong Kong, a retrospective study using both qualitative and quantitative approaches was carried out among 30 patients and 23 caregivers recruited from the Early Assessment Service for Young People with Psychosis (EASY) programme, which investigated the experience of receiving a diagnosis of psychotic disorder in young people. Young patients face a number of complex issues and challenges as the psychotic symptoms subside because they are going through a critical developmental stage while simultaneously facing specific challenges and complex issues that are related to their illness and treatment. These include concerns about the extent of their recovery, the possibility of relapse, and making sense of their illness experience. In addition, they themselves and their caretakers are likely to have strong and realistic concerns about stigmatization by peers, schools, employers and the treatment system. Understanding how young people with psychosis and their caretakers view the concept of stigma allows the possibility of developing more sensitive services guided by therapeutic optimism.

In this study, patients and caregivers did not report any enacted stigma towards the illness. However, they did report a great deal of felt stigma once the illness was made known to others. Participants expressed setbacks in many aspects of social lives in fear of potential avoidance by friends and relatives, discrimination in the workplace or during job seeking, disgrace brought about by the association with substance abuse, being the subject of gossip and treated differently, the need to keep secrets to avoid the long-term labelling effect of psychosis, and internalized stigma associated with treatment. These felt stigmas posed stress on patients and restricted them from normal engagement in society. Some experiences quoted by respondents are described below.

Being a burden to friends and relatives

The respondents felt that they would be treated differently or even avoided by friends and relatives should the diagnosis be known to others. The feeling of guilt for being a burden to others also affects patients' interpersonal relationships. Below are some accounts from patients:

> Others would avoid you if they find out that you have a psychotic illness. People with psychosis are different from other illnesses in that they don't know they're ill, although their behaviours are disturbing.

> I'm worried that if I tell my friends about my illness, they'll think I'll be their burden as I need to be taken care of.

Discrimination in job-seeking and in the workplace

The stigma of psychosis has also significant impact on the patient's career decision-making and employment opportunities. Some patients believe that discrimination in workplace is unavoidable, while others are worried about jeopardizing their chances of successfully applying for a job:

> If people find out about my illness in workplace, they'll gossip. I'll end up losing my job. Discrimination is inevitable. People will degrade your work ability. They'll have a bad impression of you and treat you differently.

> I don't want to go to job interviews as I'm worried that others will find out my illness. No one will employ someone with mental illness.

Social taboo and gossiping

Partial understanding and misconceptions of psychosis among the public exert "differentness" and rejection in society. The social taboo holds young people back from comfortably disclosing information regarding their illness. Local culture may also contribute to the "taboo" of psychosis, and studies have shown that stigma against mental illness is especially pervasive and harmful in Chinese societies (Lee et al., 2005; Pearson et al., 2003). Gossiping about mental illness is intimidating for patients, who expressed the following views about the image of psychosis in the general public in Hong Kong:

> The general public think this illness is mysterious, a social taboo. People won't talk about it in public.
>
> In overseas, people will help you if you were mentally ill. It's different in Hong Kong, where people will gossip and think that you're crazy. People in overseas are more open-minded, they respect your privacy. So, I'll be more at ease to tell others about my illness if I were overseas.

The felt needs for secrecy and concealment

One of the major dilemmas patients and caretakers face is whether to disclose the illness. Patients speculate that others would treat them differently once they find out about their illness, as they are reluctant to victimize themselves and assume a sick role. While they are aware of the potentially distressing labelling effect of the diagnosis, the need to keep a secret about their illness on the other hand adds to their cognitive load and anxiety.

> Once your friends find out about your illness, they'll treat you like a patient.
>
> I'm very reluctant to tell others. I think even when I'm totally recovered and back to normal, others will treat you differently once they know.
>
> This is a secret. My family and I have never told any friends or relatives. People may treat you differently once they find out.
>
> Mental illness is something disgraceful . . . It will not help even telling others.

Sometimes, the family is overwhelmed by enormous worries about long-term discrimination that their children might face with this diagnostic label. Most caregivers make the decision to keep the illness as a secret for fear that such a disclosure will affect the future of their children.

> All my relatives and neighbours don't know about my daughter's illness. Psychologically, I don't think I should disclose as this may affect her job seeking or chance of getting married. People will treat her differently. So, I do my best to keep it a secret.

Internalized stigma associated with treatment

Stigma can also be observed in patients and their caregivers towards themselves. For example, they tend to internalize the negative stigma of antipsychotics. The mere fact that one needs to receive medication treatment is enough to arouse uneasy feelings. This internalization of stigma may foster a vicious cycle: some of the caregivers expressed ambivalence about the effect of antipsychotics and preferred as few medications as possible. Some even have strong resistance against taking psychiatric medicine or receiving psychiatric help:

> I was so reluctant to be admitted to the psychiatric unit. I thought only seriously ill people should be in an asylum.

> [My son] said those were "medicine for the crazy" . . . Perhaps he didn't want to accept the fact that he was a crazy boy.

> I don't want others to find out that I take medications. Perhaps I don't want to accept that I'm a psychosis sufferer all along. I believe that I only have a minor problem.

> My family is strongly against psychiatric drugs. They think drugs are like dirt—if others know that you're on psychiatric drugs, they know you have mental illness. People will stay away from you just like the way they stay away from dirt.

Caregivers' Stress and Reactions

Especially for patients experiencing a first-episode psychosis, active participation of their caregivers in managing the disorder is important. How the caregivers perceive patients' experiences and handle the resultant family burden is likely to affect their emotional expression and interaction with the patients. From the above study, some patterns of caregiver reactions to the patient's diagnosis are summarized in Table 17.1.

Table 17.1
Caregivers' reactions towards the diagnosis of psychotic disorder

1. Refusal to accept the problem as a mental illness
2. Feeling worried
3. Feeling depressed
4. Self-blame

Stresses typically experienced by caregivers include persistent anxiety, persistent emotional distress, family conflicts, feelings of incapability to help, self-blame for causing treatment delays, social withdrawal, and poor emotional support.

Interestingly, a study by Lam et al. (2010) on caregiver burden revealed that many caregivers rated their experiences positively when the patients suffered from serious psychopathology. The caregiving experience was endorsed as more positive if patients had history of deliberate self-harm and longer duration of untreated psychosis. While the possible explanations for these findings are still being speculated, the same study has demonstrated promising results of early intervention on caregiver experience; among caregivers of first-episode patients, significant improvement in terms of reduced difficult behaviours and dependency of the patient, reduced feelings of loss, and increased positive personal experience were reported with early intervention.

Summary

From the patients and caregivers' account of their experience, it is obvious that stigma of psychosis remains a fact in Hong Kong, creating a major barrier to recovery and reintegration into society. Real and perceived prejudice and discrimination impact on patients and their family members' social lives, career opportunities, and psychological burden. When these distorted views are internalized, treatment and outcomes may also be negatively affected.

The issue of stigma should be addressed and tackled with high priority in the services for people with first-episode psychosis, since these services highlight the importance of reducing the duration of untreated psychosis and engaging patients and their relatives in the therapeutic alliance. Apart from targeting self-stigma in patients and families, early intervention programmes should also aim to lessen stigma in the general public in order to facilitate early detection. Furthermore, intensive family work by case managers should aim at mobilizing family members as valuable resources for long-term rehabilitation. An obstacle to mobilizing and instilling hope in relatives is the stigma attached to the family. However, reduction of stigma in the family cannot be actualized merely through transmitting the right knowledge to them. For instance, negative attitudes and perception towards the mentally ill held by patients' neighbours could bring insurmountable impacts. Destigmatization should aim at both the general public and the family. In Asia, renaming has been used as a strategy to combat stigma, for example in Hong Kong, Japan and Korea (see Chapter 2, "Early Psychosis Services in an Asian Urban Setting: EASY and Other Services in Hong Kong", Chapter 4, "Early Psychosis Intervention in an Urban Japanese Setting: Overview of Early Psychosis Services in Japan" and Chapter 5, "Overview of the Development of Services for Early Psychosis in Korea"). Continued effective anti-stigma efforts are very much needed to address the problem of stigma of psychosis (see Chapter 7, "Public Awareness Approaches in Early Psychosis"). This is obviously a long battle in changing the deep-rooted ideology in both the public and in the bearers of psychosis stigma.

References

Hayward, P., & Bright, J. A. (1997). Stigma and mental illness: A review and critique. *Journal of Mental Health, 6*(4), 345–354. doi: 10.1080/09638239718671

Lai, Y. M., Hong, C. P., & Chee, C. Y. (2001). Stigma of mental illness. *Singapore Medical Journal, 42*(3), 111–114.

Lam, M. M., Pearson, V., Ng, R. M., Chiu, C. P., Law, C. W., & Chen, E. Y. (2010). What does recovery from psychosis mean? Perceptions of young first-episode patients. *The International Journal of Social Psychiatry*. doi: 10.1177/0020764010374418

Lee, S., Lee, M. T., Chiu, M. Y., & Kleinman, A. (2005). Experience of social stigma by people with schizophrenia in Hong Kong. *British Journal of Psychiatry, 186*, 153–157. doi: 186/2/153 [pii] 10.1192/bjp.186.2.153

Link, B. G., & Phelan, J. C. (2001). Conceptualizing stigma. *Annual Review of Sociology, 27*, 363–385. doi: 10.1146/annurev.soc.27.1.363

Mueller, B., Nordt, C., Lauber, C., Rueesch, P., Meyer, P. C., & Roessler, W. (2006). Social support modifies perceived stigmatization in the first years of mental illness: A longitudinal approach. *Social Science Medicine, 62*(1), 39–49. doi: S0277-9536(05)00249-2 [pii] 10.1016/j.socscimed.2005.05.014

Ono, Y., Satsumi, Y., Kim, Y., Iwadate, T., Moriyama, K., Nakane, Y., et al. (1999). Schizophrenia: Is it time to replace the term? *Psychiatry in Clinical Neuroscience, 53*(3), 335–341. doi: 10.1046/j.1440-1819.1999.00555.x

Pearson, V., Ip, F., Hui, H., Yip, N., Ho, K. K., & Lo, E. (2003). To tell or not to tell; disability disclosure and job application outcomes. *Journal of Rehabilitation, 69*(4), 35–38.

Phillips, M. R., Pearson, V., Li, F., Xu, M., & Yang, L. (2002). Stigma and expressed emotion: A study of people with schizophrenia and their family members in China. *British Journal of Psychiatry, 181*, 488–493.

Sartorius, N. (2002). Iatrogenic stigma of mental illness. *British Medical Journal, 324*(7352), 1470–1471.

Thara, R., & Srinivasan, T. N. (2000). How stigmatising is schizophrenia in India? *International Journal of Social Psychiatry, 46*(2), 135–141.

Tsang, H. W. H., Tam, P. K. C., Chan, F., & Cheung, W. M. (2003). Stigmatizing attitudes towards individuals with mental illness in Hong Kong: Implications for their recovery. *Journal of Community Psychology, 31*(4), 383–396. doi: 10.1002/jcop.10055

18
The Phase-Specific Progress Supervision Model for Case Managers

Helen Lee

Case managers, who form a part of an allied healthcare professional specialty and those working in specialized fields such as mental health, are faced with a multitude of challenges and responsibilities of providing brokerage, assessments, and therapeutic roles to their patients. Delivering psychoeducation, coordinating services, providing supportive counselling, and formulating care plans are some of the general duties of case managers. In the Early Psychosis Intervention Programme (EPIP) in Singapore, patients are followed up by a designated case manager for a three-year period, during which a good working relationship is forged between both parties. A three-year period is a considerable amount of time, not to mention that the road to recovery is often not linear. Case managers walk together with their clients during this period, handling their crisis, boosting their self-esteem, managing their relapses and/or co-morbidities, and so forth. Such in-depth work requires great passion, maturity, commitment, and dedication of this specialized group of case managers. Burnout and exiting of the helping line can easily occur. In fact, Yalom (2001) mentioned that therapists working in specified fields, such as palliative care and psychosis, expose themselves to the risk of demoralization. In view of this, supervision plays a vital role in ensuring professional conduct, competency and more importantly in preventing unnecessary burnout.

What Is Supervision?

Definitions of supervision vary widely depending on the type of supervision relevant to each institution. In EPIP, the social work supervision model has been adopted by guide case managers. It is described as "a process, an interpersonal interaction in which one person is designated by an agency, to help another to develop profession competence, to meet organizational objectives and performance standards, to facilitate continuing professional development and to provide support to enable the fulfilment of the agency objectives and standards. The primary focus of supervision is to protect the best interests of the clients" (FRTC & SASW, 2007, p. 5).

This chapter outlines a phase-specific progress supervision model that has been heavily adapted from the integrated developmental model (Stoltenberg, McNeill, & Delworth, 1998) and strength-based supervision model (Cohen, 1999), while at the same time taking into consideration EPIP's case management model. The difficulties supervisors and supervisees face as the latter mature and progress with increasing clinical exposure are also discussed. This chapter ends with learning points and future directions.

Purpose of Supervision

Traditionally, supervision entails important components of administrative, supportive, and educational work (Cohen, 1999). In this setting, supervisors have to ensure that case managers abide with the department's as well as the hospital's standard of procedures so as to ensure thorough and competent quality patient care. Supervisors are to provide support and encouragement to supervisees so that they are motivated to strive to do better professionally and even to strive for their own personal growth. From an educational perspective, the management of caseload and skills needed are issues to consider. The tutorial mode is generally applied to new and inexperienced workers while a more consultative mode is used for more experienced supervisees (Cohen, 1999). In short, the purpose of supervision in EPIP is to enhance case managers' professional skills and clinical knowledge so as to achieve competency in providing quality patient care. Supervision also serves to encourage personal growth and development.

Case Management Model

In all early psychosis intervention programmes, the recovery process can be divided into several phases. In EPIP, the phases are categorized as acute, stabilization, stable, transfer of care, and termination. Case managers are expected to conduct a thorough assessment of patients to determine which phase of recovery they are in. Some of the general duties which case managers are cognizant of are listed in Table 18.1.

Table 18.1
Case manager's role across different phases of recovery

1. Acute phase	• Explain role and services to patients and/or family • Coordinate services • Mediate or negotiate with relevant individuals • Build rapport • Provide supportive counselling • Provide psychoeducation, if possible, on illness, symptoms, medication, and medication side-effects
2. Stabilization phase	• Assist and prepare patients to be re-integrated into school/work and community • Understand patients' explanatory model • Provide psychoeducation on the above, emphasizing medication compliance • Set goals • Identify strengths and resources and improve coping skills • Suggest ways of stress management • Watch out for comorbidity
3. Stable phase	• Revisit goal(s) • Give psychoeducation on healthy lifestyle • Prevent relapses – going through symptoms and early warning signs • Manage crisis • Report progress at one year into programme
4. Transfer of care	• Provide final revision of relapse prevention or symptoms • Refer to other services (within hospital or in the community)
5. Termination	• Write letter on transfer of care from EPIP given • Make sure that patients turn up for their first appointment • Encourage patients to reschedule appointment if they fail to turn up

A customized supervision model for EPIP case managers was developed, taking into account the EPIP case management model and adapting some of the principles and structure of the integrated developmental model and strength-based social work practice. The diagram resembles the EPIP logo.

With reference to Figure 18.1, it is expected that the staff have passion to work with young adults with first-episode psychosis. Staff members are

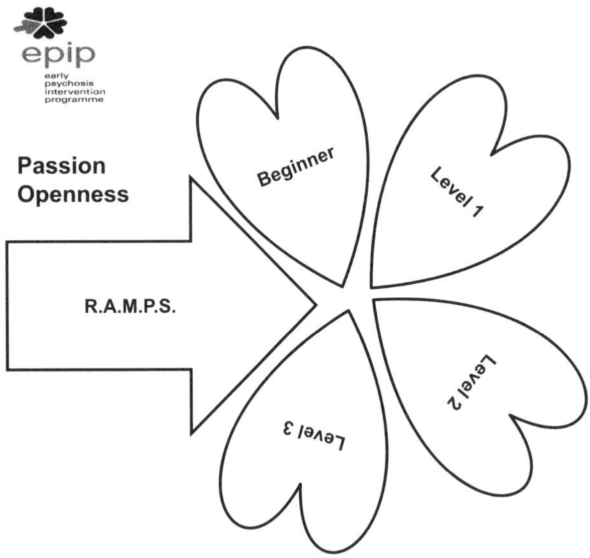

Figure 18.1

Supervision model for EPIP case managers

expected to be open-minded, as the human mind is complex and no two persons are the same. Some guiding principles for supervisors and components for evaluation of supervisees' progress follow:

Guiding Principles for Supervisors

1. Understanding of the parallel process or isomorphism. Be cognizant of the dynamics of the patient-case manager relationship and that of the supervisor-supervisee relationship. Make use of the impact of the parallel process.
2. Constant examination of the strengths of supervisees to encourage them to do the same with their patients. Analyse past successes and explore their implications for other more challenging situations.
3. Adequate attention at various levels. Take note of supervisees' progress so that sufficient support is rendered, but at the same time, challenge them to improve their skills and awareness so as to advance professionally and personally.

Components for Evaluation

EPIP case managers are evaluated against the acronym, "RAMPS". By definition, a "ramp" refers to a sloping surface between places, objects, etc. at different levels and this is analogous to the role of case managers. Such supportive handholding is not spoon-feeding but a means to lend support to patients by leveraging upon their strengths at timely intervals so as to help them achieve their goals. This is in synchrony with the supervisor-supervisee relationship. As a supervisor, the goal is to assist supervisees to reach up to different levels professionally, while at the same time facilitating their personal growth.

Hence, supervisees in EPIP are challenged and evaluated according to:

- R – Reflection: the degree of willingness to reflect on own progress professionally and at a personal level.
- A – Autonomy: ability to make independent decisions; level of self-confidence, and degree of supervision required (Powell & Brodsky, 2004)
- M – Motivation: understanding of the EPIP case management model and one's role as a case manager in EPIP, as well as having the desire to unfold both their own and patients' strengths and internal resources (Powell & Brodsky, 2004)
- P – Proactivity: competency in taking initiatives to take stock of patients' proven and potential skills in coping with adversity.
- S – Self-awareness and awareness of others: improvements shown in understanding oneself and others (cognitive and affective levels); managing anxiety and uncertainty; awareness of transference and counter-transference and responding versus reacting (Powell & Brodsky, 2004)

Supervisees' Progress

Stoltenberg (2005) charts supervisees' progress across different stages and identifies some formulae that supervisors should adopt at different phases of the supervisees' learning curve and development. This is aligned with the phase-specific recovery model, which EPIP case managers use as a guide when they work with their clients. Hence, this evaluation approach is heavily adapted from Stoltenberg (2005) to suit the profile of case managers in EPIP.

In EPIP, all newly joined case managers receive a month-long training in their orientation, comprising sit-in sessions in clinical settings and also shadowing a field supervisor. They are shown how assessments are done, the psychoeducation delivery for the condition, and how supportive counselling is conducted. New case managers also attend multidisciplinary team meetings, where new cases are presented by fellow colleagues, and clinical reviews where case managers update the progress of their respective patients. Usually, the new case managers will be assigned their new patients in the third to last week of their orientation, so that more on-the-job-training can be provided. A field supervisor is assigned to guide them through the work process and to familiarize them with the hospital system. This is conducted for a period of 6 months. During this time, the field supervisor would continue to provide guidance and support, which include case presentations and discussions, even if supervisees are already familiar with the work process. It is expected that case managers should demonstrate improvements to their clinical skills in conducting biopsychosocial assessments and develop sound case formulation of their cases by the end of the 6 months.

Below is an overview of the milestones faced by case managers as mapped across the phase-specific recovery model (Stoltenberg, 2005; Stoltenberg et al., 1998).

Beginners (≤6 months)

Case managers' characteristics and formula adopted by supervisors in general in the initial 6 months are listed in Table 18.2.

As first-episode psychosis is a specialized field, and in EPIP, case managers are the linchpins for the programme, newcomers in general experience "culture

Table 18.2
Case manager characteristics in the beginner phase

Case manager characteristics	Formula used by supervisor
Enthusiastic, innocent, ego-centric	Didactic, prescriptive
Following textbook, demanding attention	Emphasize on standard operation procedures, manual, ethical issue, boundaries, principles like "do no harm"
Motivated by anxiety	Address anxiety; be nurturing and supportive
Old habits or perceptions from previous employment	Tap on supervisee's past successes in life or work; learn from supervisees

shock" due to job expectations. Case managers are expected to have a strong desire to learn and to be able to attain levels of competency over a period of time. New case managers who have a "higher" working profile in their previous employment sometimes find themselves needing to be humble and start from scratch in learning about this specialized field. Common feedback states that they find it hard to embrace the medical model initially, especially if they came from a community setting where family intervention takes precedence.

In terms of the degree of autonomy and performance evaluation, their feedback is again diverse. In a hospital setting, a team-based approach is adopted. Aside from the case manager, there are other allied health professionals, including psychologists, social workers, and occupational therapists. Within the team, the doctor takes the lead and team-based decision-making is practised. This can be quite different in the community setting, where the diversity of professionals is less and hence the background training is more similar. New case managers who hold on tightly to past working practices will find themselves having a difficult time accepting this new environment.

As for new case managers who have just graduated from university, they are generally eager to apply what they have learned from textbooks to practice. They may be over-enthusiastic and idealistic, holding onto textbook doctrines. Realizing that not all theories can be put into practice can sometimes create confusion and disappointment. Some may find it hard to accept work practices, while others tend to wonder whether they are in the right industry. Supervisors' approach in this context must be nurturing and supportive. Lots of guidance and reassurance is indicated so that supervisees do not feel lost. Instead of treating them as totally inexperienced, appreciation of their life experiences and successes boosts their self-confidence. Allowing supervisees' to process through their disappointments without judgement and acceptance of their ambivalence ensures greater trust. This will impact the way supervisors connect with supervisees.

Level 1 (>6 months ≤2 years)

In this context, case managers enter into Level 1 when they understand and accept the working environment.

By this stage, daily work processes have become routine. Case managers are familiar with the system and able to work with their clients better. This is a stage where workers are able to undo old habits and embrace new ones. Precisely

Table 18.3
Case manager characteristics in Level 1

Case manager characteristic	Formula used by supervisor
Undo old habits and replace with new ones	Focus on case conceptualization, polish skills in case management, and use the eclectic theory
Rebellious, desirous of autonomy, confused about identity or role as a case manager	Encourage autonomy, introduce ambiguity, be supportive but also leave rooms for self-exploration and reflection; watch out for burnout
Difficulty in confronting and self-disclosing; lack of self and awareness of others, tunnelled vision, and limited treatment plan	Tap on recent success and be patient

because they are more confident in themselves, some may desire to have more autonomy. The boundary between helpers and clients may be blurred, as the former tends to make themselves readily available to clients even after office hours. The need to establish viable relationships with clients may lead to case managers constantly thinking of their clients and their interactions with them. Inevitably, an expectation of progressive recovery is created. When clients do not make linear progress, confusion over the role and identity of a case manager may surface. There may be sense of burnout and self-doubt as to whether they are in the right field. It is at this stage that they also recognize some of their own personal issues whilst working with clients. This awareness may remain at a superficial level if case managers are unwilling to address their own issues: they may feel uncomfortable in confronting the clients' underlying issues, and inevitably have tunnel vision and a limited treatment plan.

At this juncture, supervisors can assume a "push-and-hold" approach; while "pushing" them gently to face the ambiguity and their own underlying issues that may hinder their work with clients, supervisors should also be "holding" them by being supportive and patient in keeping a mindful watch for burnout signs.

In terms of skills training, the focus at this phase is on case conceptualization and formulation of treatment plans. Boundary issues are addressed and their expectations as a case manager are discussed and managed. Tapping on recent success is one way of focusing on their strengths and encouraging them to further improve their work with clients.

Level 2 (>2 years ≤3 years)

Supervisees in the field for more than two years show high levels of confidence. They tend to be less reactive and more grounded due to a higher level of awareness of self and others. They understand the isomorphism theory better, and are therefore more willing to address their own underlying issues so that they help their clients better. While some may pursue therapy, others will bring it up during supervision session about how they could carry themselves professionally. With improved knowledge, skills and awareness of self and others, they are usually more competent in mentoring junior staff (Table 18.4).

Working with supervisees at this level requires more facilitation. Supervisors usually encourage them to identify their own strengths and the improvements they have made. They would usually have established their own unique style of working with clients, and flexibility should be allowed so that they would continue to grow. Encouraging them to take on a more senior role in mentoring junior staff further encourages them to continue to learn in order to stay relevant to what they are doing.

Table 18.4
Case manager characteristics in Level 2

Case manager characteristics	Formula used by supervisor
Steering away from Level 1, more grounded due to increase in awareness of self and others	Continue to be supportive but challenge supervisees more in terms of self-discovery and management of care for their patients
Less reactive and more able to delay gratification	Allow more autonomy. Facilitate supervisees to identify own strengths and improvement, and how he or she has impacted the lives of patients
Good conceptualization, demonstrating significant improvement in knowledge and skills and showing maturity at work and ability to explore patients' inner dynamics with guidance	Tap on flexibility

Level 3 (>3 years)

Stoltenberg, McNeill, and Delworth (1998) reckon that supervision tends to be more of consultative in nature when supervisees have matured and gained higher awareness of self and others. The same is observed in EPIP; supervisees who are internally motivated and open-minded towards learning are usually mature and grounded. The delivery of supervision here is no longer didactic, but focuses on wisdom and compassion. Supervisees at this level would have the natural instinct to nurture junior staff and they are highly motivated to impart or share their knowledge and experience with others.

Table 18.5
Case manager characteristics in Level 3

Case manager characteristics	**Formula used by supervisor**
Mature professionally, able to tolerate frustration	Consultative method, peer supervision, use of humour, learning from supervisees too
High awareness of self and others with internal motivation and proactiveness to help other junior staff	Tap on wisdom

Learning Points

From the author's experience, the integrated developmental model provides a valuable structure for supervisors in terms of evaluating and motivating supervisees in their work. The concept of phase-specific progress is in sync with the case management model, which adopts different interventions depending on the patient's phase of recovery. Its principles act as a guideline for supervisees to benchmark their developmental milestones as case managers. The different levels of progress give supervisors an idea of what to expect as supervisees become more familiar and competent in their work and formulas offered provide directions to supervisors.

As case managers come from different disciplines, a limitation, exists where supervisees will still require a theoretical model to ground themselves as well as to improve their micro skills, even though case managers are not expected to conduct a full-fledged structured therapy (which are conducted by psychologists and counsellors; see Chapter 14, "The PASTE that Binds:

Culturally Relevant Psychological Interventions for First-Episode Psychosis Individuals in Singapore"). Supervisees who have no clinical practice experience may find themselves quite limited in terms of providing therapeutic benefits to their clients.

To address this limitation, EPIP case managers are now also receiving group supervisions from qualified clinical psychologists outside of the department. These include solution-focused brief therapy supervision and family systemic supervision. Supervisors are aware that they are supervising case managers, hence focusing more on therapy strategies, interviewing techniques, and eliciting strengths and resources. The idea is to provide supervisees a model to fall back on if they are doing more in-depth therapeutic work with clients other than case management.

References

A Manual on Supervision for Social Work Supervisors (2007). Published by Family Resource & Training Centre and Singapore Association of Social Workers, Singapore.

Cohen, B. Z. (1999). Intervention and supervision in strengths-based social work practice. *Families in Society: The Journal of Contemporary Human Services, 80*(5), 460–466.

Powell, D. J., & Brodsky, A. (2004). *Clinical Supervision in Alcohol and Drug Abuse Counseling: Principles, Models, Methods.* San Francisco, CA: Jossey-Bass.

Stoltenberg, C. D. (2005). Enhancing professional competence through developmental approaches to supervision. *American Psychologist, 60*(8), 857–864. doi: 2005–14550–029 [pii] 10.1037/0003–066X.60.8.85

Stoltenberg, C. D., McNeill, B., & Delworth, U. (1998). *IDM Supervision: An Integrated Developmental Model for Supervising Counselors and Therapists.* San Francisco, CA: Jossey-Bass xv, 288 pp.

Yalom, I. (2001). *The Gift of Therapy: An Open Letter to a New Generation of Therapists and Their Patients.* New York: HarperColllins.

Part IV

Support Programmes in the Community

19
Community Psychosocial Intervention in Early Psychosis

Yogeswary d/o Maniam

Overview of Psychosocial Intervention

First-episode psychosis—in the main, schizophrenia—arises often during the developmental stages of early adolescence and early adulthood (Rinaldi et al., 2010). It is also during these development stages that education, employment, self-identity, and formation of relationships tend to occur (Basset et al., 2001). Due to the impact of the illness, adolescents with early psychosis commonly experience social exclusion, low self-esteem, and decreased social and occupational functioning (Cotton et al., 2011).

The three essential elements in managing early psychosis are early recognition and assistance, initial assessment and treatment, and promoting recovery (McGorry, 2002). Programmes have to be comprehensive in supporting the needs of young people with psychosis (Bertolote & McGorry, 2005). Appropriate treatment interventions should be carried out for functional outcomes rather than just for symptom remission. Therefore, by engaging in psychosocial groups, patients can be facilitated to acquire the skills required to perform their age-appropriate roles.

In 1995, the WHO defined psychosocial rehabilitation as a comprehensive process, which strives for individuals who are impaired, disabled or handicapped by mental health problems to reach their optimal level to function independently in the community (WHO, 2001).

The primary goal of psychosocial intervention is to restore a person's ability for independent living, socialization, and effective life management. The key principles in psychosocial intervention (Hughes & Weinstein, 2000) are:

1. Hope—belief that one has control over his or her life.
2. Self-determination—empowerment required for one to actively participate and assume responsibility for making everyday life decisions.

3. Community approach—network of community support, including the community that the patient lives and works in, and the community of his or her peers.
4. Assessment and intervention needs to be individualized, activities needs to be age-specific and relevant.

The core components of psychosocial rehabilitation or intervention (Hughes & Weinstein, 2000) are:

1. Social rehabilitation—to look into social skills, social interaction, and recreation through group activities.
2. Vocational rehabilitation—to improve tolerance, concentration, instruction following, and work attitude through pre-vocational training, vocational training, and career counselling. To enhance job acquisition and retention, job placement and ongoing job support are essential.
3. Residential and housing services—to look into step-down housing and community housing for patients.
4. Education about mental illness and medications—the need for compliance, identification of relapse symptoms, and to educate patients and their family on medication side-effects.
5. Physical health.
6. Intensive case management.
7. Family support.

Distinctions in East and West Approaches

Historically, mental health services have been placed in inpatient settings but in recent years, the focus has shifted towards psychosocial rehabilitation services in the community (Pillai et al., 2010). This approach in the West, from an Indian perspective, transfers great empowerment and choice to clients to make their own decisions in treatment planning. In contrast, in the East there is still an element of the traditional approach where a team decides what is essential for the patients. However, this approach is fast disappearing and increasingly, patients are given the opportunity to make informed choices. Also, in the East, "psychosocial rehabilitation models have been developed using primary care, family support, back-up psychiatric support, community supervisors and factory rehabilitation intervention" (WHO, 2001, p. 63). There is still an element of clubhouse models and vocational training in the East whereas in the West, incorporated supported employment models such as Individual Placement and Support are commonplace.

Psychosocial Intervention in the Early Psychosis Intervention Programme (EPIP) in Singapore

In the Institute of Mental Health in Singapore, the early psychosis team adopts a multidisciplinary approach and provides early detection and intervention for individuals with early psychosis as well as those at high risk of developing psychosis, through a personalized, comprehensive, and accessible service. This facility engages patients in a variety of interventions, and one such service is Club EPIP (for individualized psychological therapy, see Chapter 14, "The PASTE that Binds: Culturally Relevant Psychological Interventions for First-Episode Psychosis Individuals in Singapore").

Club EPIP was formed in 2005, with the aim of integrating and supporting patients with early psychosis in the community. The Club focuses on functioning and psychosocial recovery. The motto of Club EPIP in 2010 was to foster greater independence, a sense of belonging, and social responsibility in individuals. The pledge that clients came up with during a focus group was, "We pledge to be *Enthusiastic* in our performance, to be *Positive* in our thoughts and speech, to be *Innovative* in our way of life, to empower our hearts, minds, and souls together to reach our goals."

Club EPIP initially functioned as a drop-in centre with regular craft activities but has now evolved to function more as an assessment centre. Social skills, work habits, quality of life, and coping mechanisms are all assessed and incorporated in the psychosocial intervention programmes conducted at Club EPIP. All current programmes have the mutual goal, to empower clients; one of the fundamental elements in the principle of recovery (Slade, 2009). The activities emphasize skills acquisition and reintegration into the community. The club is also a venue for social interaction where patients share their experiences and receive support from each other.

One of the distinctive features of Club EPIP is that group work is based on the needs and goals of the patients. Normally, a focus group allows patients to choose their activities from a range of programmes that interest them. One such focus group showed that the patients' interest leaned more towards social groups such as outings and expressive groups, probably due to their age group.

In the past, community outings were only conducted quarterly and were not linked to any other programmes. Yet, groups are now paired up with some programmes that they feel as less exciting, such as current affairs. For example, a community outing to Marina Barrage, a dam that was built to supply water to Singapore and was part of a comprehensive flood control scheme, was linked up with the current affairs group when the topic of global warming was discussed. Another example was the trip to the Singapore Zoological Gardens organized for the recovery group. Throughout the programmes, patients are often involved in planning for outings. Worksheets are given and discussed during the outings and patients are asked to write their experiences after the outings.

One of the key components assessed during outings is mobility. Community mobility activities are also carried out for patients who fear taking public transport and/or need to practise skills in social settings. The aim for these social groups goes beyond leisure exploration and attempts to create more awareness around people. The social groups promote social inclusion and social skills, give them a sense of belonging, empower them to make decisions and instil an element of fun into their life. Groups also create social identity, which is essential to mental functioning, health and well-being (University of Exeter, 2009).

Excursion to Marina Barrage: Write-up by a Client

The visit to the Marina Barrage with my fellow EPIP members was definitely a worthwhile experience and an enriching one. This visit exposed us to the importance of being self-sufficient in having adequate drinking water as well as the prevention of flooding in low lying areas of Singapore. The detailed presentation by one of the Marina Barrage's tour staff aided us in having a comprehensive understanding of the purpose of the Marina Barrage and the above mentioned topics. Coupled with state-of-the-art technology used in the presentation methods and detailed "models" and "replica" of Marina Barrage's dam in the museum, it made the learning process of Marina Barrage much more appealing and interesting. The games we played such as "Taboo!" at the "Green Roof" of Marina Barrage also made members understand each other better and it strengthened the bond between us.

Case Example 1

Mr K was a 24-year-old man whose highest educational qualification attained was Advanced-Level. He was first seen at the Institute of Mental Health in late 2007. Mr K was diagnosed with schizophrenia and anxiety disorder. He feared taking public transport and being in crowded places, as he felt that people were talking about him. He also had poor social interaction and low self-confidence.

Mr K attended Club EPIP three times a week for half-day sessions. He had poor attendance as he depended on his father to drive him there, and was unable to come if his father had other errands that day. He also had to be prompted to speak up during groups. The occupational therapist provided community mobility training for Mr K. He was taught distraction techniques such as listening to music, reading newspaper, and looking out of the window while travelling. These techniques were also tested out during the community mobility training, and processing of his experience and supportive therapy was provided at the end of each session.

Role play was also carried out with him for social situations and responding to strangers. He was also brought to malls to buy things for himself and to ask for assistance from sales assistants. Mr K also participated in current affairs and sports groups to work on his presentation skills, teamwork, and confidence and tolerance level.

Mr K was able to go back home by himself from Club EPIP and started using public transport more often to attend church and food malls. He had also shared that he was able to have dinner with his family outside without feeling self-conscious. He was also able to speak up more during programmes at Club EPIP and had reported feeling more confident about himself. To have continuity of care, Mr K was referred to a community outreach programme prior to his discharge from EPIP.

A further extension of group work at Club EPIP is the discussion groups. Discussions are normally held during current affairs and movie-screenings groups. In current affairs, patients may be gathered into smaller groups and articles handed out for review. Patients have to read the item and discuss it in their smaller groups before coming out to present in front of the larger group. At that point in time, patients are taught presentation skills (such as making eye contact with the audience, projection of voice, engaging the audience and answering questions). They are also given an option of how they wish to do their presentation (i.e. using mahjong paper or PowerPoint slides). Those in the listening role are strongly encouraged to play a proactive role during the programme. Mini assignments have been given which require patients to do some research for later discussion at Club EPIP. Occupational therapists process and notate the challenges and learning points patients have encountered during the preparation of the presentation.

At times, minor friendly debates are also conducted between the patients. Patients are taught and assessed in how to look for points, how to summarize their thoughts and how to put their points across in an acceptable manner. Patients are also asked to note points when others are presenting. Feedback is always given at the end of each presentation. There is a minute element of competitiveness in such groups mainly because of the client age group and also because they wish to be gently challenged while being in a supportive environment.

Current affairs are a vehicle for training language skills and facilitate physical and mental endurance; cognitive skills such as concentration, memory and abstract thinking also improve as do social skills.

Movies with themes of hope, recovery, and support system are screened weekly as part of the leisure programme/component or during recovery groups. At the end of the movie, a discussion is facilitated with the patients on what the storyline and themes were; which characters they identified with and why; what they thought of the ending and if they were the directors how would they end the story. In one instance, the movie *Ice-castle* was played and before the movie ended patients were asked to guess the ending. Most of them guessed that the ice skater would regain her eye-sight and continue with her career. In actual fact, the skater does progress on with her career but does not gain her full eye-sight. Patients were than asked how they felt about the ending and if they had been the skater, what kind of emotions would they have felt and could they have accomplished what she had (i.e. going on to state-level skating championships). They were also asked to come up with six word aide-memoir from the movie's themes, which were than used as personal slogans and written in a notebook provided by the Club.

Movie Themes

Haciko, A Dog's Story

Courage

About being there

Love

Punctual

Perseverance

Ice Castle

Gain confidence

Determination

Perseverance

Integrity

Fighting spirit

Teamwork

Having a goal in life

Attitude

6-word aide-memoirs

'Courage'

Dare to go. Never give up.

Courage is taking the first step.

Dare to love. Dare to hate.

Never say Die. Just proceed ahead.

Dare to say. Dare to do.

Courage is bravery and nothing else.

Swim the river without the float.

'Determination'

Try your best to do it.

Never lose hope. Just continue striving.

Believe in yourself and have faith.

Studying definitely needs determination to succeed.

Have the heart to do things.

Moving forward through rain or shine.

A winner never gives up hope.

There's a will. There's a way.

It's carrying on despite any pitfalls.

With confidence, we can fight on.

Never give up. Dare to go.

I will never give up hope.

Case Example 2

Miss B was a 17-year-old girl who had deferred her ITE education. She started attending current affairs and sports group on a regular basis. Her initial presentation in groups was that she was soft spoken and had low confidence in speaking in-front of a big group.

Miss B was encouraged to speak aloud using the articles. At a later stage, she was also given the task to write down summary points of what was discussed. Miss B started gaining her confidence and started to take on more leadership roles within the group programmes.

By the end of 6 months, she was able to lead small group discussions and had also volunteered to be a master of ceremony for the Masquerade Party organized by the patients. She was a lead singer during the performance too. Miss B has now started back at school and has been functioning well.

For consistency purposes and knowledge retention, programmes are run for two months before being changed. But sports group runs perpetually. Sports groups do not only target physical and mental endurance but they also foster teamwork, co-operation and turn-taking.

A competitive element is injected in the group and friendly matches are played, for example, fast-paced sports such as basketball, soccer, captains' ball and Frisbee. Patients are taught the basic rules of each game, which is adapted to suit the pace of the clients.

The annual sports day commenced in 2011 in line with Singapore's culture in schools and workplaces. Sports day is a common feature in most schools; competitions are a common feature in most tertiary institutions and team games are mainly played in most organizations in Singapore.

Research has also shown that exercise is beneficial in the physical and mental health domains of people with schizophrenia and that it is possible for such programmes to be conducted with these individuals (Gorczynski & Faulkner, 2010).

Cognitive remediation is carried out for patients who have cognitive decline in areas such as memory, attention, and problem solving. A bridging group has been organized and facilitated at Club EPIP, where the techniques learnt in cognitive remediation are discussed with regard to real-life situations.

Homework is then given to patients to practise these techniques, and the effects are then discussed in the following session. It is hoped that by addressing these cognitive problems, patients would be able to benefit more from other interventions and function better in social, work, and other domains. Patients are also encouraged to attend the other groups in Club EPIP to put the skills/techniques learnt during cognitive remediation into practice.

Case Example 3

Miss C was a 36-year-old woman who had a degree in electronic engineering. Her onset of illness occurred in 2008. Miss C was diagnosed with both schizophrenia and depression. She had memory problems, limited social interaction, and was slow in work. She also had difficulty sustaining employment.

Miss C started to attend Club EPIP in early 2010, initially three times a week for half-day sessions and eventually five times a week with three whole days and two half days. She went through intensive cognitive remediation three times a week for at least 1.5 hours each session for three months, and was also engaged in current affairs, sports, and creative expression groups. Her case manager and psychologist continued to give individual counselling for her during this period.

With the programmes at Club EPIP, her confidence level increased; she became more sociable with other members, and was able to complete tasks faster. She also reported that her memory had improved and she was able to solve problems more quickly with minimal prompting.

Miss C was placed in supported employment in administrative work. The occupational therapist provided intensive job coaching during her first two weeks of probation. Frequent interaction with her supervisor also took place and expectations were adjusted.

Monthly job site visits were also conducted. Miss C was also taught ways to improve her speed of work and she showed initiative in learning and applying the techniques taught in cognitive remediation to her current workplace. Continuous supported employment was given to her. Miss C was also included in all gatherings and outings of Club EPIP to further facilitate her social interaction.

Programmes such as job preparation groups and supported employment are carried out as part of the psychosocial programme in Club EPIP. They help to promote social interaction, increase confidence, improve job retention and equip patients with skills necessary to integrate into the workforce.

Since 2007, EPIP Day has been an annual event held for patients and their family members to commemorate patients and their efforts to sustain in their age appropriate roles and functioning such as returning to employment and school, or becoming a homemaker again. This event is used as a platform to encourage and motivate patients. Patients hold performances during this event, and testimonials are given to those who have shown improvements in their roles. Patients are chosen based on the following criteria:

1. Patients who have been following through all recommendations for psychosocial rehabilitation
2. Contributing to the economy and demonstrated motivation in staying well
3. Minimum three months at work
4. Integrated into school

Presenting Challenges

Many challenges are involved in working with patients with mental health problems. The most common challenge is to identify how the various programmes in Club EPIP assist patients' daily living. Many patients show a lack of pleasure or interest to participate, saying that they do not see the link or that the programmes do not seem appropriate for their age. It is therefore important to ensure that the programmes chosen for the patients are age-appropriate.

At the end of each session, patients are interviewed to ascertain how the programmes helped them either with memory, coping skills, attention activity tolerance, and/or social interaction with others. Patients may need constant reassurance, and at times, members who have been in the programme longer are called upon to give testimonials as to how they have benefited from activities.

Their motivation levels are also important. Patients may not be motivated to participate in programmes that have been repeated many times. Lack of motivation also brings about other challenges such as the inability to define goals, find meaning or overcome anxiety to meet new people. Thus, a tremendous amount of encouragement and a safe environment during initial contact is vital to promote regular attendance.

Creativity is also required in programme planning, and the programmes have to be graded according to their age and functioning ability. A range of activity levels from easy to hard needs to be provided to arouse and maintain interest.

Patients need to be empowered whenever possible. Involving patients in the planning of gatherings and outings ensures that more patients are willing to participate, as they would be more motivated to try out the programmes recommended by their peers. This inclusion also enables them to take responsibility and adopt leadership roles, thus instilling hope and increasing their self-esteem. A staff member must be available to facilitate sessions to ensure that everything goes smoothly with no negative repercussions. Fun is also added to the sessions, and patients go on field trips to nature parks and horse riding.

At times, patients who are treatment-resistant and/or symptomatic would attend Club EPIP activities. It is important that the group facilitators, namely the occupational therapist and therapy assistant, are knowledgeable about relapse symptoms and know what to do in times of crisis. As safety is crucial, all sharp objects such as knives and scissors are locked and used under close supervision. Staffs are also trained in de-escalation techniques.

At times, a small proportion of patients at Club EPIP may test boundaries with the facilitators by being persistently late for groups, speaking in other languages, and refusing to carry out the planned sessions. The facilitators should ensure that all patients are aware of the rules and regulations of the club, and that respect for everyone is paramount. Case managers may be called in to manage more difficult patients under the team's care. In any event that a patient disturbs others and/or safety is compromised, the patient would be removed from the group activity and would work individually with his/her case manager.

Conclusion

Prognosis is not just based on symptom remission but also on psychosocial functioning. This includes going back to school, rejoining the workforce or even just engaging in age appropriate activities. Thus vocational rehabilitation, supported employment model, educational interventions, cognitive remediation therapy, social groups and other psychosocial programmes should not be seen as separate services. Rather, they should integrate into the service model (Whitty et al., 2006). Social functioning and employment issues can be addressed in psychosocial group programmes, being mindful that psychosocial rehabilitation strategies change according to the different needs of the patients, where it is conducted as well as the cultural and socioeconomic conditions of the country (WHO, 2001). Thus, age appropriateness, goals and needs of patients as well as cultural and socioeconomic conditions need to be considered when planning for psychosocial programmes.

References

Basset, J., Lloyd, C., & Basset, H. (2001). Work issues for young people with psychosis: Barriers to employment. *The British Journal of Occupational Therapy, 64*, 66–72.

Bertolote, J., & McGorry, P. (2005). Early intervention and recovery for young people with early psychosis: Consensus statement. *British Journal of Psychiatry Supplement, 48*, s116–119. doi: 187/48/s116 [pii]10.1192/bjp.187.48.s116

Cotton, S. M., Luxmoore, M., Woodhead, G., Albiston, D. D., Gleeson, J. F., & McGorry, P. D. (2011). Group programmes in early intervention services. *Early Intervention in Psychiatry, 5*(3), 259–266. doi: 10.1111/j.1751-7893.2011.00277.x

Gorczynski, P. & Faulkner, G. (2010). Exercise therapy for schizophrenia. *Cochrane Database of Systemic Reviews*, 5, Art. No.: CD004412. DOI: 10.1002/14651858.CD004412.pub2

Hughes, R., & Weinstein, D. (Eds.). (2000). *Best Practices in Psychosocial Rehabilitation*. Columbia, MD: International Association of Psychosocial Rehabilitation Services.

McGorry, P. D. (2002). The recognition and optimal management of early psychosis: An evidence-based reform. *World Psychiatry, 1*(2), 76–83.

Pillai, R. R., Sahu, K. K., Matthew, V., Hazra S., Chandran, P. & Ram, D. (2010). Rehabilitation needs of persons with major mental illness in India. *International Journal of Psychosocial Rehabilitation*, 14 (2), 95–104.

Rinaldi, M., Perkins, R., McNeil, K., Hickman, N., & Singh, S. P. (2010). The individual placement and support approach to vocational rehabilitation for young people with first episode psychosis in the UK. *Journal of Mental Health, 19*(6), 483–491. doi: 10.3109/09638230903531100

Slade, M (2009). *100 Ways to Support Recovery: A Guide for Mental Health Professionals*. Rethink Recovery series: Volume 1. Retrieved 1 June 2012 from http://api.ning.com/files/G*hCgvYVbMSgn4kaBbdSXUVnfGNstJXl39JowKEgjT5XKNNd9ZGVghME04k4CT*9LjPmuyKY7WKDgFhwressOLkWKPnG4HXo/100_ways_to_support_recovery.pdf

University of Exeter (2009). Groups are key to good health. *Science Daily*. Retrieved 1 June 2012, from http://www.sciencedaily.com/releases/2009/09/090910103325.htm

Whitty, P., Lydon, C., Turner, N. & O'Callaghan, E. (2006). The influence of psychosocial rehabilitation on patients with a first episode of psychosis. *International Journal of Psychosocial Rehabilitation*, 10 (2), 17–27.

World Health Organization (2001). *The World Health Report 2001: Mental Health: New Understanding New Hope*, 19–45. Geneva: WHO.

20
The Peer Support Programme in Early Psychosis Intervention Programme (EPIP)

Suying Ang

> "Où sont les hommes?" reprit enfin le petit prince. "On est un peu seul dans le désert."
>
> "On est seul aussi chez les hommes', dit le serpent."
>
> "Where are the people?" resumed the little prince at last. "It's a little lonely in the desert . . ."
>
> "It is lonely when you're among people, too," said the snake.
>
> —*The Little Prince* (Antoine de Saint-Exupéry)

Background to Peer Support

The diagnosis of early psychosis can be a lonely experience for a young person. The illness typically strikes at the developmental stage of heightened yearnings for affiliation and intimacy. Yet, the stigma and shame of having a mental illness often results in them shunning their social support systems. Further marginalization is inadvertently caused by the medical model of diagnostic labels, which imposes a role of "mental patient", leaving a sense of otherness and disconnectedness in their lives (Mead, Hilton, & Curtis, 2001).

The provision of psychosocial interventions such as case management attempts to address this isolation through working closely with patients during the early part of the recovery process. Other adjunctive psychosocial interventions include social skills training, psychosocial clubhouses, and support groups. Peer support is a newer addition to the repertoire and emerging as a promising adjunct approach.

Peer support is essentially the process of providing encouragement, instilling hope, and sharing experiences of coping or narratives of recovery with others who are going through hardships of similar nature. The provider of peer support, by those who have gone through the process of battling the illness, has the advantage of having an "insider" perspective of what it is like to have to confront, endure, and cope with the disease. They will thus be able to show authentic empathy. This is particularly relevant in the mental health setting where self-stigmatizing beliefs are addressed through cultivating a sense of connectedness and affiliation and challenging assumptions about mental illnesses. Peer support, in other words, offers a culture of health and ability as opposed to a culture of illness and disability (Mead et al., 2001).

The stigma of mental illness, unlike in other fields such as addiction, places individuals with serious mental illness in the position where their ability to effectively offer peer support is in doubt, and this has not been caught up with earlier, despite the fact that they have been providing informal support within traditional mental health settings. Peer support services have henceforth flourished only in the 1990s, after the rise of the recovery movement by mental health consumers in the West (Davidson et al., 2006).

The recovery movement has greatly influenced how peer support relationships are viewed. While some place peer support services in the context of consumer-run self-help programmes (Mead et al., 2001), others define it as lying on a theoretical continuum between case management and mutual support programmes (Davidson et al., 2006). At one end of the continuum, the relationship with the service provider is of an intentional and one-directional nature. The other end is a naturally occurring and reciprocal relationship that is akin to friendship.

This chapter focuses on the type of support provided by peers as paid facilitators within the context of an institutional service. Having emerged from their struggles of being struck with early psychosis and having made significant functional improvements, peers offer support that involves sharing of personal experiences from a non-professional perspective, validation of experience with authentic empathy, and provision of practical advice and coping strategies to others who are still in the earlier phases of recovery. The peer support model in the Early Psychosis Intervention Programme (EPIP) is discussed, together with the learning that transpires from its application in a Singaporean context.

Description of EPIP Peer Support Programme

The Peer Support Programme, initiated by EPIP, was formally established in 2009. It is funded by the Woodbridge Endowment Fund under the Institute of Mental Health. The idea was first mooted after a participant of a support group expressed interest in helping to facilitate future support groups. Peer support groups were subsequently organized, in which a patient would co-facilitate together with a case manager. This gradually evolved to the current programme where peer support specialists are involved as paid facilitators in three main avenues of providing support, namely peer support groups, one-on-one support and group activities. The use of the word "specialist" in their title reflects their "lived experience" expertise.

Blending peer support into group work enhances the benefits of both approaches. The development of group work, originating in the West, harnesses the power of group dynamics to complement initial work with individuals (Gladding, 1991). Studies have shown that psychiatric patients who participated in support groups reported better understanding about their illness, reduced readmission rate, improved psychological functioning, and better treatment compliance (Castelein et al., 2008; Kanas, 2006). Yet, in Singapore, many people are cautious and somewhat anxious about becoming a support group member. This concern sits on top of the disempowered position that patients usually bring along at the start of the programme. To adopt the group-work approach successfully in the local setting means addressing the sense of safety. Imbuing an element of peer support through development of group norms to encourage participation can thus bridge these cultural concerns.

Inviting someone who has successfully completed a previous group to be a co-facilitator as a positive and real account of change is highly powerful, as he or she can inspire others to believe that change is also possible in their lives. The notion of universality, a therapeutic factor of group work, reminds other participants that they are not alone in their struggle with the illness. With the presence of a peer support specialist, hope flourishes. Peer support in a group setting also gives an added advantage of establishing a social network, with a peer specialist modelling appropriate social skills.

The peer support groups in EPIP are conducted in a series of four sessions, each session lasting for an hour and a half, facilitated by the peer support specialist and a case manager. Participants are recruited among existing patients who attend follow-up consultations with EPIP, and are usually identified by case managers who can recommend suitable candidates who are not in the acute phase. Group sizes range between four to twelve participants. A closed group format is preferred and will be further explained in the next section.

While every run of the peer support group is conducted with a certain thematic concern (e.g., employment, relationships, life as a student, emotions), the content of discussion is by no means structured, allowing deviation from the topic. This feature differs from the style of psychoeducation groups with its fixed agenda for imparting specific information. Participants are encouraged to bring up any pertinent issues that they may be facing, and the flow of the discussion is mainly determined by what surfaces at the moment, creating meaning in concerns that are real to them, thereby maximizing participation. Table 20.1 lists issues that are frequently brought up.

The discussion often centres around personal meanings and experiences of the illness and recovery processes. More often than not, participants' underlying hopes relate to reintegration into society, be it getting back to work, dealing with life as a student, or having meaningful interactions with others. During the process of sharing, the peer support specialist may provide insights in differentiating symptoms from behaviours, normalizing what may be perceived as an impact of the illness, offering alternative views and strategies to deal with residual symptoms and discussing a variety of social activities or even practical tips on negotiations with psychiatrists on treatment plans. These efforts strengthen self-advocacy especially for creating personal wellness plans, which are essential ingredients in peer support (Mead & Copland, 2000).

Table 20.1
Discussion topics of peer support groups

- Dealing with residual delusions or hallucinations
- Impact of medication side-effects
- Dealing with loss of interest or motivation after illness
- Struggles with comorbidities such as anxiety or depression
- Emotions (e.g., shame, fear, anger) that surface in the recovery process
- Self-identity after the illness
- Loss of self-confidence after the illness
- Sustaining work or studies
- Personal definition of recovery
- Coping and well-being
- Impact on friendships or interpersonal relationships
- Reactions of family members

Other than peer support groups, peer specialists who have the experience of facilitating at least a few runs of a support group also provide one-on-one support, either through the telephone or face-to-face. This form of peer support is initiated again by referrals from case managers. Patients identified may be those who are unable to commit to group sessions due to other commitments such as work or studies, or those who feel uncomfortable with the idea of joining a group. Phone support also allows continued support in between group sessions. Some may benefit from both modes of delivery. Others who had initial reservations of joining a group might eventually decide to do so after establishment of rapport with active encouragement from the peer support specialist.

Upon identifying people in need of support, the referring case manager will seek permission from the potential participant by signing a consent form. A referral form will also be completed and channelled through the coordinator to the peer support specialists. All peer support, one-on-one conversations are documented by the peer support specialist on a standard reporting sheet, stating in brief the theme of discussion, issues raised, the peer support specialist's input, and the plan of action. This acts as a feedback loop to the referring case manager, who can then monitor the impact of the service and follow up on the participant's concerns. The themes of discussion frequently touched on in the one-on-one peer support match those raised in support groups (see Table 20.1).

Peer specialists are also given the option to conduct activities such as board games, sports, crafts, and social skills training in Club EPIP together with the occupational therapist or case manager. This new feature provides another opportunity for peer specialists to engage with other patients, sharing their stories of recovery and coping through a more hands-on activity-based approach.

Case Managers' Criteria for Selecting Potential Peer Specialists

1. Previous participation in a peer support group
2. Interest in co-facilitating activities to help others
3. Commitment to their duties
4. Stable mental state
5. Compliant with treatment
6. Good insight into their illness

After identifying potential candidates, the case managers will bring their suggestions to the coordinator of the peer support programme. The selection will be finalized after the coordinator ascertains with the primary psychiatrist that these candidates are ready for this role in the peer support programme.

To equip peer specialists with the required skills, training in the form of debriefings, orientation, and workshops are integrated into their work. The background preparation for peer specialists may include, for example, writing of their personal accounts, which is considered a form of reimbursement for their contribution. A detailed job description can be found in Table 20.2.

In summary, the peer support specialists help fulfil EPIP's objective of promoting recovery and in particular underline these learning points that emerge from the challenges of implementing the programme.

Table 20.2
Job description of peer support specialist

(A) Peer support through group work
1. Participate in planning of peer support groups or activities with EPIP case managers or occupational therapist
2. Co-facilitate peer support groups with an EPIP case manager
3. Conduct other group activities with an EPIP case manager or occupational therapist
(B) Peer support through one-on-one work
4. Provide face-to-face support and psychoeducation to individuals
5. Provide phone support and psychoeducation to individuals
(C) Feedback and reflection
6. Participate in debriefing session with EPIP case managers
7. Participate in discussion with EPIP case managers
8. Prepare materials/content for work relating to peer support (e.g., finding relevant articles, activities for the group work, writing of personal accounts of their recovery process)
9. Provide updates on work with participants to EPIP team members (i.e., case managers)
(D) Training
10. Attend training or discussion sessions with EPIP case managers
(E) Others
11. Participate in events organized by EPIP department

Learning Points in EPIP Peer Support Programme

In recruiting participants for the peer support programme, team members are in constant communication with each other. Announcements are made for every run of the group, ideally one month in advance, so that case managers have ample time to identify and invite patients to participate. Successful persuasion of a patient to join a support group is dependent on what appeals to the individual. Generally, in Asian societies, individuals may find it daunting when told they may be sharing their experiences, especially those who feel uncomfortable in groups due to social anxiety or a lack of exposure to group work. In such cases, the invitation is positioned in a way that they may benefit from hearing others' experiences. That said, other participants are motivated by the fact that their participation may contribute to the group. The patient willingness is thus dependent on the individual case managers' powers of persuasion and encouragement, leveraging on the therapeutic alliance to convince the individual to step into the group process. Building a positive and non-stigmatized identity of the group through clear explanations of who the facilitators are and where other members come from, that they are in various stages of recovery and have a common understanding of how it is like to live with the illness, is pertinent even at the early stage of recruitment.

The location of the group activity is another important consideration, which may have a bearing on how the group dynamics evolve. The location differs from group to group, with options such as an activity room in an outpatient satellite clinic, Club EPIP in the hospital where patients regularly attend programmes on weekdays, or a hub for youth mental health located in a downtown shopping mall. A location familiar to the participants, such as Club EPIP room, will usually bring more participants. Yet, participants also give feedback on their preference for locations that are more convenient or less associated with stigma (i.e., non-clinical settings).

The choice of having a closed group, despite limiting participants in number, has been helpful, as evident from the lower dropout rate and the deeper sharing by participants. This is likely due to an increased sense of safety that is cultivated as participants become more familiar with group members over time, allowing closer bonds to be forged. It has also been observed that an open group has higher levels of turnover and lesser depth in sharing. New entrants might also restrain the development of the group dynamics as the group identity has to reform each time a new person joins. Given the brief number of sessions, a closed group is more likely to deliver the therapeutic elements, such as universality, group cohesiveness, and instillation of hope (Yalom & Leszcz, 2005).

Over the course of running the groups, this team found that group homogeneity further affects the dynamics. Although all individuals referred have received case management service from EPIP, some were at different stages of recovery, while others had a variable vocational status. Hence, factors such as age, psychopathology, and vocational status are influential when recruiting group members. This insight has resulted in designing groups with a specific theme in mind (e.g., life as a student) that allowed for some homogeneity. Issues were thus discussed in greater depth as participants would introduce current issues, which then translated into real, practical application, and learning opportunities for participants. Ensuring group homogeneity also allowed for better balance between group and personal goals that participants wish to address.

Many people enter the groups with some trepidation and have reservations about speaking up. The facilitators take careful note to create a safe environment by ensuring confidentiality when laying basic ground rules, giving frequent encouragement and appreciation for responses, as well as maintaining a warm and friendly tone. The timely use of silence by facilitators underlines the participants' responsibility to respond, as well as cultivates a group norm of being open in communication. Silence, used as a tool in this way, needs to be moderated as too much silence may create discomfort in participants.

Another related challenge, perhaps more frequently encountered in the East, is cultivating honest responses. There have been instances where participants prefer to offer politically correct answers, given their concerns about being judged by the facilitators and other group members. Again, nurturing a sense of safety helps overcome this non-disclosure. Case managers also need to emphasize how honest and open participation will benefit them during the recruitment process. Validation is also provided even when participants offer a different perspective (e.g., non-compliance to medical treatment) or disagree with a certain viewpoint. While facilitators may not confront participants who placate, the peer specialist can come in, offering differing perspectives to open up the discussion.

While goals identified by the group are beacons to guide group sessions' discussion, facilitators may go with the flow based on what salient issues participants bring to each session. The "here and now" approach is more well-received; as participants warm up in the groups, they may raise issues they feared bringing up in the initial sessions. However, a balance must also be struck, as going in different directions may scatter the focus of discussion, and lead participants to question the purpose of the group. In some cases, if participants are ready to move on after airing their issues and their related feelings or beliefs, the process can be imbued with a solution-focused approach by getting them to try out practical strategies between sessions. This is also where the peer support specialist, who was in a similar position experimenting with changes, may play a role. However, solutions introduced too early may lead to participants' over-agreement, given the compliant culture that is often observed. Practical strategies, if introduced at an appropriate time, need to be given sufficient "air-time" for discussion, especially about how comfortable the person may be when executing it.

Interestingly, most groups lacked any conflict. The theoretical framework of peer support describes how learning to confront conflicts is a way of building and deepening relationships and community (Mead et al., 2001). In group dynamics, "storming" is also an important phase of group work (Toseland & Rivas, 2001). In this case, perhaps the sessions were too short for conflict to surface? Does the Asian culture, which stresses on harmony, lead the participants to giving politically correct answers? Or does the facilitators' own discomfort with conflict downplay the likelihood of conflict arising? Was the number of sessions insufficient? While there are no clear answers to these enquiries, conflict, whether overt or covert, should be an important topic for reflection during any debriefing.

Having outlined the challenges in conducting a peer support group, the close partnership between the peer support specialist and the co-facilitating case manager is tantamount to success. While co-facilitation brings the benefits of additional attention and input from another person, it also brings the challenge of teamwork (Sharry, 2007). Hence, facilitators must invest time to come together for preparation before each session, as well as debrief to discuss group dynamics and processes, and how both felt about the session. The supporting role of the peer support specialist is not passive and is as important as taking the lead by interjecting with observations, or sharing experiences and asking relevant questions to deepen the content of discussion. At times, the peer support specialist may also adopt a leadership role while the case manager moves to the supporting role.

In individual peer support work, the peer support specialist may find him or herself in a more independent position and be required to offer one-on-one support. In such situations, they need to focus more on listening to the individuals' concerns and less on solutions. Mead, Hilton, and Curtis (2001) pointed out that being too quick to advise may result in "developing an inability to explore or re-evaluate someone's experience". The subjective experience of the recipient of support may be unfamiliar or uncomfortable to the peer support specialist who presupposes based on his or her own experience. The peer support specialist also has to be careful of over-identifying, which may result in relating to the other based on a mental patient role that is self-stigmatizing.

Hence, the peer support specialist's prior experience of running a few groups becomes vital before they adopt a more independent role. Skills involving the use of self-disclosure, use of empathy, having a compass for pain, understanding of the universality of human experience, and being comfortable with silence, learned during group work are utilized during individual conversations. The peer support specialist will also be more at ease being in a position of safe uncertainty (Mason, 2005); that they need not take on a "know-all" stance and always have solutions. Their confidence in dealing with participants' responses also develops over time until they reach the stage of skilled listening and knowing how to respond in an empathetic manner.

Support Given to Peer Support Specialists

In EPIP, as phone peer support is relatively new, close guidance is provided by the peer support coordinator through regular discussions about the phone contacts. The recording sheet that the peer specialists complete also serves as documentation to monitor issues that may surface.

The evidence is mounting that peer support specialists are pivotal to the success of the programme. In fact, they are seen as partners and time will be allocated to underlining their role, tasks, and responsibility. Besides role-related skills training, prevention of burnout is something that the coordinator should flag and notably, any slight change in scope, like rotating between running support groups and running activities or individual phone support, is always refreshing. Appreciation of the work they put in is also important. As the peer support programme becomes more established, methods of showing appreciation and recognition of their expertise will be explored.

To date, the peer support specialists have otherwise been motivated by the intrinsic rewards of being able to help others, in the process of which they find that they are able to better make sense of their own issues during recovery. This leads to greater empowerment and other benefits in the area of intrapersonal development. This reciprocity of support is reflected in one peer support specialist's words:

> Peer support group helps me to identify and share my experiences with other members within the group. I was afraid at first when I was sharing my experiences about my illness as it was something personal and hard to describe. But with the support and guidance of my facilitator, I was able to overcome my difficulty over time. It felt good and meaningful when I could also relate my own experiences with other members. I was happy that I was not alone. Peer support group helps me to address issues like relationships and friendships. Although this may sound simple, they are actually very important to people like us who are trying to recover and lead a normal, healthy life again. Sometimes, I may not be able to find immediate solutions to my problems but being able to take the courage to talk about them brings a sense of relief. I hope that other people will be able to benefit and gain confidence from peer support groups like I did.

On a final note, the peer support coordinator needs to be aware of the principles of the peer support culture and be careful not to differentiate oneself from the peer support specialists and participants. The "us" versus "them" spilt can occur easily when people are working within a medical framework in a hospital setting. The coordinator should take on a strengths-based perspective and an inclusive outlook. A systemic view of understanding the person's functioning in a larger context is helpful so as to maintain a non-clinical and growth-oriented philosophy (Mead et al., 2001), which is transferred during guidance of peer support specialists.

Future Development and Conclusion

Peer support is valuable as an adjunct to the mainstay psychosocial support of case managers. Since this is a newly established programme in EPIP, close monitoring of the processes is required and more needs to be done in looking at sustenance of the programme. Moving forward, evaluation of the programme is also necessary. Through the programme, it is hoped that participants can break through self-stigmatizing conceptions of disability, so that they no longer experience loneliness amidst the crowd in their recovery journey.

References

Castelein, S., Bruggeman, R., van Busschbach, J. T., van der Gaag, M., Stant, A. D., Knegtering, H., et al. (2008). The effectiveness of peer support groups in psychosis: A randomized controlled trial. [Multicenter Study Randomized Controlled Trial Research Support, Non-U.S. Government]. *Acta Psychiatrica Scandinavica, 118*(1), 64–72.

Davidson, L., Chinman, M., Sells, D., & Rowe, M. (2006). Peer support among adults with serious mental illness: A report from the field. [Research Support, U.S. Government, Non-P.H.S.]. *Schizophrenia Bulletin, 32*(3), 443–450. doi: 10.1093/schbul/sbj043

Gladding, S. T. (1991). *Group Work: A Counseling Specialty*. New York: Merrill.

Kanas, N. (2006). Group therapy with schizophrenia patients. [Comment Letter]. *The American Journal of Psychiatry, 163*(5), 937–938; author reply 938. doi: 10.1176/appi.ajp.163.5.937-b

Mason, B. (2005). Relational risk-taking and the training of supervisors. *Journal of Family Therapy, 27*(3), 298–301.

Mead, S., & Copland, M. E. (2000). What recovery means to us: Consumers perspectives. *Community Mental Health Journal, 36*(3), 315–328.

Mead, S., Hilton, D., & Curtis, L. (2001). Peer support: A theoretical perspective. [Review]. *Psychiatric Rehabilitation Journal, 25*(2), 134–141.

Sharry, J. (2007). *Solution-Focused Groupwork* (2nd ed.). Los Angeles, CA: Sage Publications.

Toseland, R. W., & Rivas, R. F. (2001). *An Introduction to Group Work Practice* (4th ed.). Boston: Allyn and Bacon.

Yalom, I. D., & Leszcz, M. (2005). *The Theory and Practice of Group Psychotherapy* (5th ed.). New York: Basic Books.

21
Family Work in Early Psychosis

Christopher Loh

Family Intervention

Psychosis is a major psychiatric illness that has debilitating impact on patients and their families. Providing care for patients in their home environment can be physically and emotionally demanding for the families. Numerous studies have shown caregivers of patients with psychosis experience distress and burnout (Addington et al., 2003; Barrowclough, Tarrier, & Johnston, 1996; Chen et al., 2004). Evidence suggests that some families need considerable support to prevent further deterioration in family functioning, especially when the patient is admitted to hospital (Seng & Bentelspacher, 2001).

Bowen (1978) describes the impact of serious emotional events as the "emotional shock wave", which may have ripple effects in the family over time. The effects of the illness could resonate beyond the nuclear family too. The experience of working with the families in EPIP revealed the involvement of extended family members as well. In some instances, grandparents, uncles, aunties or in-laws played essential roles in the care of the identified patient, thus making it clear that contacts with families did not merely include parents, siblings, or spouses. Patients' data collected in EPIP revealed that 92.1% of them stayed with their families, which included spouses, children, parents, siblings, and other relatives. Only 3.8% of the patients lived alone. Hence, any treatment plan must involve the family, nuclear or extended, so as to support the patients and reduce stress in the families.

Individual Psychoeducation with Families

Family psychoeducation is an essential component of the treatment process for psychosis and case managers play a crucial role in providing individual psychoeducation to patients and their families. In the case of the family, the psychoeducation can be provided with individuals or with the family as a group. Psychoeducation is done on a regular basis, especially during the initial (the first three months), mid (12th month) and end (22nd month) phases of treatment. For families of patients who require more than two years of EPIP service, psychoeducation is addressed again during discharge planning. Clearly, psychoeducation is not a one-off affair, as families need constant reminders and refreshment of their knowledge of psychosis. The frequency and intensity of psychoeducation depend largely on the needs of the families—family members may take more or less time to understand the information given during psychoeducation depending on their abilities to take in this knowledge. In our experience, there is a clear difference between the more educated families and the less educated ones in terms of their abilities to receive and understand psychoeducation. The level of understanding also depends on their acceptance of their loved one's illness. In some instances, families may find it difficult to receive psychoeducation as they may attribute the symptoms of the patients to other causes. Some examples of the reasons given by families are that the patient's "mind is too weak", he or she just needs to "be more positive", that he or she "thinks too much" or "is just stressed". Many also attribute the illness to "offending spirits". This has to do with the family's cultural beliefs, which are elaborated in Chapter 15 "Cultural Issues in Early Psychosis Management". In the course of this work, the team has come to know that the belief in spiritual invasion is somehow easier for parents to accept the bizarre behaviour displayed by their children as it externalizes the problem. Accepting that their children are suffering from a mental illness gives rise to guilt feelings as they blame themselves for not providing enough emotional support before the onset of the illness. Hence, the psychoeducation provided by case managers should be tailored to the needs of each family. Information imparted to the families is also paced carefully.

Psychoeducation provided by case managers includes the nature of psychosis, its aetiology, medication and side-effects, modes of treatment, relapse prevention, stress management, and healthy lifestyle. Materials on these topics are passed to families in the process and families are also provided with the EPIP Resource Booklet for Caregivers, which consists information on when, where, and how to seek help during a crisis. In addition, psychoeducation on depression and/or anxiety disorders will be included if it is relevant to the patient's condition. Flipcharts and relapse signature cards are also used during the educational process.

Home Visits

A home visit is conducted by every case manager for all patients, especially those who are newly accepted into EPIP. These patients could either be inpatients or outpatients. Often, families are encouraged to be present during the home visit so that case managers are able to make face-to-face contact with them. The home visit serves several purposes for the patients and families but, by and large, the objectives of the home visit are to provide psychoeducation, assess the mental state of patients, assess the side-effects of medication, build rapport with the patients and their families, contact and engage the families in the treatment, and assess family dynamics in the home environment. On some occasions, the home visit will help families encourage the unstable patients to be admitted to hospital. The visit may also occcur when crisis happens at home with the families. Such crises could include family violence, acutely unwell patients refusing medication, and other safety issues. The Mobile Crisis Team (MCT) from the Institute of Mental Health (IMH) and police are involved in these circumstances when there is a high level of risk.

Family Work during Home Leave for Inpatients

Home leave is granted for some inpatients during their ward stay. During home leave, inpatients are allowed to return home for a day or more (usually less than three days) before the treatment team and families decide on discharging the patients from the ward. The purpose of this home leave is to allow patients and families to assess their situation at home before confirming the decision for discharge. This is because some patients may experience symptoms when they are back in the home environment prematurely, or family conflict may arise when they reunite with the patient. On the other hand, some inpatients are discharged once they are stabilized without having to be granted home leave.

For some inpatients, discharge could be a challenge if families decide that they may not be able to manage the patients' behaviours or symptoms at that point in time. Thus, home leave is an opportunity for families to trial having the patient at home. During this period of time, the case manager works closely with the family to assess the situation during the home stay, via regular phone contact or home visits. After working hours, families have phone access to the night duty nurses. Case managers would work with the nurses to look at pertinent issues arising during the home leave. Issues such as medication compliance, symptoms, patients' challenging behaviours, family ability to handle the patients' condition, and family conflicts are often assessed during home leave. The benefit of home leave is that families are able to bring the patients directly to the ward if problems surface at home. This saves them any hassle of having to go through the entire admission process again.

Support Worker for Caregivers

In EPIP, a caregiver of the patient who was previously seeking treatment with EPIP, is engaged as a support worker for other caregivers. This caregiver of the former EPIP patient has shown to be of assistance to other caregivers by reaching out to existing EPIP patients' families.

This support worker is employed to assist the treating team in (1) co-facilitating the psychoeducation workshop for the caregivers of newly admitted EPIP patients (see the following section), (2) providing supportive counselling through sharing of experiences for caregivers who are experiencing caregiver's stress, and (3) providing one-to-one psychoeducation on illness, treatments, supporting patients, and crisis management to the caregivers. Such support to other caregivers can be rendered through face-to-face or phone contact. The addition of this caregiver support worker into the existing multidisciplinary team aims to better engage the patients' caregivers in the treatment process. This adjunct treatment modality seeks to promote EPIP services and encourage caregivers to support treatment for patients. Besides these stated roles, the support worker also contributes to the preparation of newsletters and outreach events.

Psychoeducation Workshop for Families

Family psychoeducation programmes have been demonstrated to improve families' perception of their overall knowledge and understanding of mental illness and its treatment (Mullen, Murray, & Happell, 2002). The literature to date suggests that family psychoeducation can reduce relapse and facilitate recovery of patients with psychiatric disabilities (Cohen et al., 2008; Dixon et al., 2001).

Further development of family psychoeducation includes a supportive element in educational group that focuses on improving caregivers' quality of life by reducing stress and burden (Solomon, 1996). Mutual support groups also enhance families' coping abilities and reduce distress and burden (Chien & Norman, 2009).

EPIP uses the caregivers' psychoeducation workshop as an adjunct treatment modality. The purpose of the educational group is to improve caregivers' knowledge of psychosis, its treatment, and caregiving. This workshop is conducted by a case manager every three months. A questionnaire has been developed to assess the caregivers' level of perceived understanding of core topics. Seven questions review the workshop content, in particular their knowledge of (1) psychosis, (2) possible causes of psychosis, (3) the medication used to treat psychosis, (4) side-effects of medication, (5) relapse, (6) their role as caregivers, and (7) community resources for caregivers. Caregivers rate their level of knowledge on each topic on a four-point Likert scale: (1) not at all good, (2) not good, (3) good, and (4) very good. The questionnaire is administered at the beginning and end of the workshop. At the end of the workshop, caregivers are also required to complete an evaluation form. This evaluation form seeks caregivers' feedback on the usefulness of the workshop and suggestions for further improvement. The questionnaires come in English and Chinese for respective workshops. Caregivers who have difficulty in understanding the questionnaire can seek help from the case managers who are conducting the workshops.

Results from the Caregivers' Psychoeducation Workshop in EPIP

Prior to every workshop, invitations are sent to the caregivers of patients newly accepted (less than three months) into EPIP. Approximately 60 invitations are sent out on each occasion. Between February and August 2009, 26 English-speaking and 32 Mandarin-speaking caregivers participated. Results from the pre- and post-tests showed improvement in the level of perceived understanding of the core topics in the workshops (see Table 21.1). Results also indicated an increase in "good" and "very good" responses.

The data collected from the caregivers' psychoeducation workshop serve as a means to evaluate the programme's effectiveness and usefulness. It is important to note that the data collected are not for clinical research purposes. A careful

Table 21.1
Results of pre-and post-tests of the caregivers' workshop in 2009

Topics	"not at all good" or "not good"		"good" or "very good"	
	Pre-test (%)	Post-test (%)	Pre-test (%)	Post-test (%)
Psychosis	84.7	9.4	14.2	69.3
Aetiology	87.6	14.0	8.1	68.8
Medication	79.2	17.6	16.6	61.0
Side-effects	84.9	14.2	17.5	64.4
Relapse	84.9	18.5	17.5	60.1
Caregiver's role	81.4	16.1	22.1	59.8
Community Resources	79.5	9.4	10.7	67.8

design of the study methods, such as the use of focus group or semi-structured interviews, is required to meet the aims of any future clinical research.

Other Family Work

Besides direct work with families as mentioned above, case managers play the role of service coordinator for families a will refer families for external services if needed. In EPIP, regular referrals are made to external programmes such as the Caregivers' Support Group and Family Link Programme at the Singapore Association for Mental Health (SAMH), Caregivers' Groups at Simei Care Centre (SCC), and events organized by the Caregivers' Association of the Mentally Ill (CAMI) and the Centre for Caregivers of Asian Women's Welfare Association (AWWA).

Families who require family therapy are referred to the Medical Social Work Department (MSW) in IMH or external family therapy services, such as SAMH and Family Service Centres (FSCs). Families who need financial assistance for the treatment are referred to the MSW in IMH as well. For families that require further social assistance, case managers may extend their service by linking them to relevant social welfare agencies. For example, some families in a dire financial situation are referred to the Community Development Council (CDC) for job and/or financial assistance.

Conclusion

In this context, most patients, especially those who are single, live with their parents and/or siblings. This team recognizes the importance of family support for patients. Hence, besides regularly educating family members about the illness, it is equally essential to link them to relevant resources to better meet their needs. Caregivers' workshops that focus on day-to-day struggles of managing their loved ones with psychosis are also valuable. On top of basic psychoeducation about psychosis, which can be done by the respective case managers, practical tips on communication and watching out for high expressed emotion are introduced in this workshop and found to be beneficial.

References

Addington, J., Coldham, E. L., Jones, B., Ko, T., & Addington, D. (2003). The first episode of psychosis: The experience of relatives. *Acta Psychiatrica Scandinavica, 108*(4), 285–289.

Barrowclough, C., Tarrier, N., & Johnston, M. (1996). Distress, expressed emotion, and attributions in relatives of schizophrenia patients. *Schizophrenia Bulletin, 22*(4), 691–702.

Bowen, M. (1978). *Family Therapy in Clinical Practice.* New York: J. Aronson.

Chen, P. S., Yang, Y. K., Liao, Y. C., Lee, Y. D., Yeh, T. L., & Chen, C. C. (2004). The psychological well-being and associated factors of caregivers of outpatients with schizophrenia in Taiwan. [Research Support, Non-U.S. Government]. *Psychiatry and Clinical Neurosciences, 58*(6), 600–605. doi: 10.1111/j.1440–1819.2004.01309.x

Chien, W. T., & Norman, I. (2009). The effectiveness and active ingredients of mutual support groups for family caregivers of people with psychotic disorders: A literature review. [Review]. *International Journal of Nursing Studies, 46*(12), 1604–1623. doi: 10.1016/j.ijnurstu.2009.04.003

Cohen, A. N., Glynn, S. M., Murray-Swank, A. B., Barrio, C., Fischer, E. P., McCutcheon, S. J., et al. (2008). The family forum: Directions for the implementation of family psychoeducation for severe mental illness. *Psychiatric Services, 59*(1), 40–48. doi: 10.1176/appi.ps.59.1.40

Dixon, L., McFarlane, W. R., Lefley, H., Lucksted, A., Cohen, M., Falloon, I., et al. (2001). Evidence-based practices for services to families of people with psychiatric disabilities. [Review]. *Psychiatric Services, 52*(7), 903–910.

Mullen, A., Murray, L., & Happell, B. (2002). Multiple family group interventions in first episode psychosis: Enhancing knowledge and understanding. [Evaluation Studies]. *International Journal of Mental Health Nursing, 11*(4), 225–232.

Seng, B. K., & Bentelspacher, C. (2001). Burden of care. *Asia Pacific Journal of Social Work, 11*, 88–105.

Solomon, P. (1996). Moving from psychoeducation to family education for families of adults with serious mental illness. [Research Support, U.S. Government, P.H.S. Review]. *Psychiatric Services, 47*(12), 1364–1370.

22
Working with Non-Governmental Organizations in Early Psychosis

Steve Tso and Simon Sai-yu Lui

The Early Assessment Service for Young People with Psychosis (EASY) in Hong Kong emphasizes close links with non-governmental organizations (NGOs) involved in providing mental healthcare to the community. In Hong Kong, NGOs provide a wide range of services. Many youth and community centres are run by NGOs where people in the local community meet and join activities. Staff members of NGOs are usually trained social workers.

NGOs are key suppliers of mental healthcare for people with early psychosis, as they:

1. refer many suspected cases of psychosis;
2. facilitate detection and identification of people with untreated psychosis in the community;
3. enhance the mental health literacy in the community;
4. assist case managers of EASY;
5. provide community support to patients with early psychosis;
6. enhance community reintegration of clients;
7. deliver rehabilitation programmes through their community and youth centres which offer easy access, less stigmatization, and can approximate real-life situations; and
8. organize group activities in a community setting that is preferable to any clinical settings.

NGO-Provided Mental Healthcare Services in Hong Kong

NGOs in Hong Kong have a long history of providing care and support to people with mental disorders. In the past, many NGOs, such as New Life Psychiatric Rehabilitation Association and the Hong Kong Mental Health

Association were more heavily involved in caring for psychosis patients discharged from psychiatric hospitals or halfway houses, by providing rehabilitation to "chronic and institutionalized" patients. Obviously, these traditional rehabilitation services are not suitable for early psychosis clients, who are young and managed mainly in outpatient clinics. In recent years, the EASY teams have worked collaboratively with different NGO youth and community centres to provide a wide range of new programmes tailor-made to the needs of early psychosis clients and their caregivers.

Community Partnership between the EASY Service and NGOs

The EASY teams collaborate actively with NGOs to deliver community programmes for EASY clients and their caregivers, and promote positive messages about mental illnesses to the general public. Since 2001, a range of therapeutic, educational, social and leisure activities have been organized.

Enhancing mental health literacy

Frequently, NGOs invite the EASY team staff to deliver talks in youth and community centres. The EASY staff members also train NGO frontline workers to deal with people with psychosis and how to engage people who are suspected to have psychosis into psychiatric services. Some of these talks are open to the general public to educate local folk to differentiate early or "prodromal" signs of psychosis from normal adolescent behaviours. These educational activities aim to enhance mental health literacy, to reduce stigma associated with the illness, and to promote early treatment of psychosis.

Early detection of untreated psychosis

NGOs are encouraged to refer suspected first-episode psychosis cases early to EASY. As some young people who are suspected to have psychosis tend to decline psychiatric assessments conducted in hospitals or clinics, the EASY team has been providing frequent nurse-led assessment sessions in a NGO centre. Those screened by the nurses to suffer from psychosis are eventually followed up at the EASY clinic.

Managing caregivers' stress

Family and caregivers play a significant role in the patient's rehabilitation and recovery process; supporting family and caregivers is therefore an important part of EASY. Family group work is a way to enhance a client's support network, and in turn minimize negative impact of the disease on the clients' families. For EASY clients, round-the-year family groups are regularly conducted collaboratively with NGO community partners. The family groups invite early psychosis clients who are at the similar stages of the illness, to join in with their caregivers. The first few sessions are usually conducted jointly by a senior psychiatrist and a medical social worker and focus on information delivery and support. The NGO workers gradually become more involved by building up support networks, and identifying other areas of need. Community and youth centres are preferred venues for these family groups in place of hospitals and clinics due to easier access, wider acceptance by caregivers, less stigmatization, better-equipped facilities, and greater availability of volunteer helpers. Moreover, clients and caregivers can benefit from other services available in those centres.

Reintegrating clients into the community through normalization

EASY clients' linkage to the community can be compromised by social withdrawal behaviours, lack of self-confidence, and other reasons. Contact with others during leisure and recreational activities in NGO-run centres provide opportunities for clients to develop and maintain "social competencies" in real-life situations rather than clinical settings, and thus promote "normalization". Clinicians also find that some clients and their families become better engaged to case managers and social workers through these community-based activities. In some deprived areas in Hong Kong where poverty is common and social support is weak (e.g. Tin Shui Wan), EASY clients, like many other young people in those communities, are generally lacking in these experiences for financial reasons. Since 2003, a range of leisure activities funded by the Social Welfare Department were organized by NGO community partners for EASY clients and their caregivers, under the "Support Scheme for Children and Youth with Early Signs of Mental Health Programme". These activities included barbeques, day camps, outdoor adventures, festival parties, sightseeing, and video making.

During their participation in volunteer services, EASY clients share their experiences with peers, improve their personal strengths and coping skills, develop an optimistic outlook for the future, and master the appropriate developmental tasks. These group programmes help young people with psychosis overcome the disruption of their normal developmental pathways caused by onset of the illness, and encourage a continuous psychosocial developmental process through peer interaction (Albiston, Francey, & Harrigan, 1998). Every year, NGO community partners invite EASY clients to participate in various volunteer activities, to help them recognize their strengths and enhance interpersonal communication skills.

Developing vocational skills and facilitating job hunting

Like other adolescents, patients with psychosis must be able to develop their vocational identity, which contributes to an overall personal identity.

Through obtaining grants from the "Enhancing Employment of People with Disabilities through Small Enterprise Project" run by the Social Welfare Department, our NGO community partners employed EASY clients in a carefully planned and sympathetic working environment. Taking the Castle Peak Hospital EASY team as an example, a training programme (爱思全接觸培訓計劃) has been organized annually by a NGO partner, Caritas Jockey Club Integrated Service for Young People (Tuen Mun), for six consecutive years. Besides promoting interpersonal skills and self-confidence, this programme provides vocational training sessions to prepare participants for job hunting and to build up their work skills and habits. "Practical sessions" are arranged, in which participants receive incentive allowances and are posted to different work settings such as restaurants and stationery shops as cooks and shop assistants. Another vocational rehabilitation service offered by NGO community partners is computer skills training (e.g., workshops on Microsoft Windows and Microsoft Office). Occupational therapists of the EASY team also actively formulate and review individualized vocational rehabilitation plans, and their recommendations are passed to NGO partners.

Managing weight gain due to medication side-effects

Recently, the NGO partners have organized aerobic dancing classes, weight reduction programmes, and talks about how to prepare a healthy diet. Clients who have overweight problems due to side-effects of drugs or unhealthy lifestyle were invited and encouraged to join.

The Future

In recent years, many leaders of NGOs in Hong Kong have become increasingly aware of the need to reform their service models. It is believed that mental healthcare services provided by NGOs should be better coordinated so as to avoid overlapping of services, and there should be a one-stop service for the sake of continuity of care. The Hong Kong government has implemented a policy to establish territory-wide integrated community centres to provide one-stop community support and social rehabilitation services for discharged mental patients, people with suspected mental health problems and their families or carers. The first of such centres, the Integrated Community Centre for Mental Wellness (ICCMW), was established in 2010 at Tin Shui Wai, a deprived area in Hong Kong. The facility is run by an NGO and offers a range of services, including drop-in services, outreach, casework/therapeutic and supportive group work, networking, a training and activity centre, outreach occupational therapy, and public education programmes. Referrals can be made to ICCMW through self-application or via doctors, social workers, and allied health workers. The services are free of charge.

Given this changing landscape of NGO-provided mental healthcare services in Hong Kong, EASY has to review and refine its model of partnership with NGOs in the near future, so as to make best use of these new and additional services.

Summary

NGOs are ideal community partners for effective management of psychosis. Collaboration with NGOs is important in order to promote mental health literacy and early detection of psychosis, to support family and caregivers, and to enhance normalization and vocational rehabilitation.

Reference

Albiston, D. J., Francey, S. M., & Harrigan, S. M. (1998). Group programmes for recovery from early psychosis. *The British Journal of Psychiatry. Supplement, 172*(33), 117–121.

Part V

Medication and Adherence Issues

23
Pharmacological Intervention in Early Psychosis

Phyllis Kwok-ling Chan and Edwin Ho-ming Lee

Questions on pharmacotherapy are frequently asked by patients and their caregivers in the treatment of early psychosis, reflecting their concern for this topic. Doctors and nurses often face questions on the following issues during psychoeducation:

- Do I need to take medication? When should it be started?
- How effective is the drug treatment? What kind of symptoms is it useful for?
- What kind of drugs should I take?
- What are the immediate and long-term side-effects?
- How to choose between the old and new drugs?
- Why do I have to continue taking drugs even when I have no symptoms?
- What are the differences between acute and maintenance treatment?
- How long will the drug treatment last?
- What is the appropriate dosage?
- What if the drug does not work?

This chapter will discuss possible answers to some of these questions based on current research and clinical knowledge.

When Should Antipsychotic Medication Be Started?

Pharmacotherapy is the core and most effective part of the comprehensive treatment care for psychosis. Pharmacotherapy has also been used in prodrome of psychosis, a stage lasting an average of five years before onset of frank psychotic symptoms (Hafner & an der Heiden, 1997). Use of antipsychotic medication in prodrome should consider the balance between effectiveness and side-effects (McGorry et al., 2009) because data on these issues are still preliminary (see Chapter 12, "Handling At-Risk Mental State"). However, there is evidence supporting the use of psychiatric treatment as soon as psychotic symptoms are identified as clinical benefits of early intervention have substantial data support (see Chapter 1, "Development of Early Intervention Services: Introduction").

Early intervention for psychosis is important because shorter duration of untreated psychosis (DUP) is associated with better outcomes (Loebel et al., 1992; McGorry et al., 2001; Scully et al., 1997; Wyatt, Green, & Tuma, 1997). Untreated psychosis is believed to be like a toxic process that can incur progressive damage to the brain (Wyatt, 1995). After each episode of psychosis, it takes longer to establish treatment response and the degree of response diminishes (Lieberman et al., 1996).

Which Medication?

Individuals with first-episode psychosis respond well to antipsychotic treatment, with as many as 80% recovering symptomatically from the initial episode (Lieberman et al., 1993; Tohen et al., 1992). In the past, the focus of antipsychotic treatment in psychosis was on positive symptomatology (Davis, Chen, & Glick, 2003). Nowadays, it is common to evaluate the pharmacological response on a number of clinical dimensions including affective symptoms (e.g. depression), cognitive symptoms (e.g. decreased attention or concentration), social impairment (e.g. lack of motivation, social withdrawal, and functional decline) and side-effects (Remington, 2003). The definition of outcome has also expanded from control of positive symptoms to other dimensions like cognition, affect, and quality of life.

However, there is no conclusive data that allow comprehensive comparison of first-generation and second-generation antipsychotics on these dimensions (Geddes et al., 2000; Jones et al., 2003; Kapur & Remington, 2000; Keefe et al., 2007). Limited data so far suggest that second-generation antipsychotics are less likely to cause negative symptoms and cognitive impairments (compared with Haloperidol in most studies), but superior efficacy for primary negative symptoms has not been supported (Kirkpatrick et al., 2000), while evidence from a controlled study for their pro-cognitive efficacy is modest (Keefe et al., 1999).

An important research finding for second-generation antipsychotics is their diminished risk of extra-pyramidal side-effects (Geddes et al., 2000; Klemp et al., 2011; Leucht et al., 1999). Data suggest the risk of tardive dyskinesia is within the range of 1% or less with one year's use of second-generation antipsychotics (Beasley et al., 1999; Tollefson et al., 1997), considerably lower than the 5% predicted following a year's exposure to first-generation antipsychotics (Glazer, Morgenstern, & Doucette, 1993). A study reported a 12-month risk of probable and persistent tardive dyskinesia of 12.3% in individuals with first-episode psychosis treated with Haloperidol at a mean dose of 2.8 mg/day (Oosthuizen et al., 2003). This is the strongest piece of evidence arguing for the use of second-generation antipsychotics as first-line treatment.

In addition, the discontinuation rates indicate that the second-generation antipsychotics may be better tolerated in general (Emsley, 1999; Lieberman et al., 2005). However, the second-generation antipsychotics have a side-effect profile that cannot be ignored: for example, weight gain associated with second-generation antipsychotics has become a significant issue (Allison & Casey, 2001; Allison et al., 1999; Nasrallah, 2003; Rummel-Kluge et al., 2010; Wirshing et al., 1999), while impaired glucose tolerance or diabetics, lipid abnormalities, cardiovascular changes (specifically QTc prolongation), etc. are of no less concern than tardive dyskinesia. On the beneficial side, the course of depression, hostility, or aggression appears to move favourably with the second generation of antipsychotic treatment.

In total there is at present a lack of compelling evidence that the second-generation antipsychotics are clinically superior in a population with first-episode psychosis (Crossley et al., 2010). Efficacy of the first-generation antipsychotics such as Perphenazine appeared to be similar to that of Quetiapine, Risperidone, and Ziprasidone (Lieberman et al., 2005). The increased risk of tardive dyskinesia with first-generation antipsychotics favour using the second-generation antipsychotics. Conversely, the risk of other side-effects, such as weight gain, diabetes, and other cardiovascular events associated with the second-generation antipsychotics counter their straight-forward acceptance as the first-line treatment.

The consensus statement on early intervention and recovery for young people with early psychosis recommended the use of second-generation versus first-generation antipsychotics according to the level of resources (World Health Organization & International Early Psychosis Association, 2004). Low-dose first-generation antipsychotic and other related medications should be available and offered routinely to people at low-level resource area. Low-dose second-generation antipsychotic medication should be available and offered routinely in medium-level resource area. Low-dose second-generation antipsychotics would be offered as medication of first choice in high-level resource area.

What Is the Appropriate Dosage and Duration of Antipsychotic Treatment?

Controlled studies have demonstrated that the recommended dose for psychosis is within the range of 3 to 12 mg Haloperidol-equivalents. Dosage higher than this does not offer any additional clinical benefits (Baldessarini, Cohen, & Teicher, 1988).

Positron emission topography (PET) studies support that antipsychotic response is optimized at a threshold of approximately 65% to 70% dopamine D_2 occupancy; that exceeding 80% leads to a substantial increase in the risk of extra-pyramidal side-effects (EPS) (Kapur et al., 1999). Using Haloperidol for comparison purposes, 2 mg results in a mean D_2 occupancy of 67%, whereas 5 mg approximates the 80% threshold associated with EPS (Kapur et al., 1996; Kapur et al., 1997). These data support a therapeutic range of approximately 2 to 5 mg Haloperidol-equivalents daily to optimise clinical response and minimize the risk of EPS.

Zhang-Wong, Zipursky, Beiser, and Bean (1999) found that 82% of their patients with first-episode psychosis were treated effectively with Haloperidol 2 to 5 mg daily. Their study allowed those who did not respond to be treated with a higher dose of 10 to 20 mg/day, but this subgroup continued to be less responsive. EPS were reported in 13% of the 2 mg group, in contrast to 55% for those who received 5 mg (Zhang-Wong et al., 1999).

According to the International Clinical Practice Guidelines for Early Psychosis (2005), examples of appropriate initial target doses for most patients are Risperidone 2 mg/day or olanzapine 7.5 to 10 mg/day. Half to two-thirds of patients can be expected to achieve a good response in positive psychotic symptoms within three weeks at the initial dose, but if necessary, the doses can be increased to 4 mg/day Risperidone or 20 mg/day Olanzapine. The level of clinical response and risk should be assessed frequently, but the dose of the antipsychotics should be increased only at widely spaced intervals if the response is inadequate, and only within the limits of sedations and emergence of EPS.

If the response is not adequate at therapeutic doses by six to eight weeks, another antipsychotic should be tried. For first-generation antipsychotics, they should be commenced at very low doses (1–2 mg Haloperidol or equivalent) and titrated very slowly within the limits of EPS. Generally, this will be a maximum of 4 to 6 mg Haloperidol or equivalent in first-episode psychosis.

As the antipsychotic should be started with a low-dose and titrating upwards very slowly over a period of several weeks, the low dose of antipsychotic medication will not have a rapid effect on distress, insomnia, and behavioural disturbances secondary to psychosis. Regular and liberal doses of benzodiazepines are essential interim components of management in many cases.

If the positive symptoms persist after a trial of two first-line antipsychotics (could be up to 12 weeks), early treatment resistance is of concern and more intensive intervention is required, including consideration of the use of Clozapine. On the other hand, in patients showing good response with stabilized symptoms, the questions of when, and under what conditions we can consider discontinuation of antipsychotics become important. Different guidelines have different recommendations for the duration of treatment (Takeuchi et al., 2012). In a local study, a group of asymptomatic patients with first-episode psychosis and at least one year of previous antipsychotic drug treatment, maintenance treatment with Quetiapine compared with placebo resulted in a substantially lower rate of relapse during the following year (Chen et al., 2010). There are further discussion in Chapter 24, "Medication Adherence: Specific Issues in Early Psychosis in Asia" and Chapter 25, "Relapse Intervention and Related Issues".

References

Allison, D. B., & Casey, D. E. (2001). Antipsychotic-induced weight gain: A review of the literature. [Research Support, Non-U.S. Government Research Support, U.S. Government, P.H.S. Review]. *The Journal of Clinical Psychiatry, 62 Suppl 7*, 22–31.

Allison, D. B., Mentore, J. L., Heo, M., Chandler, L. P., Cappelleri, J. C., Infante, M. C., et al. (1999). Antipsychotic-induced weight gain: A comprehensive research synthesis. [Research Support, Non-U.S. Government Research Support, U.S. Government, P.H.S. Review]. *The American Journal of Psychiatry, 156*(11), 1686–1696.

Baldessarini, R. J., Cohen, B. M., & Teicher, M. H. (1988). Significance of neuroleptic dose and plasma level in the pharmacological treatment of psychoses. [Research Support, Non-U.S. Government Research Support, U.S. Government, P.H.S. Review]. *Archives of General Psychiatry, 45*(1), 79–91.

Beasley, C. M., Dellva, M. A., Tamura, R. N., Morgenstern, H., Glazer, W. M., Ferguson, K., et al. (1999). Randomised double-blind comparison of the incidence of tardive dyskinesia in patients with schizophrenia during long-term treatment with olanzapine or haloperidol. [Clinical Trial Multicenter Study Randomized Controlled Trial]. *The British Journal of Psychiatry : The Journal of Mental Science, 174*, 23–30.

Chen, E. Y., Hui, C. L., Lam, M. M., Chiu, C. P., Law, C. W., Chung, D. W., et al. (2010). Maintenance treatment with quetiapine versus discontinuation after one year of treatment in patients with remitted first episode psychosis: Randomised controlled trial. *British Medical Journal, 341*, c4024. doi: 10.1136/bmj.c4024 bmj.c4024 [pii]

Crossley, N. A., Constante, M., McGuire, P., & Power, P. (2010). Efficacy of atypical v. typical antipsychotics in the treatment of early psychosis: Meta-analysis. *British Journal of Psychiatry, 196*(6), 434–439. doi: 196/6/434 [pii] 10.1192/bjp.bp.109.066217

Davis, J. M., Chen, N., & Glick, I. D. (2003). A meta-analysis of the efficacy of second-generation antipsychotics. *Archives of General Psychiatry, 60*(6), 553–564. doi: 10.1001/archpsyc.60.6.553 60/6/553 [pii]

Emsley, R. A. (1999). Risperidone in the treatment of first-episode psychotic patients: A double-blind multicenter study. Risperidone Working Group. [Clinical Trial Multicenter Study Randomized Controlled Trial]. *Schizophrenia Bulletin, 25*(4), 721–729.

Geddes, J., Freemantle, N., Harrison, P., & Bebbington, P. (2000). Atypical antipsychotics in the treatment of schizophrenia: Systematic overview and meta-regression analysis. [Meta-Analysis Review]. *British Medical Journal, 321*(7273), 1371–1376.

Glazer, W. M., Morgenstern, H., & Doucette, J. T. (1993). Predicting the long-term risk of tardive dyskinesia in outpatients maintained on neuroleptic medications. [Comparative Study]. *The Journal of Clinical Psychiatry, 54*(4), 133–139.

Hafner, H., & an der Heiden, W. (1997). Epidemiology of schizophrenia. [Comparative Study Review]. *Canadian Journal of Psychiatry. Revue Canadienne de Psychiatrie, 42*(2), 139–151.

International Early Psychosis Association Writing Group. (2005). International clinical practice guidelines for early psychosis. *British Journal of Psychiatry Supplement, 48*, s120–124. doi: 187/48/s120 [pii] 10.1192/bjp.187.48.s120

Jones, M. W., O'Reilly, P. T., McPherson, A. A., McParland, T. L., Armstrong, D. E., Cox, A. J., et al. (2003). Development, characterisation, inheritance, and cross-species utility of American lobster (Homarus americanus) microsatellite and mtDNA PCR-RFLP markers. *Genome, 46*(1), 59–69. doi: 10.1139/g02–105 g02–105 [pii]

Kapur, S., Cho, R., Jones, C., McKay, G., & Zipursky, R. B. (1999). Is amoxapine an atypical antipsychotic? Positron-emission tomography investigation of its dopamine2 and serotonin2 occupancy. [Research Support, Non-U.S. Government]. *Biological Psychiatry, 45*(9), 1217–1220.

Kapur, S., & Remington, G. (2000). Atypical antipsychotics. [Comment Editorial]. *British Medical Journal, 321*(7273), 1360–1361.

Kapur, S., Remington, G., Jones, C., Wilson, A., DaSilva, J., Houle, S., et al. (1996). High levels of dopamine D2 receptor occupancy with low-dose haloperidol treatment:

A PET study. [Clinical Trial Research Support, Non-U.S. Government]. *The American Journal of Psychiatry, 153*(7), 948–950.

Kapur, S., Zipursky, R., Roy, P., Jones, C., Remington, G., Reed, K., et al. (1997). The relationship between D2 receptor occupancy and plasma levels on low dose oral haloperidol: A PET study. [Research Support, Non-U.S. Government]. *Psychopharmacology, 131*(2), 148–152.

Keefe, R. S., Bilder, R. M., Davis, S. M., Harvey, P. D., Palmer, B. W., Gold, J. M., et al. (2007). Neurocognitive effects of antipsychotic medications in patients with chronic schizophrenia in the CATIE Trial. *Archives of General Psychiatry, 64*(6), 633–647. doi: 64/6/633 [pii] 10.1001/archpsyc.64.6.633

Keefe, R. S., Silva, S. G., Perkins, D. O., & Lieberman, J. A. (1999). The effects of atypical antipsychotic drugs on neurocognitive impairment in schizophrenia: A review and meta-analysis. [Meta-Analysis Research Support, Non-U.S. Government Research Support, U.S. Government, P.H.S.]. *Schizophrenia Bulletin, 25*(2), 201–222.

Kirkpatrick, B., Kopelowicz, A., Buchanan, R. W., & Carpenter, W. T., Jr. (2000). Assessing the efficacy of treatments for the deficit syndrome of schizophrenia. [Research Support, Non-U.S. Government Research Support, U.S. Government, P.H.S. Review]. *Neuropsychopharmacology : Official Publication of the American College of Neuropsychopharmacology, 22*(3), 303–310. doi: 10.1016/S0893-133X(99)00122-0

Klemp, M., Tvete, I. F., Skomedal, T., Gaasemyr, J., Natvig, B., & Aursnes, I. (2011). A review and Bayesian meta-analysis of clinical efficacy and adverse effects of 4 atypical neuroleptic drugs compared with haloperidol and placebo. *Journal of Clinical Psychopharmacology, 31*(6), 698–704. doi: 10.1097/JCP.0b013e31823657d9

Leucht, S., Pitschel-Walz, G., Abraham, D., & Kissling, W. (1999). Efficacy and extrapyramidal side-effects of the new antipsychotics olanzapine, quetiapine, risperidone, and sertindole compared to conventional antipsychotics and placebo: A meta-analysis of randomized controlled trials. [Comparative Study Meta-Analysis]. *Schizophrenia Research, 35*(1), 51–68.

Lieberman, J., Jody, D., Geisler, S., Alvir, J., Loebel, A., Szymanski, S., et al. (1993). Time course and biologic correlates of treatment response in first-episode schizophrenia. [Research Support, Non-U.S. Government Research Support, U.S. Government, P.H.S.]. *Archives of General Psychiatry, 50*(5), 369–376.

Lieberman, J. A., Koreen, A. R., Chakos, M., Sheitman, B., Woerner, M., Alvir, J. M., et al. (1996). Factors influencing treatment response and outcome of first-episode schizophrenia: Implications for understanding the pathophysiology of schizophrenia. [Comparative Study Research Support, U.S. Government, P.H.S. Review]. *The Journal of Clinical Psychiatry, 57 Suppl 9*, 5–9.

Lieberman, J. A., Stroup, T. S., McEvoy, J. P., Swartz, M. S., Rosenheck, R. A., Perkins, D. O., et al. (2005). Effectiveness of antipsychotic drugs in patients with chronic schizophrenia. [Clinical Trial Comparative Study Multicenter Study Randomized Controlled Trial Research Support, N.I.H., Extramural Research Support, Non-U.S. Government Research Support, U.S. Government, P.H.S.]. *The New England Journal of Medicine, 353*(12), 1209–1223. doi: 0.1056/NEJMoa051688

Loebel, A. D., Lieberman, J. A., Alvir, J. M., Mayerhoff, D. I., Geisler, S. H., & Szymanski, S. R. (1992). Duration of psychosis and outcome in first-episode schizophrenia. *American Journal of Psychiatry, 149*(9), 1183–1188.

McGorry, P. D., Harrigan, S. M., Amminger, P., Norman, R., & Malla, A. (2001). Untreated initial psychosis. [Comment Letter]. *The American Journal of Psychiatry, 158*(7), 1161–1163.

McGorry, P. D., Nelson, B., Amminger, G. P., Bechdolf, A., Francey, S. M., Berger, G., et al. (2009). Intervention in individuals at ultra-high risk for psychosis: A review and future directions. *J Clinical Psychiatry, 70*(9), 1206–1212. doi: 10.4088/JCP.08r04472

Nasrallah, H. (2003). A review of the effect of atypical antipsychotics on weight. [Review]. *Psychoneuroendocrinology, 28 Supplement 1*, 83–96.

Oosthuizen, P. P., Emsley, R. A., Maritz, J. S., Turner, J. A., & Keyter, N. (2003). Incidence of tardive dyskinesia in first-episode psychosis patients treated with low-dose haloperidol. [Research Support, Non-U.S. Government]. *The Journal of Clinical Psychiatry, 64*(9), 1075–1080.

Remington, G. (2003). Understanding antipsychotic "atypicality": A clinical and pharmacological moving target. [Review]. *Journal of Psychiatry & Neuroscience : JPN, 28*(4), 275–284.

Rummel-Kluge, C., Komossa, K., Schwarz, S., Hunger, H., Schmid, F., Lobos, C. A., et al. (2010). Head-to-head comparisons of metabolic side effects of second generation antipsychotics in the treatment of schizophrenia: A systematic review and meta-analysis. *Schizophrenia Research, 123*(2–3), 225–233. doi: S0920–9964(10)01427–1 [pii] 10.1016/j.schres.2010.07.012

Scully, P. J., Coakley, G., Kinsella, A., & Waddington, J. L. (1997). Psychopathology, executive (frontal) and general cognitive impairment in relation to duration of initially untreated versus subsequently treated psychosis in chronic schizophrenia. [Research Support, Non-U.S. Government]. *Psychological Medicine, 27*(6), 1303–1310.

Takeuchi, H., Suzuki, T., Uchida, H., Watanabe, K., & Mimura, M. (2012). Antipsychotic treatment for schizophrenia in the maintenance phase: A systematic review of the guidelines and algorithms. *Schizophrenia Research, 134*(2–3), 219–225. doi: S0920–9964(11)00619–0 [pii] 10.1016/j.schres.2011.11.021

Tohen, M., Stoll, A. L., Strakowski, S. M., Faedda, G. L., Mayer, P. V., Goodwin, D. C., et al. (1992). The McLean First-Episode Psychosis Project: Six-month recovery and recurrence outcome. [Research Support, Non-U.S. Government Research Support, U.S. Government, P.H.S.]. *Schizophrenia Bulletin, 18*(2), 273–282.

Tollefson, G. D., Beasley, C. M., Jr., Tamura, R. N., Tran, P. V., & Potvin, J. H. (1997). Blind, controlled, long-term study of the comparative incidence of treatment-emergent tardive dyskinesia with olanzapine or haloperidol. [Clinical Trial Comparative Study Randomized Controlled Trial Research Support, Non-U.S. Government]. *The American Journal of Psychiatry, 154*(9), 1248–1254.

Wirshing, D. A., Wirshing, W. C., Kysar, L., Berisford, M. A., Goldstein, D., Pashdag, J., et al. (1999). Novel antipsychotics: Comparison of weight gain liabilities. [Clinical Trial Comparative Study]. *The Journal of Clinical Psychiatry, 60*(6), 358–363.

World Health Organization, & International Early Psychosis Association. (2004). Early Psychosis Declaration: An International Consensus Statement about Early Intervention and Recovery for Young People with Early Psychosis.

Wyatt, R. J. (1995). Early intervention for schizophrenia: Can the course of the illness be altered? [Editorial]. *Biological Psychiatry, 38*(1), 1–3. doi: 10.1016/0006-3223(95)00191-I

Wyatt, R. J., Green, M. F., & Tuma, A. H. (1997). Long-term morbidity associated with delayed treatment of first admission schizophrenic patients: A re-analysis of the Camarillo State Hospital data. [Clinical Trial Randomized Controlled Trial]. *Psychological Medicine, 27*(2), 261–268.

Zhang-Wong, J., Zipursky, R. B., Beiser, M., & Bean, G. (1999). Optimal haloperidol dosage in first-episode psychosis. [Clinical Trial Research Support, Non-U.S. Government]. *Canadian Journal of pPsychiatry. Revue Canadienne de Psychiatrie, 44*(2), 164–167.

24
Medication Adherence: Specific Issues in Early Psychosis in Asia

Christy Lai-ming Hui

In psychotic disorders including schizophrenia, the risk of relapse increases five-fold upon discontinuation of treatment. This chapter discusses issues related to medication adherence in psychosis, paying particular attention to patients in the early stage of illness.

Challenges Posed in Different Stages of the Illness

With regard to medication adherence in psychosis, a variety of challenges are involved at different stages of the illness. At first presentation to clinic, most first-episode psychosis patients are experiencing full-blown hallucinations and/or delusions. During this period, things or people in the environment may carry special meanings or appear absurd to the patients, including the antipsychotic medication given to them. It is therefore not uncommon to see patients holding a sceptical attitude towards medication, which leads to non-adherence. This is especially problematic when patients lack insight into their illness.

In the remission stage as psychotic symptoms subside, the use of antipsychotics acquires a new meaning; apart from controlling symptoms in the treatment phase, it is now also used for preventing relapse in the maintenance phase of the illness, even when the patient no longer has any positive symptoms. With psychoeducation, patients are usually well-informed about the importance of maintenance medication to prevent relapse. However, despite this knowledge, non-adherence is still prevalent. A number of limiting factors make applying knowledge learned from psychoeducation into practice challenging. For example, some patients consider themselves recovered and thus free of any need for medication, just as when drugs can be stopped once the flu is gone. In a study on the perceived extent of recovery in first-episode remitted schizophrenic patients, 90% of them considered themselves not fully recovered, and "the need to continue with medication" was one of the main reasons for their subjective non-recovery (Chen et al., 2005) (see Chapter 29, "Recovery from Psychosis"). Others were disturbed by the medication side-effects. For instance, young patients may not be able to tolerate the side-effect of weight gain, even when they are also aware of the beneficial effects of medication. Stigmatization in the workplace or at school is another limiting factor for good adherence.

From time to time, patients may have many queries about medications (see Chapter 23, "Pharmacological Intervention in Early Psychosis"). Apart from basic drug information and the side-effects profile, a challenging question is when to stop taking medication. Given the complex course of psychotic disorders, there is no easy answer to this question. The important issue is to weigh costs against benefits. However, while some people can go off medication completely, others relapse despite being on medication with strong adherence.

Relapse directly affects how patients view medications, and subsequently their adherence behaviours. On one hand, some may become very pessimistic and powerless, thus unable to reflect on their own situation, and adherence is often a consequence of this sense of powerlessness. On the other hand, some may have good adherence after a relapse episode, with improved risk perception following a fear-provoking critical event. However, the heightened perceived risk may not be sustained for long, and the dread of relapse may fade with time and be overtaken by the "default" risk perception. Therefore, continuous efforts are needed throughout the course of treatment to maintain insight.

Tip 1

Perceived risk is often highest after critical events, so it is an opportune timing to educate patients regarding the importance of medication adherence soon after a relapse. However, staff should always bear in mind that this sense of importance will gradually decrease with time. This highlights the view that medication adherence intervention should not be seen as something one-off, but as an ongoing long-term, interactive programme.

Adherence Attitudes and Behaviours

The classification of adherence into attitude and behaviour guides different intervention strategies. Social psychology suggests that attitude does not always equate with behaviours. Thus, a patient's awareness of the benefits of medication and the importance of adherence does not necessarily mean that he or she will take the medications as prescribed in view of the likely challenges.

Tip 2

Even if the patient reaffirms his or her faith in medications, adherence should not be taken for granted, as attitude does not always lead to subsequent behaviour of taking medication.

Non-adherent behaviours can be further divided into intentional and unintentional. Some patients simply forget to take medications occasionally when they are, for example, studying too hard for an examination or rushing to work in the morning. However, some patients skip or stop medications on purpose, and it is crucial for staff to explore the reasons behind these behaviours.

Tip 3

Differentiating non-adherent behaviours into intentional and unintentional informs intervention strategies. In handling intended non-adherence, the focus should be on knowledge and reasoning, whereas for unintended non-adherence, different delivery methods or reminder systems may be indicated.

The process of attitude formation is a dynamic one, which changes from time to time during the course of the illness. Inpatients who have just started taking medications, their perception of them could be shaped by intensive psychoeducation, and thus should be handled with great care. A vicious cycle develops if poor adherence leads to a relapse, which in turn results in demoralization and loss of hope, as well as further negative feelings towards medications.

Tip 4

Grab the chance to deliver psychoeducation to patients with recent onset of a psychotic disorder before they experience any relapse and feel demoralized.

Why Is Medication Non-Adherence Difficult to Detect?

Non-adherence behaviour can be assessed directly and indirectly. One obvious way is to ask patients directly and assess the self-report. The answer they provide is often a result of many interacting factors, for instance, how tactful the interviewer is when asking the question, the rapport between the two parties, and the mental state of the patient. In particular, the response depends on how willing the patients are to tell the truth. First, patients may be afraid of the consequences, which include possible re-hospitalization or depot medication. Second, patients who feel better may want to experiment stopping medication on their own to avoid stigma associated with regular intake of antipsychotics, and see if they could get away with it, despite the risk of relapse as advised. In this case, patients would be reluctant to reveal their hidden agenda to others. An adherence judgement based on patients' own account is thus limited in many ways.

Tip 5

A programme to manage relapse and non-adherence is essential, which should involve the patient making an informed decision about maintenance medication and being supported by the clinical team in that decision.

Tip 6

Establishing good long-term rapport with patients can facilitate accurate verbal reports from them about medication adherence.

Apart from direct questioning, non-adherent behaviours can be probed by indirect questioning techniques. However, too much probing may hamper rapport. Some other measures are therefore suggested to help estimate medication adherence. One of them is the device of Medication Event Monitoring System (MEMS), which records the date and time of every opening of medication bottles. However, the number of times the medication bottle is opened is not necessary equivalent to the number of pills taken every day, as the system can be cheated by simply opening the bottle without taking any pill. Biological measures, such as blood tests, also do not guarantee accurate assessment, as results can be affected by different individual absorption rates. Reports from family members can sometimes help detect non-adherence.

Tip 7

There is no single method that could perfectly detect non-adherence, and each test has its own limitations; a combination of methods is often more revealing.

A Case Study of Non-Adherence in Psychosis Patients in Hong Kong

Although there is no perfect way of detecting non-adherence, it is nevertheless worth knowing how skilled clinicians are in noticing non-adherence behaviours. A study was carried out to help understand the cardinal issues of the problem (Hui et al., 2006). A self-administered adherence questionnaire was used to detect non-adherence. To facilitate self-reporting and minimize under-reporting, patients filled in the questionnaires in the absence of their clinicians, and were reassured that clinicians would have no knowledge about their answers.

The study included 484 schizophrenic patients aged 18 to 65 years from four outpatient clinics in Hong Kong. Patients were asked to complete a self-rated questionnaire, the Medication Adherence Rating Scale (MARS), while clinicians completed a questionnaire with some items overlapping with MARS; their results were then compared. Patients were further divided into an early group (illness duration of less than five years) and chronic group (illness duration of more than five years) to examine the potential issues involved in different disease stages. In summary, results suggest that clinicians generally underestimated non-adherence attitude (e.g., feeling embarrassed about medications) in both early (38% vs. 21%) and chronic patients (22% vs. 16%) and did not recognize the non-adherence behaviours in early, but not chronic, patients (Table 24.1).

In this study, sensitivity and specificity rates were also used to explore how accurate clinicians were in identifying patients with non-adherence behaviours. In early psychosis patients, sensitivity rate for "forgetting to take medication" was 0.35, which means that clinicians can identify one-third of patients who have forgotten to take medication. Specificity rate was 0.82, meaning that clinicians can identify about 80% of patients who have not forgotten to take medication. In general, for both early and chronic psychosis patients, the overall sensitivity was low for clinicians' detection of non-adherence behaviours, while the specificity was high (Table 24.2).

Table 24.1

Ratings on Medication Adherence Rating Scale

	Patients' Self-reports		Clinicians' Perceptions	
	Early	Chronic	Early	Chronic
Attitude item				
Feel embarrassed about medication	38%	22%	21%	16%
Behaviour items				
Forget to take medication	38%	17%	25%	17%
Decide to stop medication	25%	14%	13%	27%

Note: Early group: n = 229; Chronic group: n = 255

Table 24.2

Sensitivity and specificity of clinicians' detection of non-adherent behaviours

	Early Group (n=229)		Chronic Group (n=255)	
	Sensitivity	Specificity	Sensitivity	Specificity
Forget to take medication	0.35	0.82	0.30	0.86
Decide to stop medication	0.32	0.93	0.29	0.73

Tip 8

Clinicians may under-recognize non-adherence behaviours in patients. The situation is far more serious in patients who have been ill for only a short period of time. Compared with the detection of overall non-adherence rate in a group of patients, more work is needed to facilitate identification of individuals with non-adherent behaviours.

Conclusion

In Chinese culture, clinicians are generally perceived as authoritative figures. With most patients believing in their clinicians and dutifully complying with their advice and requests, non-adherent behaviours in Chinese patients may appear a lesser problem compared with that in the West. Nevertheless, approximately 40% of schizophrenic patients in Hong Kong have problems of non-adherence associated with forgetting to take medication. This finding is similar to that reported by Coldham, Addington, and Addington (2002) in a Western population. It is also acknowledged that with possible under-reporting when using a self-administered questionnaire, the 40% non-adherence rate may be an underestimation of non-compliance to medications in early psychosis patients. To sum up, non-adherence is an important issue worldwide that should not be neglected by early intervention services.

References

Chen, E. Y., Tam, D. K., Wong, J. W., Law, C. W., & Chiu, C. P. (2005). Self-administered instrument to measure the patient's experience of recovery after first-episode psychosis: Development and validation of the Psychosis Recovery Inventory. [Validation Studies]. *The Australian and New Zealand Journal of Psychiatry, 39*(6), 493–499. doi: 10.1111/j.1440–1614.2005.01609.x

Coldham, E. L., Addington, J., & Addington, D. (2002). Medication adherence of individuals with a first episode of psychosis. [Research Support, Non-U.S. Government]. *Acta Psychiatrica Scandinavica, 106*(4), 286–290.

Hui, C. L., Chen, E. Y., Kan, C. S., Yip, K. C., Law, C. W., & Chiu, C. P. (2006). Detection of non-adherent behaviour in early psychosis. [Research Support, Non-U.S. Government]. *The Australian and New Zealand Journal of Psychiatry, 40*(5), 446–451. doi: 10.1111/j.1440–1614.2006.01821.x

Part VI

Handling Specific Challenges

25
Relapse Intervention and Related Issues

Christy Lai-ming Hui

Having a psychotic disease is unlike other illnesses in the sense that it significantly alters a person's normal experience. As the metaphor "fish is the last to discover water" goes, the ability to perceive reality is so basic a process that seems effortless and unnoticeable to most of us. Thus, it is hard to imagine how a person functions when this ability is disturbed.

This chapter explores an important aftermath of psychosis, namely relapse after a first episode of psychosis. Special attention will be given to relapse rates, relapse predictors, and maintenance medication to prevent relapse. Local prospective data of patients with first-episode psychosis are discussed to illustrate the relapse.

Relapse

Patients pass through different stages in the course of their illness. After an initial episode of psychosis, some patients experience a complete remission when the positive symptoms subside; others may go into a stable condition with some residual symptoms. The likelihood of relapse (i.e., re-emergence of psychotic symptoms) varies, and may be related to the level of residual or subthreshold symptoms. On one hand, both residual and subthreshold symptoms have a role in heightening the risk for relapse. On the other hand, environmental factors such as the extent of social support and stress levels may either instigate or prevent a relapse from occurring. The complex interactions between these internal and external factors may serve as a framework for understanding relapse in psychosis.

Costs of Relapse

The costs of relapse can be tremendous to patients, their families, and society as a whole. At the societal level, more support would be needed for mental health service because of the increased hospitalizations and treatment costs. Within the family, apart from the psychological distress, the financial burden may also be great, especially if the patient is the breadwinner in the family. To patients, there may be a need for re-admission to the psychiatric ward, resulting in disruptions in their work and social life, which are sometimes irreversible. The anxiety and frustrations faced by the patients can be devastating, altering their perceptions of the illness and future recovery. The re-experience of psychotic symptoms can be highly distressing too, particularly in patients who have just "settled" from their first-episode psychosis and were hoping that the illness would not return.

Relapse Rates

Relapse rates in first-episode patients from both naturalistic and controlled studies illustrate how common relapse is following the first episode. However, the reported rates vary among studies, depending on subject selection, follow-up periods, research design, and definition of relapse. In general, five-year relapse rates were found to be around 70% to 82% (Robinson et al., 1999; Shepherd et al., 1989; The Scottish Schizophrenia Research Group, 1992), and that for two years ranged between 47% and 70% (Crow et al., 1986; Johnstone et al., 1986; Johnstone et al., 1990; Sartorius et al., 1986; The Scottish Schizophrenia Research Group, 1992).

Longitudinal follow-up studies provide meaningful data in which the pattern of changes during the course of the illness can be detected. That said, long-term follow-up studies are difficult to implement, as they are expected to have a high patient dropout rate and require intensive resource input. The Nottingham study by Mason et al. (1996) followed up first-episode patients for 13 years. They found that after an initial episode, the course was relatively stable with no major deterioration or amelioration, but the relapse rate was 82%. Another 20-year follow-up study in Madras confirmed that most of the patients (n=61) had multiple relapses, with or without complete remission in between (Thara, 2004).

Relapse Predictors

Predictors of relapse have been studied intensively for their important implications in clinical intervention. Ideally, with these predictors, clinicians can better identify those patients who are at risk of relapse. However, most studies on relapse predictors have been carried out in chronic rather than first-episode patients; the former may be a biased sample with over-representation of patients with repeated relapses.

Among first-episode studies, substantial empirical evidence shows that expressed emotion (Linszen, Dingemans & Lenior, 1994) and medication non-adherence (Crow et al., 1986; Csernansky & Schuchart, 2002; Gitlin et al., 2001; Kane et al., 1982; Linszen et al., 1994; Rabiner, Wegner & Kane, 1986) predict relapses. A study in Hong Kong also confirmed the role of medication non-adherence in first-episode patients (Chen et al., 2005).

Predictors of relapse also include younger age (Csernansky & Schuchart, 2002; Gilbert et al., 1995; Hershon, Kennedy & McGuire, 1972; Prien, Cole & Belkin, 1969; Rassidakis et al., 1970; Zander et al., 1981), longer duration of untreated psychosis (Crow et al., 1986), substance abuse (Csernansky & Schuchart, 2002; Linszen et al., 1994) and poorer premorbid functioning (e.g., poor adaptation and social withdrawal) (Kane et al., 1982; Rabiner et al., 1986; Robinson et al., 1999). Relapse is also associated with persistent negative and disorganization symptoms (Linszen et al., 1994), affective symptoms (Rabiner et al., 1986) and residual psychopathology (Csernansky & Schuchart, 2002; Doering et al., 1998).

Maintenance Medication: For How Long?

As mentioned above, medication non-adherence is a strong and consistent predictor of relapse in psychosis. In other words, there is a high chance of relapse in patients who do not take their medication as prescribed.

While this may immediately lead to issues such as improving medication compliance and detecting non-adherence behaviours, a cardinal question should be asked first: "For how long does the medication have to be taken to prevent a relapse?" At present, in general clinical practice, the advice is simply medication needs to be continuous. There is little research to address this seemingly simple question as to how long medication should be continued, despite the fact that this is a question encountered by clinicians and other mental health workers on a daily basis. More recently, a randomized controlled study in Hong Kong has provided data for consideration, which will be discussed in the next section.

In general, it is common practice to advise patients to continue taking medication for a longer, often unspecified period of time, even if their positive symptoms have subsided. However, considerations should be given to the side-effects associated with lifelong medication, and the fact that although maintenance medication reduces the chance of relapse, it does not guarantee being free from relapses. Some patients may also try to stop the medication on their own against the clinician's advice. On the other hand, in selected patients who demonstrate good recovery, a planned trial of stopping medication may be carried out, with regular monitoring of at least two years after the withdrawal (National Institute for Health and Clinical Excellence, 2009). With early intervention services, patients and clinicians are more open to discussing this latter option of planned discontinuation. In a study in Hong Kong comparing an early intervention group with a standard care group, although the same relapse rate has been observed, the early intervention group had nevertheless fewer days of hospitalization, milder symptoms, fewer suicides, and disengagement (Chen et al., 2011), suggesting that the event of a relapse may not be as devastating an experience with careful monitoring and good support.

Relapse Prevention Studies in Hong Kong

In 1997, a study investigated the relapse rates and potential relapse predictors in a sample of first-episode patients in Hong Kong (Chen et al., 2005). A total of 93 patients were followed up for three years to regularly assess their psychopathology, cognitive functions (e.g., working memory, verbal memory, executive function), medication adherence, and relapse. Although this study did not directly address the important question of duration of maintenance medication, it is one of the few studies that looked into cognitive predictors of relapse in first-episode psychosis.

Data from the study showed that 60% (n=55) of patients experienced no relapse during the three years of follow up. The cumulative relapse rate was 21% (n=19) in the first year, which increased to 33% (n=31) by the end of the second year, and 40% (n=37) by the end of the third year. Of these patients, 27% (n=25) experienced a single relapse and 13% (n=12) experienced two or more relapses. Using a logistic regression model to explore the potential predictors for relapse, it was found that perseverative errors in the Wisconsin Card Sorting Test and medication non-adherence were significant predictors of relapse.

A more recent randomized controlled relapse prevention trial has been completed in Hong Kong to address the question of whether antipsychotics can be discontinued after a stable period of maintenance treatment. In this study, 178 first-episode patients who had fully remitted and taken medications for more than one year were followed up for another year; half of the patients were randomized into a maintenance group, and half into a placebo group (i.e., medication discontinuation). Results showed that the relapse rate after discontinuation was high (79%) compared with patients who continued treatment (41%). The findings supported maintenance treatment even in well-stabilized patients beyond one year of treatment (Chen et al., 2010).

Summary

The exploration of risk factors and processes involved in relapse is important. Discussion so far has highlighted the significant role of medication adherence in preventing relapse in first-episode psychosis. Besides, the cognitive predictor (perseverative errors) identified suggested that error correction based on feedback system might be an important process. Further empirical work has to be carried out before the results can be applied to clinical use with patients to predict relapse.

Although the high relapse rate in first-episode patients may be depressing, some patients do function well without continued medication; and that with careful monitoring, a relapse may not be as disruptive and frightening an experience to patients and families. This fact is a hopeful sign.

References

Chen, E. Y., Hui, C. L., Dunn, E. L., Miao, M. Y., Yeung, W. S., Wong, C. K., et al. (2005). A prospective 3-year longitudinal study of cognitive predictors of relapse in first-episode schizophrenic patients. *Schizophrenia Research, 77*(1), 99–104. doi: S0920-9964(05)00086-1 [pii]10.1016/j.schres.2005.02.020

Chen, E. Y., Hui, C. L., Lam, M. M., Chiu, C. P., Law, C. W., Chung, D. W., et al. (2010). Maintenance treatment with quetiapine versus discontinuation after one year of treatment in patients with remitted first episode psychosis: Randomised controlled trial. *British Medical Journal, 341*, c4024. doi: 10.1136/bmj.c4024bmj.c4024 [pii]

Chen, E. Y., Tang, J. Y., Hui, C. L., Chiu, C. P., Lam, M. M., Law, C. W., et al. (2011). Three-year outcome of phase-specific early intervention for first-episode psychosis: A cohort study in Hong Kong. *Early Intervention in Psychiatry*. doi: 10.1111/j.1751-7893.2011.00279.x

Crow, T. J., MacMillan, J. F., Johnson, A. L., & Johnstone, E. C. (1986). A randomised controlled trial of prophylactic neuroleptic treatment. [Clinical Trial Randomized Controlled Trial]. *The British Journal of Psychiatry: The Journal of Mental Science, 148*, 120–127.

Csernansky, J. G., & Schuchart, E. K. (2002). Relapse and rehospitalisation rates in patients with schizophrenia: Effects of second generation antipsychotics. [Research Support, Non-U.S. Government Research Support, U.S. Government, P.H.S. Review]. *CNS drugs, 16*(7), 473–484.

Doering, S., Muller, E., Kopcke, W., Pietzcker, A., Gaebel, W., Linden, M., et al. (1998). Predictors of relapse and rehospitalization in schizophrenia and schizoaffective disorder. [Multicenter Study]. *Schizophrenia Bulletin, 24*(1), 87–98.

Gilbert, P. L., Harris, M. J., McAdams, L. A., & Jeste, D. V. (1995). Neuroleptic withdrawal in schizophrenic patients: A review of the literature. [Meta-Analysis Research Support, U.S. Government, Non-P.H.S. Research Support, U.S. Government, P.H.S.]. *Archives of General Psychiatry, 52*(3), 173–188.

Gitlin, M., Nuechterlein, K., Subotnik, K. L., Ventura, J., Mintz, J., Fogelson, D. L., et al. (2001). Clinical outcome following neuroleptic discontinuation in patients with remitted recent-onset schizophrenia. [Clinical Trial Randomized Controlled Trial Research Support, U.S. Government, P.H.S.]. *The American Journal of Psychiatry, 158*(11), 1835–1842.

Hershon, H. I., Kennedy, P. F., & McGuire, R. J. (1972). Persistence of extra-pyramidal disorders and psychiatric relapse after withdrawal of long-term phenothiazine therapy. [Clinical Trial Controlled Clinical Trial]. *The British Journal of Psychiatry: The Journal of Mental Science, 120*(554), 41–50.

Johnstone, E. C., Crow, T. J., Johnson, A. L., & MacMillan, J. F. (1986). The Northwick Park Study of first episodes of schizophrenia. I. Presentation of the illness and problems relating to admission. *The British Journal of Psychiatry: The Journal of Mental Science, 148*, 115–120.

Johnstone, E. C., Macmillan, J. F., Frith, C. D., Benn, D. K., & Crow, T. J. (1990). Further investigation of the predictors of outcome following first schizophrenic episodes. *The British Journal of Psychiatry: The Journal of Mental Science, 157*, 182–189.

Kane, J. M., Rifkin, A., Quitkin, F., Nayak, D., & Ramos-Lorenzi, J. (1982). Fluphenazine vs. placebo in patients with remitted, acute first-episode schizophrenia. [Clinical Trial Randomized Controlled Trial Research Support, U.S. Government, P.H.S.]. *Archives of General Psychiatry, 39*(1), 70–73.

Linszen, D. H., Dingemans, P. M., & Lenior, M. E. (1994). Cannabis abuse and the course of recent-onset schizophrenic disorders. [Research Support, Non-U.S. Government]. *Archives of General Psychiatry, 51*(4), 273–279.

Mason, P., Harrison, G., Glazebrook, C., Medley, I., & Croudace, T. (1996). The course of schizophrenia over 13 years. A report from the International Study on Schizophrenia (ISoS) coordinated by the World Health Organization. [Research Support, Non-U.S. Government]. *The British Journal of Psychiatry: The Journal of Mental Science, 169*(5), 580–586.

National Institute for Health and Clinical Excellence (Ed.). (2009). *Schizophrenia. NICE Clinical Guideline 82*. London: National Institute for Health and Clinical Excellence.

Prien, R. F., Cole, J. O., & Belkin, N. F. (1969). Relapse in chronic schizophrenics following abrupt withdrawal of tranquillizing medication. [Clinical Trial Controlled Clinical Trial]. *The British Journal of Psychiatry: The Journal of Mental Science, 115*(523), 679–686.

Rabiner, C. J., Wegner, J. T., & Kane, J. M. (1986). Outcome study of first-episode psychosis. I: Relapse rates after 1 year. *The American Journal of Psychiatry, 143*(9), 1155–1158.

Rassidakis, N. C., Kondakis, X., Papanastassiou, A., & Michalakeas, A. (1970). Withdrawal of antipsychotic drugs from chronic psychiatric patients. [Clinical Trial]. *Bulletin of the Menninger Clinic, 34*(4), 216–222.

Robinson, D., Woerner, M. G., Alvir, J. M., Bilder, R., Goldman, R., Geisler, S., et al. (1999). Predictors of relapse following response from a first episode of schizophrenia or schizoaffective disorder. [Research Support, Non-U.S. Government Research Support, U.S. Government, P.H.S.]. *Archives of General Psychiatry, 56*(3), 241–247.

Sartorius, N., Jablensky, A., Korten, A., Ernberg, G., Anker, M., Cooper, J. E., & Day, R. (1986). Early manifestations and first-contact incidence of schizophrenia in different cultures. A preliminary report on the initial evaluation phase of the WHO Collaborative Study on determinants of outcome of severe mental disorders. [Comparative Study Research Support, Non-U.S. Government Research Support, U.S. Government, P.H.S.]. *Psychological Medicine, 16*(4), 909–928.

Shepherd, M., Watt, D., Falloon, I., & Smeeton, N. (1989). The natural history of schizophrenia: A five-year follow-up study of outcome and prediction in a representative sample of schizophrenics. [Research Support, Non-U.S. Government]. *Psychological Medicine. Monograph Supplement, 15*, 1–46.

Thara, R. (2004). Twenty-year course of schizophrenia: The Madras Longitudinal Study. [Research Support, Non-U.S. Government]. *Canadian Journal of Psychiatry. Revue Canadienne de Psychiatrie, 49*(8), 564–569.

The Scottish Schizophrenia Research Group. (1992). The Scottish first episode schizophrenia study. VIII. Five-year follow-up: Clinical and psychosocial findings. The Scottish Schizophrenia Research Group. [Clinical Trial Comparative Study]. *British Journal of Psychiatry, 161*, 496–500.

Zander, K. J., Fischer, B., Zimmer, R., & Ackenheil, M. (1981). Long-term neuroleptic treatment of chronic schizophrenic patients: Clinical and biochemical effects of withdrawal. *Psychopharmacology, 73*(1), 43–47.

26
Suicide and Self-Harm Behaviour in Early Psychosis

Edwin Pui-fai Pang

Suicide and Psychosis

Suicide has a strong association with psychosis and contributes to its high mortality. In a meta-analysis conducted in 1997, Harris and Barraclough (1997) showed that the overall suicide risk for schizophrenia was 8.5 times that of the general population. As with other disorders, precise identification of risk factors may assist clinicians in managing suicide risk among patients with psychosis. For this purpose, researchers have been looking into the risk factors, using a broad array of methodological designs of various scientific rigours. Hawton et al. (2005) conducted a systematic review of cohort and case-control studies to provide valid estimates of risk factors for suicide in schizophrenia. The authors categorized selected studies to reflect the strength of study design according to the international standard set forth for systematic review (Sackett, Haynes & Tugwell, 1991). They revealed that while sharing similar risk factors for suicide with the general population, patients with schizophrenia might possess certain specific risk factors for suicide. The suicide risk is related less to the core psychotic features of the disorder and more to affective symptoms, agitation or motor restlessness, and to awareness that the illness is affecting their mental functioning.

Risk Factors for Suicide in Psychotic Disorders

Socio-demographic factors

A greater suicide risk is associated with the male gender. It was estimated that about 60% to 90% of suicides in schizophrenia were committed by men

(De Hert, McKenzie & Peuskens, 2001; Drake et al., 1984; Heila et al., 1997). Advanced age is associated with suicide in the general population but not as robustly in schizophrenia patients. The risk of suicide appears to peak during young adulthood (Breier & Astrachan, 1984; Drake, Gates & Cotton, 1986; Heila et al., 1997; Roy, 1982). White people are more at risk than their non-white counterparts (Drake et al., 1984; Roy, 1982; Westermeyer, Harrow & Marengo, 1991). Married and cohabiting individuals are at lower risk, although being single or divorced is not a robust risk factor (Hawton et al., 2005). No association was found with religious denomination and employment status (Hawton et al., 2005).

Personal, social, and family history

Higher education is associated with greater risk. In a study by Drake et al. (1984), 73% of suicide victims suffering from schizophrenia had completed college education. Social isolation such as living alone and recent loss events increased suicide risk among schizophrenia patients (Hawton et al., 2005). Stressful life events and loss were not consistently identified as predictors of suicide in schizophrenic patients (Chan, Chen & Chan, 2003). A family history of depression is correlated with suicide risk, and the same applies to family history of suicide (De Hert et al., 2001).

Clinical characteristics

Diagnosis

The paranoid subtype of schizophrenia is generally believed to be more prevalent among suicide victims with schizophrenia. Fenton (2000) postulated that the relatively higher premorbid functioning and shorter course of illness experienced among patients with this subtype might partially explain their over-representation in suicide victims.

Symptoms

The association between positive symptoms and suicide risk remains inconclusive, as seen from the conflicting results of four previous studies (De Hert et al., 2001; Havaki-Kontaxaki, 1994; Hu, Sun & Lee, 1991; Taiminen, 1994). In fact, hallucinations and delusions are paradoxically associated with a reduced risk of suicide (Hawton et al., 2005). The findings appear to be at odds with the clinical impression that command hallucinations might cause patients to commit suicide (Barraclough et al., 1974; Planansky & Johnston, 1973).

Similar to positive symptoms, results of a meta-analysis concerning negative symptoms are not conclusive. Westermeyer et al. (1991) were able to demonstrate higher severity of negative symptoms among suicidal patients with schizophrenia as compared to non-suicidal patients. In contrast, Fenton (2000) found a protective effect with flat affect, social withdrawal, and poverty of speech. Affective symptoms such as agitation, sense of hopelessness, worthlessness, and fear of mental disintegration were associated with suicide (Drake et al., 1986; Steblaj, Tavear & Dernovsek, 1999). Although it was suggested that improvement of insight into one's own illness and its consequences might lead to depression (Chan, Yip & Au, 2005), there was considerable heterogeneity in study results in respect of insight in predicting suicide (Hawton et al., 2005). Concerning treatment adherence, suicide risk was considerably increased in individuals poorly engaged with treatment (De Hert et al., 2001; Drake et al., 1986; Roos, Boraine & Bodemer, 1992; Steblaj et al., 1999).

Suicidal attempts

A history of attempted suicide strongly increases the risk of subsequent suicide, based on the results of a systematic review of 22 studies (Hawton et al., 2005). Suicide was shown to be linked to both past and recent suicidal ideation. In a study conducted by Drake and Ehrlich (1985), 73% of suicide victims with history of schizophrenia had harboured suicidal ideation prior to the act.

Comorbid disorders and behaviour

Depression is strongly associated with suicide in schizophrenia (Cheng, Leung & Lo, 1990; De Hert et al., 2001; Havaki-Kontaxaki et al., 1994; Hu et al., 1991; Roy, 1982). Both current and past episodes of depression indicate higher risk. Suicide risk is considerably increased in the presence of drug misuse or dependence (Casadebaig & Phillipe, 1999; Modestin, Zarro & Waldvogel, 1992; Roos et al., 1992; Shah & Ganescvaran, 1999). In respect of alcohol misuse or dependence, the association with suicide risk is less conclusive (Hawton et al., 2005).

Personality variables

Among the personality traits in patients with schizophrenia, impulsivity is associated with elevated risk (Brown et al., 1991; Williams, Davidson & Montgomery, 1980). Data from Hong Kong suggest that suicidal ideation is positively correlated with more stressful life events, more hopelessness, a more negative future outlook, higher cognitive impulsivity, poorer internal locus of control, as well as survival and coping beliefs, and fear of social disapproval (HKU Study on Suicidal ideation in Early Psychosis Youths, 2010).

High-risk period

Evidence suggests that schizophrenia patients are more likely to take their lives during the early phase and within the first ten years of illness (Caldwell & Gottesman, 1992; Mortensen & Juel, 1993). As with patients suffering other forms of mental illness such as depression, schizophrenia patients admitted as hospital inpatients are at high risk of suicide (Stanard, 2000). The suicide risk tends to extend beyond discharge (Appleby et al., 1999). The National Confidential Inquiry into Suicide and Homicide in the UK pointed out that a quarter of all deaths occurred within the first three months of discharge from a psychiatric hospital. Hong Kong data have shown that the suicidal ideation rate among young patients with early psychosis nearly doubles that of their healthy counterparts (40.5% and 21.1% respectively), once again highlighting the importance of early intervention, especially for young people suffering from psychosis.

Self-Harm Behaviours in Early Psychosis

Few studies have examined suicide and parasuicide in early psychosis. There is a marked difference in suicide rates between the first-episode and chronic schizophrenia patient groups. Between 15% and 26% of psychotic patients made at least one suicide attempt by their first treatment contact, and between 2% and 11% had at least one more attempt during their first year of treatment (Addington et al., 2004; Nordentoft et al., 2002; Verdoux et al., 2001).

Predictors for Self-Harm among Patients with Early Psychosis

Demographic characteristics in general fail to predict self-harm behaviour among patients with early psychosis (Addington et al., 2004; Verdoux et al., 2001). This can be related to the small sample size of existing studies and the relatively low prevalence rate for this outcome measure. Strong baseline predictors of self-harm behaviour include:

- previous history of parasuicide (Verdoux et al., 2001)
- milder positive symptoms at baseline (Verdoux et al., 2001)
- longer duration of first admission for psychosis (Verdoux et al., 2001)
- greater depression at first admission (Addington et al., 2004)
- previous history of substance use (Verdoux et al., 2001)

Approaches to Risk Assessment

Risk assessment can be defined as the process of identifying and studying hazards to reduce the probability of their occurrence (Hart, 1998). Suicide risk factors can be categorized as static, dynamic, and future (Bouch & Marshall, 2005). Static risk factors may be historical and are likely to endure for years, while dynamic risk factors tend to fluctuate in both duration and intensity, and future risk factors refer to those that may be anticipated (see Table 26.1).

How to Engage Patients in Revealing Their Suicidal Ideation?

Potentially suicidal patients seldom spontaneously express their psychological distress and suicidal thought. Healthcare professionals therefore need to handle this issue tactfully with skill and care, through establishing a strong therapeutic relationship with patients and building up effective communication channels.

Empathy

Empathy is the ability to put oneself in others' shoes to understand their feelings and the frame of mind behind those feelings that impinges upon them. To achieve this, it is desirable to focus on the patients' expressions, both verbal and non-verbal.

Table 26.1
Static, dynamic and future risk factors for suicide

Static factors	Dynamic factors	Future factors
• History of self-harm • Seriousness of previous suicidality • Previous hospitalization • History of mental disorder • History of substance use disorder • Personality disorder/ traits • Childhood adversity • Family history of suicide • Age, gender, and marital status	• Suicidal ideation, communication, and intent • Hopelessness • Active psychological symptoms • Treatment adherence • Substance use • Psychiatric admission and discharge • Psychosocial stress • Problem-solving deficits	• Access to preferred method of suicide • Future service contact • Future response to drug treatment • Future response to psychosocial intervention • Future stress

Open-ended questions

Open-ended questions facilitate patients' elaboration of their own problems using their own frame of mind, thus avoiding premature interpretation and interruption (e.g., "How can I help you?", "Could you tell me what brings you here today?").

Reflective listening

This encompasses the ability to show understanding of what patients have said and how they feel (e.g., "When you talked about the 'voice' that has been troubling you, I could sense that you were very upset about it"). There are two levels of reflection: on the content itself and the emotion behind the content.

Non-verbal cues

Non-verbal cues include three aspects: physical, emotional, and interpersonal. Physical cues include the patient's appearance, body-built, and level of energy; emotional cues include the patient's facial expression, eye contact, tone of speech, and posture; and interpersonal cues are the way the patient relates to the worker.

Preliminary Screening for Suicide Risk

Several questions may be asked to preliminarily screen for suicide risk in patients. For example, "Have you had the feeling that life would be better off dead?", "Have you ever had the idea that life is not worth living?", "Have you ever come up with any idea of taking your own life?", "Have you actually done anything to take your life?"

Summary

Although suicide is by and large a relatively uncommon event even in disorders such as psychosis, its occurrence will always be a tragedy not only to the deceased but also to the surviving family and society at large.

Suicide is a potentially preventable outcome among patients with psychosis. The main factors to be taken into account are the clinicians' and workers' sensitivity and communication skills in detecting the suicide risk factors, which are often elusive at the outset. Clinicians and workers need also to understand the dynamic nature of suicide risk factors and the importance of systematic evaluation in any patient with psychosis.

References

Addington, J., Williams, J., Young, J., & Addington, D. (2004). Suicidal behaviour in early psychosis. [Research Support, Non-U.S. Government]. *Acta Psychiatrica Scandinavica, 109*(2), 116–120.

Appleby, L., Dennehy, J. A., Thomas, C. S., Faragher, E. B., & Lewis, G. (1999). Aftercare and clinical characteristics of people with mental illness who commit suicide: A case-control study. [Research Support, Non-U.S. Government]. *Lancet, 353*(9162), 1397–1400. doi: 10.1016/S0140–6736(98)10014–4

Barraclough, B., Bunch, J., Nelson, B., et al. (1974). A hundred cases of suicide: Clinical aspects. *British Journal of Psychiatry, 125*, 355–373.

Bouch, J., & Marshall, J. J. (2005). Suicide risk: Structured professional judgement. *Advances in Psychiatric Treatment, 11*, 84–91.

Breier, A., & Astrachan, B. M. (1984). Characterization of schizophrenic patients who commit suicide. *The American Journal of Psychiatry, 141*(2), 206–209.

Brown, L. K., Overholser, J., Spirito, A., & Fritz, G. K. (1991). The correlates of planning in adolescent suicide attempts. *Journal of American Academy of Child and Adolescent Psychiatry, 30*, 95–99.

Caldwell, C. B., & Gottesman I. I. (1992). Schizophrenia-a high risk factor for suicide: Clues to risk reduction. *Suicide and Life Threatening Behaviour, 22*, 479–493.

Casadebaig, F., & Philippe, A. (1999). Mortality in schizophrenic patients: Three-year follow-up of a cohort. *Encephale, 25*, 329–337.

Chan, H., Chen, E. Y., & Chan, R. C. (2003). Suicide in Schizophrenia. *Medical Progress, 30*, 9–15.

Chan, K. P. M., Yip, P. S. F., & Au, J. (2005). Charcoal-burning suicide in post-transition Hong Kong. *British Journal of Psychiatry, 186*, 67–73.

Cheng, K. K., Leung, C. M., Lo, W. H., et al. (1990). Risk factors of suicide among schizophrenics. *Acta Psychiatrica Scandinavica, 81*, 220–224.

De Hert, M., McKenzie, K., & Peuskens, J. (2001). Risk factors for suicide in young people suffering from schizophrenia: A long-term follow-up study. *Schizophrenia Research, 47*(2–3), 127–134.

Drake, R. E., & Ehrlich, J. (1985). Suicide attempts associated with akathisia. *American Journal of Psychiatry, 142*, 499–501.

Drake, R. E., Gates, C., & Cotton, P. G. (1986). Suicide among schizophrenics: A comparison of attempters and completed suicides. [Comparative Study]. *The British Journal of Psychiatry: The Journal of Mental Science, 149*, 784–787.

Drake, R. E., Gates, C., Cotton, P. G., & Whitaker, A. (1984). Suicide among schizophrenics: Who is at risk? *The Journal of Nervous and Mental Diseases, 172*(10), 613–617.

Fenton, W. S. (2000). Depression, suicide, and suicide prevention on schizophrenia. *Suicide and Life Threatening Behaviour, 30*, 34–49.

Harris, E. C., & Barraclough, B. (1997). Suicide as an outcome for mental disorders. A meta-analysis. [Meta-Analysis Research Support, Non-U.S. Government]. *The British Journal of Psychiatry: The Journal of Mental Science, 170*, 205–228.

Hart, S. D. (1998). The role of psychopathy in assessing risk for violence: Conceptual and methodological issues. *Legal and Criminological Psychology, 3*, 123–140.

Havaki-Kontaxaki, B. J., Kontaxakis, V. P., Protopappa, V. A., et al. (1994). Suicides in a large psychiatric hospital: Risk factors for schizophrenic patients. *Bibliotheca Psychiatrica, 165*, 63–71.

Hawton, K., Sutton, L., Haw, C., Sinclair, J., & Deeks, J. J. (2005). Schizophrenia and suicide: Systematic review of risk factors. [Research Support, Non-U.S. Government Review]. *The British Journal of Psychiatry: the Journal of Mental Science, 187*, 9–20. doi: 10.1192/bjp.187.1.9

Heila, H., Isometsa, E. T., Henriksson, M. M., Heikkinen, M. E., Marttunen, M. J., & Lonnqvist, J. K. (1997). Suicide and schizophrenia: A nationwide psychological autopsy study on age-and sex-specific clinical characteristics of 92 suicide victims with schizophrenia. [Research Support, Non-U.S. Government]. *The American Journal of Psychiatry, 154*(9), 1235–1242.

Hong Kong University. *HKU Study on Suicidal Ideation in Early Psychosis Youths*. (2010). Hong Kong: The University of Hong Kong, Li Ka Shing Faculty of Medicine.

Hu, W. H., Sun, C. M., Lee, C. T., Peng, S. L., Lin, S. K., Shen, W. W. (1991). A clinical study of schizophrenic suicides. 42 cases in Taiwan. *Schizophrenia Research, 5*, 43–50.

Modestin, J., Zarro, I., & Waldvogel, D. (1992). A study of suicide in schizophrenic in-patients. *British Journal of Psychiatry, 160*, 398–401.

Mortensen, P. B., & Juel, K. (1993). Mortality and causes of death in first admitted schizophrenic patients. *British Journal of Psychiatry, 163*, 183–189.

Nordentoft, M., Jeppesen, P., Abel, M., Kassow, P., Petersen, L., Thorup, A., et al. (2002). OPUS study: Suicidal behaviour, suicidal ideation and hopelessness among patients with first-episode psychosis. One-year follow-up of a randomised controlled trial. [Clinical Trial Randomized Controlled Trial Research Support, Non-U.S. Government]. *The British Journal of Psychiatry. Supplement, 43*, s98–106.

Planansky, K., & Johnston, R. (1973). Clinical setting and motivation in suicidal attempts of schizophrenics. *Acta Psychiatrica Scandinavica, 49*, 680–690.

Roos, J. L., Boraine, H., & Bodemer, W. (1992). Suicide in psychiatric patients. [Sefmoord by pasiente met skisofrenie.]. *South African Medical Journal, 81*, 365–369.

Roy, A. (1982). Suicide in chronic schizophrenia. *The British Journal of Psychiatry: The Journal of Mental Science, 141*, 171–177.

Sackett, D. L., Haynes, R. B., & Tugwell, P. (1991). *Clinical Epidemiology*. Boston: Little, Brown and Co.

Shah, A., & Ganescvaran, T. (1999). Suicide among psychiatric in-patients with schizophrenia in an Australian mental hospital. *Medicine, Science, and the Law, 39*, 251–259.

Stanard, R. P. (2000). Assessment and Treatment of Adolescent Depression and Suicidality. *Journal of Mental Health Counseling, 22*(3), 204.

Steblaj, A., Tavcar, R., & Dernovsek, M. Z. (1999). Predictors of suicide in psychiatric hospital. *Acta Psychiatrica Scandinavica, 100*, 383–388.

Taiminen, T. J., & Kujari, H. (1994). Antipsychotic medication and suicide risk among schizophrenic and paranoid inpatients: A controlled retrospective study. *Acta Psychiatrica Scandinavica, 90*, 247–251.

Verdoux, H., Liraud, F., Gonzales, B., Assens, F., Abalan, F., & van Os, J. (2001). Predictors and outcome characteristics associated with suicidal behaviour in early psychosis: A two-year follow-up of first-admitted subjects. [Research Support, Non-U.S. Government]. *Acta Psychiatrica Scandinavica, 103*(5), 347–354.

Westermeyer, J. F., Harrow, M., & Marengo, J. T. (1991). Risk for suicide in schizophrenia and other psychotic and nonpsychotic disorders. [Comparative Study Research Support, Non-U.S. Government Research Support, U.S. Government, P.H.S.]. *The Journal of Nervous and Mental Diseases, 179*(5), 259–266.

Williams, C., Davidson, J., & Montgomery, I. (1980). Impulsive suicidal behaviour. *Journal of Clinical Psychology, 36*, 90–94.

27
Comorbid Substance Abuse in Early Psychosis

Sherry Kit-wa Chan and Kathy Po-man Chan

Substance misuse is prevalent among clients suffering from first-episode psychosis. Figures from the West have shown prevalence ranging from 20% to 53% (Addington & Addington, 2007; Barnett et al., 2007; Cantwell et al., 1999; Hambrecht & Hafner, 1996; Wade et al., 2006). Although less common among first-episode clients in Hong Kong, a significant proportion of the clients suffer from comorbid substance abuse. Based on the cohort of clients from the Early Assessment Service for Young People with Psychosis (EASY) programme, about 12% of clients have recently used illicit substances prior to their contact with EASY. This habit presents particular problems to the service, as comorbid substance use is associated with poorer medication adherence (Wade et al., 2006), higher rates of relapse (Linszen, Dingemans, & Lenior, 1994; Wade et al., 2006), poorer treatment response (Green et al., 2004; Wade et al., 2006; Wade et al., 2007), higher rates of suicide attempts (Kamali et al., 2000), more aggressive incidents (Dumais et al., 2011; Fazel et al., 2009; Milton et al., 2001) and poorer outcomes in symptoms and functioning (Cantor-Graae, Nordstrom, & McNeil, 2001; Wade et al. 2006; Wade et al., 2007). In addition, clients with a history of substance abuse, particularly males, have an earlier onset of psychotic illness. All these scenarios pose great challenges to the service for young, first-episode psychosis clients.

Substance Abuse among EASY Clients

In a similar way to data from the West, cannabis is the most commonly abused substance among young psychotic clients in Hong Kong. About half of the EASY clients who abuse drugs use cannabis with or without other substances. In Hong Kong, ecstasy and ketamine abuse is prevalent among young substance abusers. Not surprisingly, over one-third of substance-using EASY clients have used these two psychoactive drugs. Amphetamine, another common drug of abuse, is used by about one-third of EASY clients.

Relationship between Psychosis and Substance Misuse

The mechanism underlying the frequent comorbidity of substance abuse and psychotic disorders remains unresolved. Two main hypotheses have been proposed (Linszen & Lenior, 1999):

1. Vulnerability hypothesis: substance misuse contributes to the development of psychotic symptoms, or precipitates signs and symptoms in individuals who later become psychotic.
2. Self-medication hypothesis: clients with psychosis may attempt to alleviate the distressing symptoms of the illness, or the side-effects of medication, through the use of illicit substances.

A study by Hambrecht and Hafner (1996) has shown that both hypotheses are true for different populations. In their study, one-third of schizophrenic clients have longstanding substance abuse prior to the onset of initial symptoms, while another third clearly started their substance use after the onset of illness. When treating first-episode clients with substance abuse problems, these two possibilities should always be considered. Apart from the two hypotheses, the common sharing of underlying biological, personality and environmental factors between psychosis and substance misuse disorder has been suggested recently (Lubman, King, & Castle, 2010).

Drug-Induced Psychosis versus Psychosis with Comorbid Substance Abuse

Differentiation between drug-induced psychosis and psychosis with comorbid substance abuse is often difficult. In general, psychotic symptoms usually emerge immediately or soon after the use of substances, and these psychotic symptoms are usually short-lived once the substance use ceases. One recent study has suggested that those with drug-induced psychosis are likely to have higher level of insight, more severe hostility and anxious symptoms than those with primary psychosis (Fraser et al., 2012). Nevertheless, the boundary is often not as clear. The relationship of effects of each substance and the emergency of psychotic symptoms tends to vary.

Assessment

Detecting the substance use problem is crucial while assessing young clients with psychosis. Substance abuse is often under-recognized, especially in the early phase of treatment, as clients commonly would not volunteer the condition. An open and non-judgemental approach must be adopted during assessment. The initiation, development and progress of the substance abuse, including previous abstinence and relapse, should be evaluated, and its relationship with the psychotic illness ascertained. Abuse and psychological and/or physical dependence should also be established. Different degrees of severity call for different treatment strategies. The clients' own perception of why they take the substance, its subsequent effects and their level of motivation for any changes should be key areas for assessment. Furthermore, a detailed assessment of the psychosocial environment is essential for treatment planning. As an example, marital or family stress, peer culture, comorbid depression, and disengagement from work or school are all potential barriers for the client to abstain from substance use. Looking for potential strengths and resources, and areas for enhancement are vital. For example, a client who is motivated to work may significantly benefit from having a stable job. Not only will the job reduce his unengaged time, his aspiration to keep his job may be a powerful factor to keep him abstinent. On the other hand, clients who are easily influenced by peers may need strengthening of their assertive skills during treatment. Last but not least, a thorough medical history and physical examination should be conducted especially to look for any physical complications of substance use. Indiscreet use of toxicology screening should be avoided, although this investigation can be helpful at times to monitor drug use and determine the role of substances.

Service Model of Dual Diagnosis

Due to the complexity of the needs of clients with dual diagnosis and poorer long term prognosis, different service models have been established to better cater for their needs. A recent review study (Wisdom, Manuel, & Drake, 2011) suggested about half of the clients abstained or significantly reduced substance use after becoming engaged in the first-episode psychosis treatment programme. The specialized substance abuse programme did not provide additional benefit at the initial stage. However, the authors consider that the heterogeneous nature of this group of clients suggests a diversity of needs, implying that a stage-approach would be more effective. Provision of specialized substance abuse service at later stages would be helpful to individuals with persistent substance abuse.

Early Psychosis Prevention and Intervention Centre (EPPIC) Service Model

In many countries, including Hong Kong, services for first-episode psychosis and substance abuse are often separated; this fragmentation of service may be undesirable. Youths who abuse substances usually have little interest to treat their abuse problems. Psychotic clients with substance abuse problems are even more likely to default follow-up consultations and not adhere to treatment if they are to attend two separate services. Various well-resourced centres, such as the Early Psychosis Prevention and Intervention Centre (EPPIC) in Australia, have made initial efforts to set up integrated programmes targeting young psychotic clients with comorbid psychosis and substance abuse (Addington, Leriger, & Addington, 2003). At EPPIC, a specialty group called the Stopping Substances Group was set up within the first-episode psychosis service for those with ongoing substance use problems (Addington et al., 2003). In that explanatory model, certain individuals have a vulnerability to psychotic disorders, for example a "sensitive brain", which may be a result of genetic, neurodevelopmental, intrauterine, or perinatal insults. These factors have made the brain less resilient to certain kinds of stress compared with other individuals; substance misuse is one of these stressors. This model places emphasis on psychosis being a brain disease, with evidence supportive of substances being detrimental to the condition. Thus, the focus on avoiding substances is not one of disapproval or moral judgement. Rather, it is an issue of working with clients who have a specific disease and eliminating a behaviour that potentially compromises improvement or long-term outcomes. The Australian group believes that this is an important stance to take when dealing with these young clients. Moreover, substance misuse is not only counted as a comorbid disorder, but also a risk factor for psychosis-vulnerable individuals. Hence, psychoeducation is not only provided to psychotic youths with comorbid substance problems, but to all clients, with the intention to prevent the use of substances among clients out of an attempt to self-medicate to alleviate symptoms.

Service Model for EASY Clients

Youths attending EASY with comorbid substance abuse problems tend to have higher rates of disengagement, higher chances of non-compliance to treatment, and more relapses. For them, social and family supports are often less available. Their sleep hours may also be irregular they are more likely to have more physical complaints. Despite the usually flexible appointment for these clients, they still have a relatively high rate of disengagement. All these are difficult issues for case managers to handle. Due to limited human resources, with each case manager having a caseload exceeding 100 cases, case managers often cannot provide more intensive support and follow-up actions. Trying to fill the service gap, some of the EASY centres have close and active liaison with non-governmental organizations (NGOs) specializing in drug abuse services. The NGO social workers, with ample experience in working with clients with substance abuse problems, normally adopt a proactive outreach approach, have expertise in engaging young drug users, and provide specialized treatment and social programmes for youths abusing substances.

The joint effort has shown initial promising results. Some clients have become better engaged with the service and medical attendance and compliance to treatment have also been improved. Skills and devotion of NGO workers is an invaluable asset to the service. To enhance communication, regular meetings are held between the different service teams to discuss the management and progress of individual clients. Clients with predominant and severe substance use problems, accompanied by a short-lived or remitted drug-induced psychotic episode, may be referred to the substance abuse services for managing their substance use disorders.

Pharmacological Treatment of the Dually Diagnosed

Psychotic clients who abuse substances respond differently to conventional antipsychotics compared with those who do not. Bowers et al. (1990) found that schizophrenic clients who abused substances showed a poorer response to fixed doses of Haloperidol and Perphenazine. They postulated that such problems might be related to substance-induced alterations in the mesolimbic dopaminergic system, which is associated with motivational states and is implicated in reinforcing the actions of most drugs of abuse. Studies have also shown a higher incidence of neuroleptic-induced movement disorder and tardive dyskinesia in schizophrenic clients abusing alcohol and other substances (Dixon et al., 1992; Olivera, Kiefer, & Manley, 1990; Potvin et al., 2006). Schizophrenic clients who abused stimulants were also found to receive higher dose of conventional antipsychotics during hospitalization than those who did not (Day, Georgiou, & Crome, 2008). All these issues alert clinicians to pay special attention to the dose and choice of antipsychotics and the monitoring of side-effects.

Studies have shown that Clozapine has a favourable response in the dually diagnosed and moderate substance abuse was found not to alter the clinical response to Clozapine (Buckley et al., 1994). Moreover, reduction in substance abuse was reported in schizophrenic clients with comorbid substance use treated with Clozapine (Buckley et al., 1994; Marcus & Snyder, 1995; Tsuang et al., 1999). Nevertheless, these findings have been observed among more chronic schizophrenic clients rather than first-episode psychosis clients. There are few data available on the latter and very little evidence from large randomized controlled studies. The benefits of Clozapine in this population may be related to many factors: a low propensity for extra-pyramidal side-effects, neuroleptic-associated dysphoria, altered mesolimbic dopaminergic tone, selective antagonism of central serotonergic receptors, potential effects on negative symptoms, increased medical monitoring, and treatment contact during Clozapine therapy, which enables detection of noncompliance and enhance therapeutic alliance (Buckley, 1998). Despite interests in other atypical antipsychotics, thus far there has been little solid evidence for their effectiveness in this group of clients based on a recent review (Lubman et al., 2010). Last but not least, depot injection has been very useful in clinical experience in these clients who have a tendency to erratic medication adherence.

Role of the Case Manager

Although the meta-analysis of 25 randomized controlled trials did not support the effectiveness of any single psychosocial intervention for this group of clients (Cleary et al., 2008), an integrated approach has been advocated (Lubman et al., 2010). The case manager has an essential role as a link between the services and programmes. Besides, the case manager plays a key role in the therapeutic engagement process. As mentioned above, engagement of these clients can be notoriously difficult, demanding more persistence, and enduring flexibility and additional skills. A close working relationship with social workers specialized in substance abuse treatment or other professionals working with the client is important to enhance integration of different services and programmes. Together with that, involvement of the family is essential as clients with more supportive families often have more regular medical attendance and fewer relapses of using substances. Enhancing social and occupational functioning of the client is also beneficial in sustaining abstinence or reducing substance use.

Drug Counselling

There are various levels of drug counselling. Following the model of the Stopping Substances Group, the case manager may adopt the goals listed below, in collaboration with the client:

1. Assessment and psychoeducation. The effects of drugs, dependence, and withdrawal are explained to clients and families. Risks of continuing the substances in the context of a psychotic illness are emphasized. The client is engaged with a commitment to reduce or abstain from drug use.
2. Goal setting for harm reduction and/or abstinence. The goals should be appropriate and realistic. In cases where abstinence is not practical, harm reduction should be considered.
3. Assessing push and pull factors. Reasons for the clients' drug use and their attitude towards quitting are explored. Barriers to quitting are also identified.
4. Developing strategies to help change drug-use behaviours. Relevant skills are taught. For instance, if substance use prevails among the peers, the client has to learn to say "no". In some situations, he/she may have to change the social network. Thus, a new social environment and social skill training will be pertinent.
5. Reasons for relapse are explored. High-risk situations are identified with contingency plans.

References

Addington, J., Leriger, E., Addington, D. (2003). Symptom outcome 1-year after admission to an early psychosis program. *Canadian Journal of Psychiatry, 48*(3), 204–207.

Addington, J., & Addington, D. (2007). Patterns, predictors and impact of substance use in early psychosis: A longitudinal study. *Acta Psychiatrica Scandinavica, 115*(4), 304–309.

Barnett, J. H., Werners, U., Secher, S. M., Hill, K. E., Brazil, R., Masson, K., et al. (2007). Substance use in a population-based clinic sample of people with first-episode psychosis. *The British Journal of Psychiatry, 190*(6), 515–520.

Bowers, M. B., Jr., Mazure, C. M., Nelson, J. C., & Jatlow, P. I. (1990). Psychotogenic drug use and neuroleptic response. [Research Support, Non-U.S. Government Research Support, U.S. Government, P.H.S.]. *Schizophrenia Bulletin, 16*(1), 81–85.

Buckley, P., Thompson, P. A., Way, L., & Meltzer, H. Y. (1994). Substance abuse and clozapine treatment. [Research Support, Non-U.S. Government Research Support, U.S. Government, P.H.S.]. *The Journal of Clinical Psychiatry, 55 Supplement B*, 114–116.

Buckley, P. F. (1998). Substance abuse in schizophrenia: A review. [Research Support, Non-U.S. Government Review]. *The Journal of Clinical Psychiatry, 59 Supplement 3*, 26–30.

Cantor-Graae, E., Nordstrom, L. G., & McNeil, T. F. (2001). Substance abuse in schizophrenia: A review of the literature and a study of correlates in Sweden. [Research Support, Non-U.S. Government Review]. *Schizophrenia Research, 48*(1), 69–82.

Cantwell, R., Brewin, J., Glazebrook, C., Dalkin, T., Fox, R., Medley, I., et al. (1999). Prevalence of substance misuse in first-episode psychosis. [Research Support, Non-U.S. Government]. *The British Journal of Psychiatry: The Journal of Mental Science, 174*, 150–153.

Cleary, M., Hunt, G., Matheson, S., Siegfried, N., & Walter, G. (2008). Psychosocial treatment programs for people with both severe mental illness and substance misuse. *Schizophrenia Bulletin, 34*(2), 226–228.

Day, E., Georgiou, G., & Crome, I. (2008). Pharmcological management of substance misuse in psychosis. In *Substance Misuse in Psychosis: Approaches to Treatment and Service Delivery*, edited by H. L. Graham, A. Copello, M. J. Birchwood and K. T. Mueser. West Sussex, London: John Wiley & Sons.

Dixon, L., Weiden, P. J., Haas, G., Sweeney, J., & Frances, A. J. (1992). Increased tardive dyskinesia in alcohol-abusing schizophrenic patients. [Research Support, U.S. Government, P.H.S.]. *Comprehensive Psychiatry, 33*(2), 121–122.

Dumais, A., Potvin, S., Joyal, C., Allaire, J., Stip, E., Lesage, A., et al. (2011). Schizophrenia and serious violence: A clinical-profile analysis incorporating impulsivity and substance-use disorders. *Schizophrenia Research, 130*(1–3), 234–237.

Fazel, S., Gulati, G., Linsell, L., Geddes, J. R., & Grann, M. (2009). Schizophrenia and violence: Systematic review and meta-analysis. *PLoS Medicine, 6*(8), e1000120.

Fraser, S., Hides, L., Philips, L., Proctor, D., & Lubman, D. I. (2012). Differentiating first episode substance induced and primary psychotic disorders with concurrent substance use in young people. *Schizophrenia Research*.

Green, A. I., Tohen, M. F., Hamer, R. M., Strakowski, S. M., Lieberman, J. A., Glick, I., et al. (2004). First episode schizophrenia-related psychosis and substance use disorders: Acute response to olanzapine and haloperidol. *Schizophrenia Research, 66*(2), 125–135.

Hambrecht, M., & Hafner, H. (1996). Substance abuse and the onset of schizophrenia. [Clinical Trial Research Support, Non-U.S. Government]. *Biological Psychiatry, 40*(11), 1155–1163. doi: 10.1016/S0006-3223(95)00609-5

Kamali, M., Kelly, L., Gervin, M., Browne, S., Larkin, C., & O'Callaghan, E. (2000). The prevalence of comorbid substance misuse and its influence on suicidal ideation among in-patients with schizophrenia. [Research Support, Non-U.S. Government]. *Acta Psychiatrica Scandinavica, 101*(6), 452–456.

Linszen, D. H., Dingemans, P. M., & Lenior, M. E. (1994). Cannabis abuse and the course of recent-onset schizophrenic disorders. [Research Support, Non-U.S. Government]. *Archives of General Psychiatry, 51*(4), 273–279.

Lubman, D. I., King, J. A., & Castle, D. J. (2010). Treating comorbid substance use disorders in schizophrenia. *International Review of Psychiatry, 22*(2), 191–201.

Marcus, P., & Snyder, R. (1995). Reduction of comorbid substance abuse with clozapine. [CommentLetter]. *The American Journal of Psychiatry, 152*(6), 959.

Milton, J., Amin, S., Singh, S. P., Harrison, G., Jones, P., Croudace, T., et al. (2001). Aggressive incidents in first-episode psychosis. [Research Support, Non-U.S. Government]. *The British Journal of Psychiatry: The Journal of Mental Science, 178*, 433–440.

Olivera, A. A., Kiefer, M. W., & Manley, N. K. (1990). Tardive dyskinesia in psychiatric patients with substance use disorders. *The American Journal of Drug and Alcohol Abuse, 16*(1–2), 57–66.

Potvin, S., Pampoulova, T., Mancini-Marie, A., Lipp, O., Bouchard, R., & Stip, E. (2006). Increased extrapyramidal symptoms in patients with schizophrenia and a comorbid substance use disorder. *Journal of Neurology, Neurosurgery & Psychiatry, 77*(6), 796–798.

Tsuang, J. W., Eckman, T. E., Shaner, A., & Marder, S. R. (1999). Clozapine for substance-abusing schizophrenic patients. [Case Reports Letter]. *The American Journal of Psychiatry, 156*(7), 1119–1120.

Wade, D., Harrigan, S., Edwards, J., Burgess, P., Whelan, G., & McGorry, P. (2006). Substance misuse in first-episode psychosis: 15-month prospective follow-up study. *The British Journal of Psychiatry, 189*(3), 229–234.

Wade, D., Harrigan, S., McGorry, P. D., Burgess, P. M., & Whelan, G. (2007). Impact of severity of substance use disorder on symptomatic and functional outcome in young individuals with first-episode psychosis. *The Journal of Clinical Psychiatry, 68*(5), 767–774.

Wisdom, J. P., Manuel, J. I., & Drake, R. E. (2011). Substance use disorder among people with first-episode psychosis: A systematic review of course and treatment. *Psychiatric Services, 62*(9), 1007–1012.

28
Handling Patients with Negative Symptoms

Wing-chung Chang and Cindy Pui-yu Chiu

Manifestations of Negative Symptoms

People suffering from first-episode psychosis are often bewildered by the extraordinary experiences evolving around them, being helplessly entwined by events, which often bring turmoil into their lives. Positive psychotic symptoms may be readily understood by patients and caregivers as symptoms of an illness, whereas negative symptoms (including blunted affect, poverty of speech, avolition, apathy, and lack of social drive) are usually less easily accepted as part of the pathological process.

Case Vignette 1

"He was a bright boy, being described by teachers to be inquisitive and helpful. He was always busy with sports and extracurricular activities [mother takes out a photo from her purse showing the patient in a wide grin with his parents in front of a cake]. Now he barely does any talking and is rather impatient with us. He spends hours in his room and seems to prefer solitude. In the past he was rather picky with his clothing but now he wears the same old jacket every day. He eats a lot but hardly notices what he is eating. There is little which interests him." (Mother of Sam, 23 years old)

When positive symptoms subside with treatment, some patients may be left with a residual state or deficit state where negative symptoms predominate.

In fact, negative symptoms have long been regarded as a core feature of schizophrenia (Bleuler, 1950; Kirkpatrick et al., 2006; Kraepelin, Barclay, & Robertson, 1919). Unlike positive symptoms, negative symptoms remain an unmet therapeutic need, and are associated with poor functional outcomes (Harvey et al., 2006; Ventura et al., 2009) and limited responses to pharmacotherapy (Murphy et al., 2006).

Negative symptoms in the mild form may limit the patients' personal effectiveness as they go back to work or study. They would be less enthusiastic, look detached, and may have problems in communicating or mixing with others. They may no longer find enjoyment in their work and some may feel frustrated about the changes. Those with more prominent negative symptoms may have problems with self-care or lack motivation to return to work, leading to deterioration in functional status. In any case, an individual's recovery process is affected adversely and such diminished self-efficacy further decreases one's self-esteem. Caregivers who witness such changes may show concern. They may render the patients responsible for such changes, interpreting such behaviours as sloth or laziness. Some caregivers may react by being permissive and overprotective while others may set strict standards and criticize or act with hostility. This scenario of high expressed emotions is undesirable with consequent escalated conflicts within the family and increased risk of psychotic relapse.

What Contributes to Negative Symptoms?

Certain subtypes of schizophrenia, particularly simple schizophrenia, have pronounced negative symptoms. Numerous studies examining relationship of duration of untreated psychosis (DUP) and psychopathology in first-episode psychosis showed that prolonged DUP was associated with more severe negative symptoms at both initial presentation and follow-up (Malla et al., 2002; Marshall et al., 2005; Melle et al., 2004; Perkins et al., 2005). Several previous reports also demonstrate that patients with long DUP may have a higher likelihood of developing persistent negative symptoms (Chang et al., 2011; Chang et al., 2012; Edwards et al., 2002; Malla et al., 2005). It should, however, be noted that some investigators have suggested that it was duration of untreated illness (DUI) rather than DUP that was related to worse outcome on negative symptoms (Harris et al., 2005; Jeppesen et al., 2008). Poor premorbid adjustment, male sex, schizophrenia diagnosis and psychotic illness of neurodevelopmental origin have also been found to be related to more prominent negative symptoms (Chang et al., 2011a; Chang et al., 2011b; MacBeth & Gumley, 2008; Murray et al., 1992; Roy et al., 2001).

Differential Diagnosis of Negative Symptoms

Negative symptoms can be conceptualized and classified as primary versus secondary symptoms. Differentiating primary from secondary negative symptoms is of utmost clinical significance as the apparent negative symptoms can be much improved if secondary sources are correctly identified and properly treated.

Concerning the source of secondary negative symptoms, persecutory delusions and heightened suspiciousness with consequent social avoidance and preoccupation may mimic negative symptoms. Depression, another differential diagnosis, should show other depressive features alongside lack of interest and motivation such as biological symptoms and negative cognitions upon detailed history taking. Medications used to treat the illness may cause sedation and extra-pyramidal signs which resemble negative symptoms. Such medication side-effects can be very disabling and should be minimized as far as possible. Individuals with a history of stimulant use may complain of depression and concentration and motivation problems. Environmental deprivation and protracted hospitalization (i.e., institutionalization effect on chronic patients) may also contribute to volitional impairment, lack of social drive and diminished emotion expression. Those with a poor premorbid status such as low IQ, which may be revealed by a poor school or employment record, may have a lower functional status upon recovery and lead one to suspect the individual as having negative symptoms.

Case Vignette 2

June, a 25-year-old secretary, complained of feeling dull and unmotivated. June revealed her feelings after much prompting, "It was difficult going back to my office after several weeks of unexplainable absence . . . my colleagues might have guessed, since I had been speaking inappropriate things before I was admitted to hospital. They were very nice, giving me few tasks that were extremely easy, like checking emails. However, I didn't enjoy going to work anymore. I just did not want to do anything. I lost interest in my children and seldom initiated games with them. I could sleep reasonably well but felt tired easily in the day. I preferred to be on my own at lunch. There were times when I felt like crying because things were not the same anymore. It was then when I realized I might not get back to my old self anymore." June improved with the addition of antidepressants and psychotherapy.

Management

Early intervention

In an early psychosis service, individuals range from having little to almost no negative symptoms to a few extreme cases of gross self-neglect, prominent apathy, and marked social withdrawal. Nonetheless, negative symptoms should be checked for and treated promptly. Management aims at early and timely intervention at the initial stage of psychotic illness so as to shorten treatment delay and to reduce the risk of developing persistent negative symptoms. A flexible referral system that minimizes potential obstacles and delays in the pathway to care is one way of getting at this issue.

Role of case managers

The case managers often act as the advocate by engaging with patients and their families with the service, overseeing any needs, and being the key persons to facilitate liaison among the professionals taking care of the patient. They also give advice on treatment and offer psychoeducation. Periodic review at team meetings allows orchestration of efforts, as well as a broader perspective, hence better planning for treatment.

Medication

With regard to medication, side-effects such as sedation, neuroleptic-related dysphoria, and Parkinsonism should be avoided by cautious dose titration to minimize secondary source of negative symptoms. Research suggested that second-generation antipsychotics (SGAs) may be more effective than first-generation ones (FGAs) in treating negative symptoms. It is, however, also argued that the apparent greater reduction in severity of negative symptoms with SGAs over FGAs may mainly be attributable to minimizing antipsychotic-induced side-effects, in particular Parkinsonism features, by the former treatment (Davis, Chen, & Glick, 2003; Correll, Leucht, & Kane, 2004; Leucht et al., 2009).

Psychoeducation

Psychoeducation, including recognition of the negative symptoms, for caregivers is crucial for proper acknowledgement of the problem, realistic expectations, and appropriate attitudes. Care should be taken to avoid self-blame in patients and hostility from caregivers out of frustration and misunderstanding. Case managers have an eminent role in this work as they liaise closely with patients' families.

Tailored care plan

A tailored care plan, appropriate for the individual's capability, is devised to gently stimulate and maintain the level of activity achieved. Over-enthusiasm and excessive stimulation should be avoided while small steps and patience should be kept in mind for inducing changes. Balancing the instillation of hope, rebuilding self-confidence, and goal-setting are also important considerations. Achievable goals and reward for effort paid are implemented through psychological interventions and behavioural modification techniques.

Rehabilitation

Rehabilitation is a key treatment component in facilitating functional improvement. For school-aged patients, close liaison with teachers and school social workers not only provides important information about how the patients are doing at school, but also helps prepare the person prior to perceived stressful periods such as examinations. Advice on possible functional impairments such as concentration difficulties, drug side-effects, and negative symptoms could enhance the school's understanding and acceptance of ill students. Special arrangements such as trying to resume school by half days at the initial stages may also help the student adjust to school life.

Community day services

Services provided by NGOs help extend rehabilitation beyond the hospital and into the community, with less stigmatizing effects (see Chapter 22, "Working with Non-Governmental Organizations in Early Psychosis"). These services are tailored to the needs of the young patients and assist caregivers as well. Social skills training, occupational training, engagement in a social club, psychoeducational talks, parents groups, self-help groups are just a few examples of these contributions.

Relapse prevention

Relapse prevention is crucial to reduce risks of chronic illness, which is associated with persistent primary negative symptoms or deficit syndrome, at least in a subset of patients with schizophrenia. Depending on the individuals' treatment response, the duration of medication can vary. However, it is generally recommended that maintenance medication should be continued for an additional year after the first episode (see Chapter 25, "Relapse Intervention and Related Issues"). Education about the importance of drug compliance and relapse prevention is of paramount importance (see Chapter 24, "Medication Adherence: Specific Issues in Early Psychosis in Asia").

Case Vignette 3

"Sam was not willing to take his medication even after explanation. He would become sulky and shut himself in his room. We tried different methods at home to help with his condition, but did not succeed. Eventually, he agreed to try taking his medication after talking with the case manager, in the hope of being able to study overseas once he recovered. After several visits, he was willing to spend more time at the community centre and joined some of the groups. Sometimes he would leave after a short time, but recently he was able to stay till the group ended. He seldom talked with others, but hung out with another young man who also did not talk much but liked video games, like himself. Sometimes he would go to the videogame arcade with others. He is still not quite his old self, but he is already making visible progress. I used to think that he was just being lazy, but now I understand that he is mentally ill. I hope he will continue to improve." (Mother of Sam, 23 years old)

Service Provision and Role of Professionals

Clinical team level

Case management is useful to identify people with greatest needs, and to provide timely intervention to shorten the duration of untreated psychosis. Caregivers and patients need to be motivated to stay engaged with the service and treat the illness vigorously to minimize disruptions to work or school. Comorbidities such as mood or substance misuse need to be taken care of. Families are to be actively involved to instil hope in the early stage of illness. Rehabilitation programmes, tailored to individual needs, and case discussion meetings match needs with services and review individual cases regularly in order to revise diagnosis and make periodic clinical ratings to mark longitudinal changes.

On a macro level

Public education on symptoms including negative symptoms, as well as campaigns to enhance public knowledge and reduce stigma, are valuable. Through removal of these potential obstacles to care, the duration of untreated psychosis might be further reduced. Regular reviews of service delivery also monitor effectiveness and ensure best-practice is maintained.

References

Bleuler, E. (1950). *Dementia Praecox*. New York: International Universities Press.

Chang, W. C., Hui, C. L., Tang, J. Y., Wong, G. H., Lam, M. M., Chan, S. K., & Chen, E. Y. (2011a). Persistent negative symptoms in first-episode schizophrenia: A prospective three-year follow-up study. [Research Support, Non-U.S. Government]. *Schizophrenia Research, 133*(1–3), 22–28. doi: 10.1016/j.schres.2011.09.006

Chang, W. C., Tang, J. Y., Hui, C. L., Chiu, C. P., Lam, M. M., Wong, G. H., et al. (2011b). Gender differences in patients presenting with first-episode psychosis in Hong Kong: A three-year follow up study. [Research Support, Non-U.S. Government]. *The Australian and New Zealand Journal of Psychiatry, 45*(3), 199–205. doi: 10.3109/00048674.2010.547841

Chang, W. C., Hui, C. L., Tang, J. Y., Wong, G. H., Chan, S. K., Lee, E. H., & Chen, E. Y. (2012). Impacts of duration of untreated psychosis on cognition and negative symptoms in first-episode schizophrenia: A 3-year prospective follow-up study. *Psychological Medicine*, doi.: 10.1017/S0033291712002838.

Correll, C. U., Leucht, S., Kane, J. M. (2004). Lower risk for tardive dyskinesia associated with second-generation antipsychotics: A systematic review of 1-year studies. *American Journal of Psychiatry 161*, 414–425. doi: 10.1176/appi.ajp.161.3.414

Davis, J. M., Chen, N., Glick, I. D. (2003). A meta-analysis of the efficacy of second-generation antipsychotics. *Archives of General Psychiatry, 60*(6), 553–564. doi: 10.1001/archpsyc.60.6.553

Edwards, J., Harrigan, S. M., McGorry, P. D., & Amminger, P. G. (2002). Duration of untreated psychosis (DUP) and outcome in schizophrenia. [Comment Letter]. *Psychological Medicine, 32*(3), 563–564.

Harris, M. G., Henry, L. P., Harrigan, S. M., Purcell, R., Schwartz, O. S., Farrelly, S. E., et al. (2005). The relationship between duration of untreated psychosis and outcome: An eight-year prospective study. [Research Support, Non-U.S. Government]. *Schizophrenia Research, 79*(1), 85–93. doi: 10.1016/j.schres.2005.05.024

Harvey, P. D., Koren, D., Reichenberg, A., & Bowie, C. R. (2006). Negative symptoms and cognitive deficits: What is the nature of their relationship? [Research Support, N.I.H., Extramural Research Support, Non-U.S. Government Research Support, U.S. Government, Non-P.H.S.Review]. *Schizophrenia Bulletin, 32*(2), 250–258. doi: 10.1093/schbul/sbj011

Jeppesen, P., Petersen, L., Thorup, A., Abel, M. B., Ohlenschlaeger, J., Christensen, T. O., et al. (2008). The association between pre-morbid adjustment, duration of untreated psychosis and outcome in first-episode psychosis. [Randomized Controlled Trial Research Support, Non-U.S. Government]. *Psychological Medicine, 38*(8), 1157–1166. doi: 10.1017/S0033291708003449

Kirkpatrick, B., Fenton, W. S., Carpenter, W. T., Jr., & Marder, S. R. (2006). The NIMH-MATRICS consensus statement on negative symptoms. [Consensus Development Conference, NIH]. *Schizophrenia Bulletin, 32*(2), 214–219. doi: 10.1093/schbul/sbj053

Kraepelin, E., Barclay, R. M., & Robertson, G. M. (1919). *Dementia Præcox and Paraphrenia*. Edinburgh: E. & S. Livingstone.

Leucht, S., Corves, C., Arbter, D., Engel, R. R., Li, C., Davis, J. M. (2009). Second-generation versus first-generation antipsychotic drugs for schizophrenia: A meta-analysis. *Lancet, 373*(9657), 31–41. doi: 10.1016/S0140–6736(08)61764-X

MacBeth, A., & Gumley, A. (2008). Premorbid adjustment, symptom development and quality of life in first episode psychosis: A systematic review and critical reappraisal. [Review]. *Acta Psychiatrica Scandinavica, 117*(2), 85–99. doi: 10.1111/j.1600–0447.2007.01134.x

Malla, A., Norman, R., Scholten, D., Manchanda, R., & McLean, T. (2005). A community intervention for early identification of first episode psychosis: Impact on duration of untreated psychosis (DUP) and patient characteristics. [Research Support, Non-U.S. Government]. *Social Psychiatry and Psychiatric Epidemiology, 40*(5), 337–344. doi: 10.1007/s00127–005-0901–6

Malla, A. K., Norman, R. M., Manchanda, R., Ahmed, M. R., Scholten, D., Harricharan, R., et al. (2002). One-year outcome in first episode psychosis: Influence of DUP and other predictors. [Research Support, Non-U.S. Government]. *Schizophrenia Research, 54*(3), 231–242.

Marshall, M., Lewis, S., Lockwood, A., Drake, R., Jones, P., & Croudace, T. (2005). Association between duration of untreated psychosis and outcome in cohorts of first-episode patients: A systematic review. *Archives of General Psychiatry, 62*(9), 975–983. doi: 62/9/975 [pii]10.1001/archpsyc.62.9.975

Melle, I., Larsen, T. K., Haahr, U., Friis, S., Johannessen, J. O., Opjordsmoen, S., et al. (2004). Reducing the duration of untreated first-episode psychosis: Effects on clinical presentation. [Clinical Trial Controlled Clinical Trial Multicenter Study Research Support, Non-U.S. Government Research Support, U.S. Government, P.H.S.]. *Archives of General Psychiatry, 61*(2), 143–150. doi: 10.1001/archpsyc.61.2.143

Murphy, B. P., Chung, Y. C., Park, T. W., & McGorry, P. D. (2006). Pharmacological treatment of primary negative symptoms in schizophrenia: A systematic review. [Review]. *Schizophrenia Research, 88*(1–3), 5–25. doi: 10.1016/j.schres.2006.07.002

Murray, R. M., O'Callaghan, E., Castle, D. J., & Lewis, S. W. (1992). A neurodevelopmental approach to the classification of schizophrenia. [Review]. *Schizophrenia Bulletin, 18*(2), 319–332.

Perkins, D. O., Gu, H., Boteva, K., & Lieberman, J. A. (2005). Relationship between duration of untreated psychosis and outcome in first-episode schizophrenia: A critical review and meta-analysis. [Meta-Analysis Research Support, N.I.H., Extramural Research Support, Non-U.S. Government Review]. *The American Journal of Psychiatry, 162*(10), 1785–1804. doi: 10.1176/appi.ajp.162.10.1785

Roy, M. A., Maziade, M., Labbe, A., & Merette, C. (2001). Male gender is associated with deficit schizophrenia: A meta-analysis. [Meta-Analysis Research Support, Non-U.S. Government]. *Schizophrenia Research, 47*(2–3), 141–147.

Ventura, J., Hellemann, G. S., Thames, A. D., Koellner, V., & Nuechterlein, K. H. (2009). Symptoms as mediators of the relationship between neurocognition and functional outcome in schizophrenia: A meta-analysis. [Meta-Analysis]. *Schizophrenia Research, 113*(2–3), 189–199. doi: 10.1016/j.schres.2009.03.035

Part VII

Recovering from Early Psychosis

29
Recovery from Psychosis

Chi-wing Law

The development of antipsychotics in the 1950s marked the turning point in the treatment of psychosis. Since then, there has been a progressive increase in expectations for treatment outcomes in psychotic disorders. In the pre-1960s era, the goal of treatment was simply "improvement in self-care and reduction in aggression and self-injury". With time, this goal has changed to "deinstitutionalization" in the 1960s and 1970s, and to "reduction of recidivism and minimization of positive symptoms" in the 1980s. From the 1990s onward, the ultimate goal of the treatment of psychosis has advanced to the "increase in periods of stabilization, minimization of negative symptoms and reduction of side-effect burden".

Nowadays, the long-term management aim of psychosis should at least include optimization of quality of life, helping clients to regain their former level of independence, encouragement of integration into the society, as well as minimization of relapse (Taylor et al., 2005). In promoting recovery especially in people with early psychosis, services should be enabling rather than disabling, ultimately aspiring to healing and recovery. Clients need encouragement and sufficient support to retain or regain full participation in society (Bertolote & McGorry, 2005).

Remission and Recovery

In clinical research, attempts have been made to define criteria for remission of psychosis. A proposed definition of remission from the illness process is absence of symptoms, or presence of only minimal symptoms, in major psychopathology dimensions including psychotic symptoms (delusions, hallucinations, and unusual thought content), disorganization (conceptual disorganization and mannerisms or posturing), and negative symptoms (blunted affect, social withdrawal, and lack of spontaneity) for more than six months (Andreasen et al., 2005). The concept of recovery, however, seems to be more vaguely defined. Recovery refers not only to the client being free from symptoms, but also returning to reasonable functioning levels. Remission is considered a necessary but not sufficient step towards recovery, which is a higher hurdle and longer-term goal. Possible future definition of recovery is expected to be operationalized in the sense of moving forward and rebuilding one's life and is likely to incorporate improvements in other areas, such as empowerment, quality of life, and psychosocial functioning (van Os et al., 2006). Another effort to standardize the criteria of recovery was proposed by Liberman et al. (2002). Their definition includes both a clinical criterion, which specifies the limit of Brief Psychiatric Rating Score (BPRS) score for different items, and a functioning criterion, which specifies participation in occupational and social aspects of life. Bellack (2006) has commented that this definition of recovery suggests that total symptom remission is not absolutely necessary for recovery; instead, it can be attained even with mild to moderate symptoms. It is possible that some people have periods of good functioning while also having intermittent exacerbations of clinical symptoms.

Clients undergoing the process of recovery need to face a number of challenges as their active symptoms remit. These complex issues include the appraisal of the extent of recovery and the possibility of relapse, as well as making sense of the illness episode and its treatment (Andresen, Oades, & Caputi, 2003; Sells, Stayner, & Davidson, 2004). These interconnected issues, on the other hand, are potentially open to the influence of prior knowledge about the illness, personality of the client in the premorbid state, sociocultural influences, experiences of the illness process, as well as psychoeducational messages delivered by the intervention team during the process of treatment (Roe et al., 2004; Sells et al., 2004; Strauss, 1994; White et al., 2000).

Discrepancy in Expectations

The meanings and expectations of recovery from psychosis could differ among different clients, caregivers, and health professionals. Even among different health professionals, their focus in the recovery process could also vary. Clinicians would be more concerned about symptom control, degree of medication side-effects, etc., whereas other disciplines such as social workers may be paying more attention towards the clients' employment and relationship with others. The expectation of recovery would also be constantly changing during different phases of the illness.

In everyday clinical practice, health professionals do not often raise the issue of recovery during the interview session. On the other hand, clients and their caregivers may be expecting more discussion in this aspect, but find it hard to raise this issue in a brief clinical follow-up session with clinicians. Moreover, clients with significant residual and negative symptoms, and thus most in need of rehabilitation, could paradoxically be the ones most easily neglected in a busy clinic, as they seldom make active requests. The process of recovery in this group of clients is likely to worsen further as a consequence.

In clinical practice, the discrepancy between health professionals and their clients in the expected degree of recovery can significantly influence the treatment alliance. This gap could lead to great disappointment and distress in clients and caregivers, which in turn result in major obstacles in their path of rehabilitation. As a result, health professionals need to be particularly aware of any debilitating depressive and anxiety symptoms. Such discrepancy in expectations is well illustrated in Case Vignette 1.

Case Vignette 1

Alan suffered from the first episode of psychosis nine months ago, with prominent psychotic symptoms including auditory hallucinations and reference delusions at onset. He was 23 years old at the time and had graduated from university the previous year. He had been working as a clerical worker for six months before the onset, and reported satisfactory initial work performance. He was dismissed from his job around the time of illness onset due to deteriorating and unsatisfactory work performance, and became socially withdrawn and stayed at home. After he had received psychiatric treatment five months ago, his positive symptoms improved, and he has completely remitted with regular medication. He now spends most of his time going to places such as libraries and shopping malls.

His case doctor and case manager started discussing with him about job-hunting plans. Alan, however, showed strong hesitation in the discussion, and was reluctant to start planning or attempt job seeking despite repeated persuasions. On further enquiry, Alan admitted that he lacked confidence in any attempt to find a job. He did not consider himself recovered yet because he still needed to take regular medications and attend regular follow-ups in the psychiatric clinic. More than that, his father shared a similar view: he could accept Alan as a "normal person" only after he could "get rid of" further medication treatment and follow-ups. Before that, he was still considered "sick" and vulnerable to any kind of stress, including attempts at job-hunting.

This case scenario is not uncommon in everyday clinical practice in an early assessment and treatment service programme for clients suffering from first-episode psychosis. To many of the clients and caregivers, recovery from a psychotic disorder is an "all-or-none" process. The termination of regular medication treatment is often regarded as the "benchmark" of recovery.

Distorted View of Recovery

Many clients believe that, as long as one is in need of regular medication, he or she is still "fragile" and unable to tolerate the "normal" levels of stress. Many believe that only when the regimen of regular medication stops with no further chance of relapse, is an individual considered a "normal person". They believe that the normal facets and planning of life, including employment, marriage, and having children, etc., could only commence from this time onward.

This distorted belief towards recovery may bring about two major problems. First, the progressive pathway to engagement in rehabilitation towards recovery would likely be delayed and prolonged as a consequence. The potential presence of features such as negative and depressive symptoms, which are commonly encountered in this phase of illness as the positive symptoms subside, would further complicate the problem. Second, as a reaction to this belief, clients are likely to terminate their maintenance medications prematurely. Together with the false sense of security that cessation of medication treatment means getting rid of their illness permanently, the chance of relapse is even higher.

To help clients and caregivers acquire a more accurate concept of recovery, the use of physical illness as analogy, such as recovery from a lower limb fracture, may be a reasonable attempt. It is illogical to expect a client who has just undergone an operation for his leg fracture to participate in practising for a marathon game at this stage. He inevitably needs to go through the gradual process of practising walking with a frame, with sticks, then walking unaided slowly by himself, before he could finally train for a marathon. Careful balance and timing of this rehabilitation process is required. On the one hand, it would be disappointing and even detrimental to the recovering client if this process was hurried. On the other hand, if the client simply "waits" in bed expecting to suddenly leap out of bed one day and win a marathon, he would never succeed either.

Patricia Deegan (1993), who suffered from schizophrenia at the age of 17 and subsequently received her doctorate in psychology, is today one of the strongest advocates in the recovery movement. She wrote that "recovery is a process, not an end point or destination. In many ways, everyone who seeks healing is in transit, always trying to move forward. The journey itself maybe what heals us, not whether we reach a set destination. Everyone's recovery journey is different and deeply personal, and hope is central to recovery" (Deegan, 1993). This is probably the most accurate and positive message regarding the process of recovery that could be channelled to the clients.

"Persistent" Nature of Psychosis

Acceptance of the chronic nature of the illness presents another challenge for psychoeducation, particularly the notion of partial recovery (when compared with the premorbid state of clients), as well as the prevalence of relapses, used as a justification for regular maintenance medication. These issues are particularly difficult to address in this group of relatively young clients, with most of them probably having had enjoyed good physical health in the past.

Discussions with clients and their caregivers to reach consensus on reasonable goals to define recovery is essential to avoid over-optimistic or over-pessimistic expectations. Again, the use of common physical illness analogies such as hypertension, epilepsy, or near-sightedness could be useful. With this in mind, the focus of the endpoint of recovery is shifting from "no need to see a doctor" towards leading a relatively normal life while bearing the "burden" of needing ongoing medication. Understandably, the acceptance of having a chronic and possibly lifelong illness could be difficult. How this message is disseminated progressively with time, adjusting to the appropriate phase of the illness, is important. Therapists need to be alert to potential problems that may develop during this process, including secondary depressive symptoms and suicidal ideas (see Chapter 26, "Suicide and Self-Harm Behaviour in Early

Psychosis"). Moreover, other issues such as possible side-effects of medications and stigmatization of chronic psychiatric problems are important sequelae that also need to be addressed in the discussion.

Employment of Patients

The issue of employment for clients recovered from psychosis is a complicated one, which involves interplay between social and economic pressures that clients face, the labour market, as well as the psychological and social barriers to working. Barriers to getting employment include stigma, discrimination, fear of loss of benefits, and a lack of appropriate professional help. On the other hand, working is correlated with positive outcomes in social functioning, symptom levels, quality of life, and self-esteem, though a clear causal relationship has not been established (Marwaha & Johnson, 2004).

Subjective Cognitive Impairment

In the course of recovery in clients suffering from psychosis, subjective cognitive impairment can be easily and commonly neglected by clinicians. Compared with active psychotic symptoms, negative symptoms, or medication side-effects (e.g., extra-pyramidal signs, which are relatively prominent and less difficult to spot), subjective cognitive impairments largely rely upon clients' own experience and descriptions to be noticed. As seen in the Case Vignette 2, these dimensions are sometimes difficult to capture by commonly used objective cognitive assessments.

Case Vignette 2

Ann was a 25-year-old lady who suffered from first-episode psychosis more than one year ago. Before the onset of her illness, Ann used to have an outgoing personality with lots of peers as friends and was active in social activities. During her active psychotic state, she developed various reference and persecutory delusions towards her friends. These symptoms have remitted completely now. Nevertheless, after this psychotic episode, Ann could not get along with her friends as well as in her premorbid state. She kept on feeling that her thoughts and reactions were not as fluent and efficient as they had been before the onset of her illness. Because of such experiences, she often felt anxious being with her friends. She always felt "inferior" in front of her peers, and that they often regarded her as "silly" owing to her perceived residual disability. Various objective neurocognitive assessments were carried out longitudinally and they showed no obvious deficit. The results were explained to Ann but she simply could not accept them. She often feels upset about her "persistent disability" and sometimes avoids social activities with friends.

Studies reveal that clients' reported memory and attention issues do not correspond to objective neurocognitive measures. On the other hand, subjective depressive symptoms are strongly correlated with subjective neurocognitive complaints (Moritz, Ferahli, & Naber, 2004). However, subjective cognitive dysfunction has been found to be a strong predictor of poor symptomatic outcomes in clients with first-episode psychosis (Moritz et al., 2000). Furthermore, given that neurocognitive disturbances are important determinants of functional outcome variables such as psychosocial and work functioning (Brekke et al., 1997; Gold et al., 2002; Green, 1996), neurocognitive dysfunction reported by clients should still be taken seriously even when unverified by clinicians or psychometric tests.

Social Anxiety

Case Vignette 2 also reveals the common difficulty of social anxiety experienced by clients recovering from psychotic episodes. Whether it is a distinct feature at this stage of illness or secondary to residual reference delusion is sometimes difficult to distinguish. Studies show that about one-third of clients with first-episode psychosis met clinical diagnostic criteria for social phobia (Voges & Addington, 2005). Individuals with anxiety disorders tend to overestimate the probability of a negative outcome and underestimate their ability to cope, as did Ann. These distorted thoughts might focus on the anticipation of rejection, disapproval, or embarrassment. It is thus reasonable to expect that poor social functioning in clients with psychosis is positively correlated with social anxiety (Blanchard, Mueser, & Bellack, 1998).

A number of mechanisms may underlie social anxiety, which could be intrinsic to the illness of psychosis itself or, alternatively, developmental and related to the early social isolation and withdrawal that occurs long before the onset of psychotic symptoms. Third, it could be a reaction to the process of psychosis in terms of a loss of social contacts, or a coping strategy in response to perceived threats or other symptoms, such as positive symptoms, negative symptoms, or depression. These need to be distinguished during subsequent evaluations with the clients in order to implement an appropriate strategy for illness management.

Personal Significance of Symptoms

Case Vignette 3

Mary was a 29-year-old lady who suffered first-episode psychosis. One of the distinctive features of her psychotic episode was that she had prominent auditory hallucinations as part of her symptoms. The "origin" of her hallucination was believed to be a young man, an ex-colleague of Mary. She had a crush on this young man but failed to start any relationship with him. Thus, in some way, she actually enjoyed the companion of the voices and perceived "him" as her virtual boyfriend. In the process of recovery, her auditory hallucination subsided gradually, but she had a rather mixed feeling towards that outcome. On one hand, after psychoeducation and treatment, she realized these voices were unreal and should be well controlled with medications. On the other hand, she felt somewhat desperate as the voices lessened as it resembled a termination of a romantic love affair. She could not help having the impulse from time to time to search for her ex-colleague in order to "clarify" the issue.

The experience of Mary in Case Vignette 3 reveals that the symptoms could have highly personal meaning for the client. To the therapist, the remission of symptoms seems undoubtedly a relief to the clients, which, however, could be grief from the client's perspective. Without in-depth understanding of the client, such experiences could never be revealed. It is true that the removal of active symptoms can bring about a remission of the illness, but in some clients this may not be a pleasant experience at all. In this case, the probable underlying, deep-rooted problems of Mary, including her deficits in handling social and particularly heterosexual relationships, needed to be dealt with before she could enjoy a satisfactory recovery from her illness.

Summary

The meaning of recovery is highly individualized and can vary among different people and in different aspects. Apart from the core symptoms and course of the illness, recovery is affected by numerous contributing factors including the client's premorbid functioning, personality, coping strategies, core personal beliefs, as well as influences from others around them. Achieving a consensus among clients and various disciplines on recovery that is most beneficial and applicable to the client is a difficult but vital task in the treatment process.

The process of psychosis itself is not necessarily a "trauma" or detrimental event to clients. Some could view it in a positive way and perceive it as a chance for personal growth. Recovery could be redefined as "the development of new meaning and purpose as one grows beyond the catastrophe of mental illness" (Anthony, 1993). From a more positive perspective, the growth in recovery could be seen in terms of grieving for what is lost, understanding what has happened, and discovering the meaning of life (Coleman, 1999).

References

Andreasen, N. C., Carpenter, W. T., Jr., Kane, J. M., Lasser, R. A., Marder, S. R., & Weinberger, D. R. (2005). Remission in schizophrenia: Proposed criteria and rationale for consensus. [Review]. *The American Journal of Psychiatry, 162*(3), 441–449. doi: 10.1176/appi.ajp.162.3.441

Andresen, R., Oades, L., & Caputi, P. (2003). The experience of recovery from schizophrenia: Towards an empirically validated stage model. [Research Support, Non-U.S. Government Review]. *The Australian and New Zealand Journal of Psychiatry, 37*(5), 586–594.

Anthony, W. (1993). Recovery from mental illness: The guiding vision of the mental health service system in the 1990s. *Psychosocial Rehabilitation Journal, 16*, 11–23.

Bellack, A. S. (2006). Scientific and consumer models of recovery in schizophrenia: Concordance, contrasts, and implications. *Schizophrenia Bulletin, 32*(3), 432–442. doi: sbj044 [pii] 10.1093/schbul/sbj044

Bertolote, J., & McGorry, P. (2005). Early intervention and recovery for young people with early psychosis: Consensus statement. *The British Journal of Psychiatry. Supplement, 48*, s116–119. doi: 10.1192/bjp.187.48.s116

Blanchard, J. J., Mueser, K. T., & Bellack, A. S. (1998). Anhedonia, positive and negative affect, and social functioning in schizophrenia. [Research Support, Non-U.S.

Government Research Support, U.S. Government, P.H.S.]. *Schizophrenia Bulletin, 24*(3), 413–424.

Brekke, J. S., Raine, A., Ansel, M., Lencz, T., & Bird, L. (1997). Neuropsychological and psychophysiological correlates of psychosocial functioning in schizophrenia. [Research Support, U.S. Government, P.H.S.]. *Schizophrenia Bulletin, 23*(1), 19–28.

Coleman, R. (1999). *Recovery: An Alien Concept*. Gloucester: Handsell Publishing.

Deegan, P. E. (1993). Recovering our sense of value after being labeled mentally ill. *Journal of Psychosocial Nursing and Mental Health Services, 31*(4), 7–11.

Gold, J. M., Goldberg, R. W., McNary, S. W., Dixon, L. B., & Lehman, A. F. (2002). Cognitive correlates of job tenure among patients with severe mental illness. [Comparative Study Research Support, Non-U.S. Government Research Support, U.S. Government, P.H.S.]. *The American Journal of Psychiatry, 159*(8), 1395–1402.

Green, M. F. (1996). What are the functional consequences of neurocognitive deficits in schizophrenia? [Review]. *The American Journal of Psychiatry, 153*(3), 321–330.

Liberman, R. P., Kopelowicz, A., Ventura, J., & Gutkind, D. (2002). Operational criteria and factors related to recovery from schizophrenia. *International Review of Psychiatry, 14*(4), 256–272. doi: Doi 10.1080/0954026021000016905

Marwaha, S., & Johnson, S. (2004). Schizophrenia and employment: A review. [Review]. *Social Psychiatry and Psychiatric Epidemiology, 39*(5), 337–349. doi: 10.1007/s00127-004-0762-4

Moritz, S., Ferahli, S., & Naber, D. (2004). Memory and attention performance in psychiatric patients: Lack of correspondence between clinician-rated and patient-rated functioning with neuropsychological test results. [Comparative Study]. *Journal of the International Neuropsychological Society: JINS, 10*(4), 623–633. doi: 10.1017/S1355617704104153

Moritz, S., Krausz, M., Gottwalz, E., Lambert, M., Perro, C., Ganzer, S., et al. (2000). Cognitive dysfunction at baseline predicts symptomatic 1-year outcome in first-episode schizophrenics. *Psychopathology, 33*(1), 48–51.

Roe, D., Chopra, M., Wagner, B., Katz, G., & Rudnick, A. (2004). The emerging self in conceptualizing and treating mental illness. [Review]. *Journal of Psychosocial Nursing and Mental Health Services, 42*(2), 32–40.

Sells, D. J., Stayner, D. A., & Davidson, L. (2004). Recovering the self in schizophrenia: An integrative review of qualitative studies. [Review]. *The Psychiatric Quarterly, 75*(1), 87–97.

Strauss, J. S. (1994). The person with schizophrenia as a person. II: Approaches to the subjective and complex. [Research Support, Non-U.S. Government Research Support, U.S. Government, P.H.S.]. *The British Journal of Psychiatry. Supplement*(23), 103–107.

Taylor, M., Chaudhry, I., Cross, M., McDonald, E., Miller, P., Pilowsky, L., et al. (2005). Towards consensus in the long-term management of relapse prevention in schizophrenia. [Research Support, Non-U.S. Government Review]. *Human Psychopharmacology, 20*(3), 175–181. doi: 10.1002/hup.675

van Os, J., Burns, T., Cavallaro, R., Leucht, S., Peuskens, J., Helldin, L., et al. (2006). Standardized remission criteria in schizophrenia. [Review]. *Acta Psychiatrica Scandinavica, 113*(2), 91–95. doi: 10.1111/j.1600–0447.2005.00659.x

Voges, M., & Addington, J. (2005). The association between social anxiety and social functioning in first episode psychosis. *Schizophrenia Research, 76*(2–3), 287–292. doi: 10.1016/j.schres.2005.01.001

White, R., Bebbington, P., Pearson, J., Johnson, S., & Ellis, D. (2000). The social context of insight in schizophrenia. [Research Support, Non-U.S. Government]. *Social Psychiatry and Psychiatric Epidemiology, 35*(11), 500–507.

30

Concepts of Recovery in Early Psychosis: A Cognitive Linguistic Approach

Eric Yu-hai Chen

The concepts of "recovery" and "remission" are often differentiated in the literature. While remission has a more stringent definition and emphasizes symptoms, the concept of recovery is broader with more demanding criteria. This chapter will first discuss some definitions of recovery and remission commonly used in clinical and research settings, and then explore subjective ideas of recovery and the potential use of a tool to reconcile differences. Thirdly, the cognitive linguistic approach to the concept of recovery will be considered before a review of some experiential aspects of psychosis including reality judgement, sealing over and integration approaches.

Defining "Recovery" and "Remission" Clinically

Based on the definitions by the Recovery in Schizophrenia Working Group in the US (Andreasen et al., 2005), remission is a necessary but not sufficient condition for recovery. This working group adopted a broad symptom dimension to define recovery in that it does not only look at positive symptoms such as hallucinations and delusions, but also takes into consideration the negative symptoms. Furthermore, rather than requiring a patient to be completely symptom-free to qualify as having recovered, improvement in positive and negative symptoms is also considered. Another criterion of recovery pertains to the patients' functioning, including the vocational, social, and family roles they are able to play. Also, patients have to maintain such improved state of being and functioning for a certain time period to qualify for "recovery".

Robinson's commonly used concept of recovery (Robinson et al., 2004) embraces two dimensions, namely, symptom remission and psychosocial functioning. On the symptom remission dimension, the positive symptoms presented have to be no worse than mild, and negative symptoms no worse than moderate. On the psychosocial functioning dimension, the patients' role functioning, daily living, as well as social functioning are considered. On the other hand, the more stringent Torgalsborn's criteria require no hospitalization for five years, psychosocial functioning within a normal range (Global Assessment Scale score >65), and no or low-dosage of medication. Torgalsborn's conceptualization is among one of the few that takes medication (or rather the cessation of medication) into consideration when conceptualizing recovery.

Clinical Construct of Recovery

Robinson's approach represents a medical model of recovery, which is viewed as an outcome. This can be compared with the "consumer model" of recovery, which emphasizes that recovery is an ongoing process of positive adaption (Bellack, 2006). The underlying philosophy in the medical model adopts a natural science perspective. However, natural science has certain limitations when it comes to comprehending human experience. Natural sciences emphasize the reliability of measurements of certain major constructs and data obtained are used to explain the phenomena under scrutiny. This approach does not adequately capture patients' experience and personal hardships they face. If a line is to be drawn on a set of data to define recovery, the exact position of the line is necessarily somewhat arbitrary: if the criteria are too stringent with too few patients qualifying for recovery, the situation can be frustrating. It is equally unrealistic if the criteria are so lenient that most of the patients are considered having recovered. Also, such quantification does not take into account the patients' own conceptualization and expectation about recovery, overlooking a possible misalignment between clinicians' and patients' expectations.

Subjective Ideas about Recovery

While understanding the concept of recovery from a clinical perspective belongs to a natural science endeavour, subjective experience of illness is not fully accessible using conventional empirical techniques from natural sciences, including positivist social sciences. In order to gain a more complete understanding of this concept, the natural science approach has to be complemented by more engaging access to subjective experience.

One approach to evaluating subjective ideas about recovery is to employ the methodology derived from ethnography field studies, which emphasizes an experience-centred (interpretive) rather than an explanation-centred (rationalist) framework. In this approach, the subjective components of recovery can be described in "etic" and "emic" terms. Etic descriptions employ categories from outside, such as clinical terms; while emic descriptions use categories from the subjects, such as patients' spontaneous accounts. It is noteworthy that every emic account inevitably has its etic components when, for instances, researchers reconstruct the meaning of patients' accounts, or when clinical dialogue exerts its influence on patients' expressions and thoughts. Subjective accounts of recovery are often highly individualized and difficult to compare across subjects.

The Psychosis Recovery Inventory

As both the clinical approach and subjective approach to recovery have their strengths and drawbacks, an attempt has been made to bridge qualitative data and quantitative methodology. The development of the Psychosis Recovery Inventory (Chen et al., 2005) involved two stages. In the first stage, a qualitative exploration was employed to capture emic ideas and thus emphasize the subjectivity of recovery; in the second stage, basing on the ideas derived from the first stage, a quantitative instrument was derived for surveying a more representative sample. The inventory developed in this manner comprises three subscales, with a total of 28 items self-rated by participants for recovery and relapse judgement combined with two subsections—misattribution and residual problems. Simple language is used wherever appropriate to avoid ambiguity.

Study results showed that few respondents thought they had fully recovered. They admitted that, to a certain degree, they had not yet returned to their previous state. Pursuing respondents' perception as to what was missing for their recovery, patients typically reported that they still had problems in cognitive, social, occupational, and medication aspects. Importantly, cognitive and medication issues were rated as more important than social and occupational ones. However, these two areas were exactly those most often neglected in similar studies. On the cognitive level, many patients complained about slowness in response and poor concentration and memory. Patients also thought that they fell short of recovery simply because they were still on medication and, interestingly, this perception did not change even if the medication they were taking did not have any significant side-effects.

Conceptual Misalignment and Consequences

Conceptual misalignment of recovery arises among clinicians and patients often hampers communication causing some patients to retreat and avoid any discussion on recovery altogether. Two forms of misalignment are possible. First, from a clinical perspective, the clinician may feel that the patient has already recovered (e.g., no signs of delusions and hallucinations on rating scales) but the patient does not feel that way (e.g., still complaining about slower response than before), increasing the patient's mistrust and feeling that the clinician is not able/willing to help him or her anymore. Second and conversely, the patient believes that he or she has already recovered while the clinician does not. This situation often happens when medication issues are involved. In this case, the patient may manifest undesirable responses such as disengagement, non-adherence, demoralization, and a poor sense of agency. In particular, patients who have the best insight may abide by clinicians' advice to adhere to treatment simply because they trust the authority of clinicians, without internalizing an understanding for the role of medication, resulting in demoralization and even depression. Worst still, with conceptual misalignments, clinicians and patients may fail to communicate on some key issues that need to be addressed; important dimensions that are often overlooked include medication, relapse, need for maintenance therapy, subjective cognitive dysfunction, and attribution. Such a misalignment between clinicians and patients can sometimes be ascribed to a lack of suitable vocabulary and concepts to communicate the complex issues associated with a psychotic illness.

One particular issue is the use of medications for relapse prevention, which may be at odds with patients' concept of recovery. As discussed in Chapter 31 ("Experiential Aspects of Recovery in Early Psychosis"), stopping medication and follow-up clinic visits are key criteria of subject recovery. In view of this prevailing expectation, together with the side-effects of medications, the possibility of medication discontinuation in remitted patients is a question that many clinicians and patients ponder. No consensus has been reached about the appropriate length of maintenance medication after the first year of treatment. Yet, a recent randomized controlled trial in Hong Kong clearly demonstrated that maintenance medication beyond one year of stabilization still cuts relapse rate nearly by half (79% vs. 41%) in patients with well-controlled psychosis (Chen et al., 2010). While this fact may be more difficult to reconcile with the subjective idea of recovery that many patients hold, this trial highlighted the need to re-consider a recovery concept that is more useful and meaningful with an appreciation of the nature of a psychotic illness.

Cognitive Linguistic Exploration of the Concept of Recovery

In everyday communication, a word in the mind refers to an object in the external world, and the audience can link the word to the concept being discussed. Unfortunately, this simple representation of the process of communication is inadequate in several ways. First, concepts do not exist in our mind like a dictionary loaded onto our brains via education. Instead, these concepts are closely linked to our everyday life. Some linguists even propose that the words people use are based on some image schemas, which are so fundamental that we are not always aware of their existence (Lakoff, 1990; Lakoff & Johnson, 2003). One example of such image schemas is the container image schema, which gives people the concept of "inside" and "outside" (see Figure 30.1). Through a process called metaphorical projection, people extend such basic image schema to abstract constructs, such as some "states" concepts like "out of trouble", "in a coma", "fell into depression", and "in remission", describing abstract states by using spatial words. Nevertheless, when talking about recovery, this kind of spatial representation of a state is seldom used. For example, people rarely say "in recovery", implying that something more than "a state" is involved in the concept of recovery.

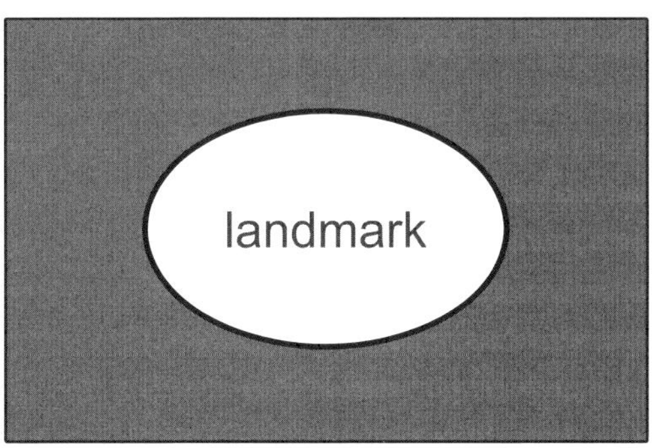

Figure 30.1

Container image schema

Another image schema is the path image schema, whose most primitive form consists of a source, a goal, and a unidirectional path linking the two. This schema is often used to describe people's actions and goals, whether attainable or not (Figure 30.2). The concept of "recovery" may align better with a "goal" schema rather than a "state" schema as a starting point.

Figure 30.2

Path image schema

According to semantics, words are not used to simply denote meaning as if they merely appear in dictionaries. Instead, a word triggers a bundle of related concepts and adopts meaning only if understood in the context of the matrix of related concepts. For instance, in order to explain what an aorta is, it is meaningless to describe its properties such as diameter and location. Instead, the explanation must describe the aorta in the context of the whole circulatory system. Thus, a word in isolation is meaningless until it is placed in the frame or domain in which it exists (connotation). Some ideal cognitive models emphasize the prototypicality effects of concepts. For instance, whenever the concept of "mother" comes to mind, some associated concepts and knowledge domains such as birth, genetic relationship, upbringing, marital status, gynaecology, etc. flow in. If the definition does not take all these domains into consideration, elements of the concept will be missed. Applying these principles to the concept of recovery, some domains associated with the concept of recovery might include concepts such as health, healing, illness, cure, remission, full recovery, rehabilitation, and normality.

Use of metaphors

Metaphors are unidirectional mappings across conceptual domains; specifically, the mapping points from a source domain (which is concrete and experience-near) to a target domain (which is abstract). For example, sometimes people say they get lost during a conversation. The concept of getting lost originally comes from finding a way out in terms of spatial orientation. By describing the confusion during a conversation in the form of getting lost in spatial orientation, the physical action of finding a way out is metaphorically applied to the abstract concept of getting out of a confused conversation. One prerequisite of a metaphor is that the mappings it brings about should reflect the cognitive typology of the source domain, which is consistent with the inherent structure of the target domain. The major problem concerning recovery is that a full metaphor of the concept is lacking. Cognitive linguistics use the event structure metaphor to describe life events as components of a journey, in which states are locations, change is motion, causes are forces, purposes are destinations, means are paths, and difficulties are impediments to motion (Table 30.1).

Table 30.1
The journey metaphor of life events

Journey (source domain)	Life event (target domain)
Locations	States
Motion	Change
Forces	Causes
Destinations	Purposes
Paths	Means
Impediments to motion	Difficulties

The term "recovery" is often associated with concepts such as "reclaiming lost ground" and "returning to a previous state". In Chinese, the word "recovery" can be translated in different ways. For example, the Cantonese phrase *ho fan* (好返) in Cantonese relates to a complete return to a previous state, while the Chinese phrase *kang fu* (康復) relates to one's improving from chronic illness with possible residual impact.

An image schema of recovery often involves a spatial metaphor underlying the concept, with states (previous and present states) as positions, movement as changes, and a return movement as recovery. This simple concept of recovery represents a return to a previous state, assuming that (1) there is a clear representation of a previous state; (2) there is a clear representation of a perturbation; (3) the presence of a removable cause; and (4) the process is a reversible one. Too often, this simple recovery model is employed by default because most young adults only have experiences of conditions that fit such model (e.g., infection, accidental injuries), and lack other "experience-near" concepts for more complex disorders at a young age.

Undoubtedly, this simple recovery model has a number of limitations. First, it is not always easy to clearly describe a previous state or to distinguish the original and perturbed states. For patients with an acute onset of illness, this task may be easier; but for those with a progressive and gradual onset, it is very difficult to clearly define the state prior to the onset. Second, most of the causes involved are not removable and life experiences are fundamentally irreversible. Such a simple recovery model is inadequate in the sense that it fails to take into account some distinctive features of psychotic illnesses. For example, according to the stress-vulnerability model, mental illnesses (including psychotic ones) are ascribed to a combination of internal and external causative factors.

"Journey of time": Fallacy of the spatial metaphor

It is also inadequate to describe psychosis in terms of "states of being" because the course of the illness often lasts for weeks or even months, which is unidirectional in nature. Once a patient has gone through a certain stage of the illness, the course is irreversible and it is impossible to return to a "previous state". Even the healthy person would have changed substantially after months. Thus, it is more appropriate to describe the course of the illness in terms of a unidirectional journey, rather than a change in states of being.

Self as an experiencing agent

The experience of an illness is an intrinsic part of the patient, that is, the self being the agent experiencing the illness. Patients with psychosis are unique in the sense that the illness itself distorts the experiencing agent, thus rendering psychosis special and difficult to manage. If it were just physical pain, the person suffering from the pain remains the intact experiencing agent, however severe the pain might be, as it is external to the agent. However, in the case of psychosis, the affliction distorts the fundamental core of the experiencing self, thus complicating the situation.

Authority to judge reality

People usually regard the reality they experience as fundamental and take it for granted; but for psychotic patients, because of the reality distortion capacity of psychosis, this is not the case. As their symptoms remit, some patients feel the implications of not having the ultimate authority to judge the reality around them; instead, they now have to accept the possibility that one day their reality is to be better judged by the clinicians and others. Such a loss in authority can be demoralizing and devastating for patients' autonomy and dignity. However, this does not necessarily dictate failure or hopelessness. If patients have the foresight of the possibility of losing their autonomy and get prepared accordingly, failure is not inevitable.

"Sealing over" versus integration

Some patients attempt to "delete" the experience of the illness from their personal narratives, pretending that they did not happen. These attempts aim to maintain the continuity of healthy experience on the part of the patients, but whether this way of coping should be encouraged needs further discussion. On the contrary, some patients tend to remember or even regret their period of illness indefinitely, leaving some perpetual form of blemish.

Patients may also find it demoralizing to realize that, after the onset of their illness, many aspects of life are out of their control, and even the nature of their selves has been distorted to a certain extent. However, their hope lies in the fact that the future is yet to be determined and possibilities of adaptation remain to unfold. Thus, the key issue becomes how patients adapt to the new game rules of life; whether they try to ignore, surrender, or grasp the new rules is an important determinant of recovery.

Take Chinese calligraphy as a cultural metaphor, in most cases the calligrapher is able to control his or her own writing. However, if suddenly a slip occurs due to a change in the texture of the writing paper, the resulting imperfection can be irreversible and distressing. One way of coping with these imperfections is to ignore them and continue the writing (as in the case of sealing over). Another way to cope with the situation however is to accept the slip as it is and incorporate the slip into the gestalt of subsequent writing, making use of the future strokes to enhance the overall coherence and aesthetics of the integral piece. This task of incorporating imperfections is definitely more difficult.

However, if the patient can accept these challenges, knowing that illnesses are inevitable vulnerabilities of human life, the results can be growth not only in health, but also in relation to a challenging illness, attaining a resilience that is even more profoundly human.

References

Andreasen, N. C., Carpenter, W. T., Jr., Kane, J. M., Lasser, R. A., Marder, S. R., & Weinberger, D. R. (2005). Remission in schizophrenia: Proposed criteria and rationale for consensus. [Review]. *The American Journal of Psychiatry, 162*(3), 441–449. doi: 10.1176/appi.ajp.162.3.441

Bellack, A. S. (2006). Scientific and consumer models of recovery in schizophrenia: Concordance, contrasts, and implications. *Schizophrenia Bulletin, 32*(3), 432–442. doi: sbj044 [pii] 10.1093/schbul/sbj044

Chen, E. Y., Hui, C. L., Lam, M. M., Chiu, C. P., Law, C. W., Chung, D. W., et al. (2010). Maintenance treatment with quetiapine versus discontinuation after one year of treatment in patients with remitted first episode psychosis: Randomised controlled trial. *British Medical Journal, 341*, c4024. doi: 10.1136/bmj.c4024 bmj.c4024 [pii]

Chen, E. Y., Tam, D. K., Wong, J. W., Law, C. W., & Chiu, C. P. (2005). Self-administered instrument to measure the patient's experience of recovery after first-episode psychosis: Development and validation of the Psychosis Recovery Inventory. [Validation Studies]. *The Australian and New Zealand Journal of Psychiatry, 39*(6), 493–499. doi: 10.1111/j.1440-1614.2005.01609.x

Lakoff, G. (1990). *Women, Fire, and Dangerous Things*: University of Chicago Press.

Lakoff, G., & Johnson, M. (2003). *Metaphors We Live By*. Chicago: University of Chicago Press.

Robinson, D. G., Woerner, M. G., McMeniman, M., Mendelowitz, A., & Bilder, R. M. (2004). Symptomatic and functional recovery from a first episode of schizophrenia or schizoaffective disorder. [Research Support, U.S. Government, P.H.S.]. *The American Journal of Psychiatry, 161*(3), 473–479.

31
Experiential Aspects of Recovery in Early Psychosis: Focus Group Findings

May Mei-ling Lam

Importance of Subjective Experience

Young people who have suffered from a first episode of psychosis have high rates of remission if treated adequately and comprehensively. Despite this, more than 33% of clients are readmitted to the hospital within six months, 55% within two years and 80% within five years following the treatment of their first episode of psychosis. Given these alarming relapse rates, it is important to develop ways of intervention during the initial recovery period in order to reduce the risk of recurrence. This cannot be achieved without understanding the complex issues associated with increased risk of relapse. These include poor adherence to medication (see Chapter 24, "Medication Adherence: Specific Issues in Early Psychosis in Asia"), increased substance use (see Chapter 27, "Comorbid Substance Abuse in Early Psychosis"), impaired insight and understanding of the illness, emotional stress, and the subjective recovery experience. The current clinical focus observes a client's behaviour and interpreting it in terms of clinical models, instead of adopting an approach that starts from valuing and respectfully understanding the person's experience from his or her perspective. Not much research has looked into what recovery is and what it means to people with first episode of psychosis. Qualitative studies on the subjective perspective of recovery experience with individuals with a first episode of psychosis are few.

Early psychosis services recognized some of the shortfalls of traditional services and endeavour to provide a comprehensive and individually focused approach that tailors treatment to the needs of young people. This chapter will look at the subjective experience of these young people in making sense of the psychotic experiences and recovery as promoted by early psychosis services. The concept of recovery is briefly discussed, followed by the young person's subjective perspective on what is "good" service that helps the individual to recover from psychotic disorders, so as to shed light on therapeutic strategies and actions that are likely to aid the recovery process.

What Is Recovery?

Recovery is a concept unique to each individual and may have different meanings for different people. It is also not static; as the person grows and achieves his or her goals and dreams, he or she may feel that a greater level of recovery is reached. Recovery is essentially a transitional state of mind where people feel at ease with themselves so that they can respect, love, and appreciate themselves and others, as well as the world they live in.

The recovery concept was originally used in the physical disability movement in America. Since then, it has been widely used by mental health professionals. Anthony (1993) suggests that the concept of recovery for severe mental health problems is multidimensional. In this model, social and psychological recovery processes are as important as clinical recovery. Clinical recovery is defined by a reduction of symptoms, such as auditory hallucinations and delusions. On the other hand, social recovery includes development of meaningful social roles and relationships, involvement in vocational activities, and access to safe and clean housing, while psychological recovery is the process of developing ways to understand and manage psychotic experiences and to regain the maximum sense of life structure.

These distinctions are important as current services and research focus too heavily on clinical recovery. However, if a person can recover socially and psychologically, clinical recovery may be less relevant to the person's quality of life. Definition of recovery includes dimensions of self-esteem, adjustment to disability, empowerment, and self-determination. "For some of us, recovery means learning to cope with our difficulties, gaining control of our lives, achieving our goals, developing our skills and fulfilling our dreams." The eight principles listed in Table 31.1 are adapted by Anthony (1993), who describes them as important in understanding a recovery-based approach to serious mental health problems.

Experience of Early Psychosis Clients

Psychosis is often, although not always, experienced as a personal disaster with a potentially damaging mix of secondary trauma and loss. This is particularly

Table 31.1
Eight principles of recovery described by Anthony (1993)

Each person's recovery is different:
1. Recovery requires other people to believe in and stand by the person. Other people's opportunities play an important part in enabling the person to walk through this recovery journey.
2. Recovery does not mean cure. It does not mean complete disappearance of difficulties.
3. Recovery can occur without professional help. Service users hold the key to recovery.
4. Recovery is an ongoing process. During the recovery journey, there will be growth and setbacks, times of big changes, and times of little changes.
5. Recovery from the consequences of mental distress (stigma, unemployment, poor housing, etc.) can sometimes be more difficult than recovery from the distress and confusion itself.
6. People who have recovered or are recovering from confusion or distress have valuable knowledge about recovery and can help others who are recovering.
7. A recovering vision does not require a particular view of the mental health problems.

important in young adolescents recovering from their first-episode of psychosis at an early psychosis service. As it is, young individuals are going through their golden developmental stage in life, yet at the same time, they are facing specific challenges and complex issues related to their illness and treatment experiences, such as appraisal of the extent of their recovery and the risk of relapse.

There are a number of key developmental tasks the individual is facing at this stage of life, such as identity formation, which may be profoundly affected by the onset of illness. The person's self-esteem may be battered by the psychotic experience and the self-stigma associated with being a psychiatric client. At the time when their peers are testing and achieving independence, young people recovering from psychosis are being monitored and treated by a range of health professionals. Additionally, vocational or educational opportunities may be either lost or delayed. As a result of their illness, young clients may have difficulties relating to and reintegrating with their peer groups. The experience of psychosis, the treatment, and the responses from others after the psychotic episode are potentially traumatic experiences, which can change a person's way of construing themselves, their environment, and their future.

Three questions are particularly important for gaining better understanding of the psychotic and recovery experience in people with first-episode psychosis so as to shed light on promoting recovery processes:

1. What is the subjective experience of a psychotic disorder?
2. What is the personal impact of psychosis?
3. How does one cope with the illness?

These questions were explored in a focus group conducted in an early psychosis centre in Hong Kong. Qualitative research methods were particularly suitable for exploring subjective views on these issues, putting the attention on the individuals and their perspectives of the world. The lived experiences of those being studied or their accounts of it served as a basis for data analysis.

Focus groups are commonly used as a form of qualitative research method in the sociology of health and illness. Compared with individual interviews, focus groups allow access to research participants who may find one-on-one, face-to-face interaction intimidating. This may be particularly true for young people with first-episode psychosis, who may be reminded of their therapeutic relationships in individual interviews and thus adjust their communications to this familiar interaction setting, expecting to get help through an expert's knowledge and advice. This pilot study, on the contrary, seeks to explore among those who have experienced the illness, placing them in the role of experts with knowledge and experience essential to advancing the theoretical understanding of recovery.

In addition, focus groups create multiple lines of communication, thus offering participants a safe environment where they can share experiences, ideas, and beliefs with empathic people. The familiar atmosphere is helpful in facilitating statements on difficult and unpleasant topics such as stigma. Moreover, the interaction among group participants often reduces the amount of interaction between the moderator and individual members of the group. In this way, the group dynamics decrease the influence of the researcher over the interview process and hence assign a more prominent role to participants' opinions. The group setting has also a synergistic effect: the group dynamics stimulate thinking and verbal contributions. Focus groups are also considered to be a less direct method, which is more appropriate to elicit responses that better reflect social realities of the participants.

Using this qualitative approach to explore the experiential aspects of recovery in early psychosis clients (Lam et al., 2010), data obtained from the focus group were analysed manually, with the interview deconstructed sentence by sentence to identify key themes in line with the topic guide, as well as new categories emerging from the data. As the data were coded, further themes emerged; these were then combined and sorted into significant and meaningful areas, and frequency counts were done for the major themes. The identified themes were presented and discussed among the early psychosis research team.

Main Themes from Focus Group Discussions

From the statements of the focus group participants, four main themes were identified: understanding of psychosis and psychotic experience, normalization, stigma, and optimistic view of recovery.

Understanding of psychosis and psychotic experience

Only one participant in the focus group believed that she had "schizophrenia", while most participants (three out of six) believed that they had "early psychosis", which was viewed as a less serious illness with less labelling than "schizophrenia". The term "schizophrenia" literally means an irreversible "splitting of mind", which is often associated with a negative public image (see Chapter 17, "Experience of Stigma in Early Psychosis Patients and Caregivers"). One participant thought she had "mental nervousness" and believed that it was the very beginning of "early psychosis". Another participant thought she suffered from mixed anxiety and depression. Anxiety, depression, and "mental nervousness" were perceived by the participants to be more positive and well accepted by the public.

One participant understood her psychotic illness as "too high a dopamine level in the brain, which makes me not able to sense things that I can normally sense". This biological brain disease model may have a positive and protective effect on her as it reduces the public perception that clients are personally responsible for bringing about their own illness, that is, to dispel the belief that clients can control their illness. In contrast to other chronic physical illnesses, psychotic disorders are perceived to be more mysterious, less understood, and more debilitating. One participant accounted that "mental illness is much more mysterious because its cause is unclear . . . nobody knows how to really treat it. I feel that illness such as high blood pressure is more straightforward to treat, with some kind of a standard course to follow. But mental illness is more complicated, every case has a different story. The experience is different."

The feelings of "loss", "uncertainty", and "fear" associated with the experience of losing touch with the reality emerged as subthemes. One client commented that "it was so real. It was as close as you and me now, but I couldn't touch it, but I could hear somebody talking, yet I couldn't touch him." One method to try to distinguish the hallucinations from reality was to "touch" and see if it was real, thus dispelling what could not be "touched". Other strategies that participants tried to distinguish psychotic experience from reality included joining others in conversations to avoid the paranoia of being talked about. Others should try to be direct and clear in their communications and avoid instigating suspicion and paranoia, and "avoid holding private conversations that exclude me in my presence". The unpredictable course of illness and the burden of fear of relapse create a lot of uncertainties for participants, who are facing developmental challenges such as continuing studies, finding a life partner, or having children. The mere mentioning of the illness induces concern and anxiety in some participants that affect their normal life, including the loss of confidence to re-enter the workforce.

Recovery: Being normal, no medication

In contrast to the medical focus of symptomatic recovery in controlling psychotic symptoms, participants' perception of recovery includes being able to "concentrate", "focus", and be "responsive"; able to have a "normal reaction speed" and to "think clearly". Recovery means "one could think like others, have normal routines in life like others, and have normal social relationships as opposed to self-imposed isolation from others". For the participants, recovery also means being engaged with others such as friends and families, to maintain a "sense of being a normal member of the community" such as joining community voluntary work, engaging in social and recreational activities, and being "able to hold down a job", "follow lectures", "get married", and "have babies". Participants believe that having the opportunities to carry out valued activities that contribute to and introduce one to the world of others can enable them to be less preoccupied with their own inner world.

A university student viewed recovery as "being normalized again in thoughts and activities; being the same as others, eat and sleep like others, and work like others. It means having a normal life—to cook, sleep, exercise and go out. All very natural." Another university graduate thought that she is "almost fully recovered". "I'm almost fully recovered 'cos I'm pretty much doing the stuff I want to be doing . . . my family tells me that I'm now the same as before, such as my personality. I'm talking as much as I used to. My behaviour is back to the way it was, and I'm smiling again. I'm having a normal social life again, being myself again, my old self . . . And now I'm much quicker with responses. Now I'm online as usual, like I used to be. I do ICQ to train my reaction time, to seek out friends to hang out, to chat and be myself again; other than the medication side-effects, there is no difference." Another unemployed university graduate was concerned about medications, that "the side-effects make me feel sick. I can't concentrate. [The medications] make me irritable about gaining so much weight."

Most participants did not think that they were fully recovered because of their continued need for medications and follow-up visits with psychiatrists. While all participants were on atypical antipsychotics, they all expressed negative views on taking medications. Perceived side-effects of medications such as "impaired concentration", "dizziness", "mental dullness", "slowness in response", and "weight gain" were significant and recurring concerns of the participants. Concerns such as not being able to bear children while on medications were also raised in the focus group discussion. One participant accounted, " I feel that if I'm still on medications, then I'm not cured yet." The continued need for medications and concentration difficulties emerged as a consistent theme in their accounts of recovery, which has reduced the participants' confidence in re-entering the workforce. "I'm still on medications and this reduces my work performance a lot. I tried a few jobs but couldn't stay with them. I couldn't focus, so I had to quit."

The treatment of psychosis is experienced as having a negative impact on the participants' social relationships. The medication side-effects such as weight gain, emotional and generalized cognitive blunting may be noticed by others as visible signs of illness. This may lead to avoidance of social contact as clients are no longer capable of concealing the illness. In addition, side-effects may undermine morale, reducing confidence levels as body image is an important source of self-esteem, particularly for young adolescents. This further complicates interactions with their social environment and efforts to establish new social contacts as a large share of previous social interactions has been disrupted. Therefore, the risk of disability caused by medications needs to be considered and compared with the increased risk of psychotic experiences.

In contrast to the psychiatrists' perspective that recovery means that symptoms are under control and the person is compliant with treatment, for these participants, psychosis is the mind's way of coping with extreme trauma and conflict, emotional abandonment, and social isolation. Recovery is about finding one's true self and one's gifts and talents. In this sense, recovery has little to do with symptoms and illness, and has more to do with a personal outlook about the future and having a valued role; that is, with positive relationships and perceptions of the true self in relation to other people, and respect for the self and other people.

Stigma

Participants talked a great deal about stigma. Subjective feelings of stigma, even in the absence of any overt discrimination, emerged as a major theme in the focus group discussion among young people with first-episode psychosis. The participants' feeling of stigma was often related to the psychotic diagnosis. One aspect of stigma common to all participants was anxiety about how to manage information regarding illness and whether to disclose it or not to friends, family, and prospective employers and colleagues. Concealment of illness from colleagues, friends, and relatives (except immediate household family members) was reported by all participants in the focus group. Participants desired to avoid talking about their illness with others as they tried to be "normal, not being reminded" and at the same time maintain "secrecy and privacy".

The perceived consequences of subjective stigma and fear of disclosure included being "rejected", "gossiped", "treated differently", "discriminated in workplace", and "put on travel restrictions". One participant believed that having a psychotic illness was like being a "criminal", whose record would be shown on his/her passport and on whom travel restrictions were imposed. One participant shared, "I don't want to be the subject of gossip, in general. If my illness is disclosed, I'll just be gossiped about more, other people will distant you, reject you, they will have a different attitude, think differently, or talk in a different way; not everybody understands; putting yourself in their shoes, you'd probably do the same."

If necessary, participants would use an edited version of the illness experience that they perceived to be less stigmatizing, as opposed to revealing the true diagnosis, to explain their absence during periods of illness, for example, "I just told them I was burnt out during that time." The employment situation for people suffering from psychotic illness is further complicated by the dilemma as to whether or not to reveal the illness to potential employers. Honest information about psychiatric history in job application forms or interviews may result in failure of application in the first place, while wrong information or concealment of the illness involves danger of dismissal should the truth come to light. Regardless of this risk, participants preferred to keep the illness to themselves and explained periods of prolonged absence with functional diagnosis such as "burnout". Commonly, in daily clinical practice, clients do ask for a "fake diagnosis" and the use of "general" hospital stamps on sick leave certificates in an attempt to conceal the illness.

Concern about disclosure of illness emerged as a major subtheme in this study. Managing a discreditable identity, such as being a psychotic client, can be a powerful source of anxiety. Participants' attempts to avoid disclosure may result in stress, isolation, and a sense of shame. The feeling of being stigmatized can occur in the absence of any direct discrimination.

Positive experience of recovery

It is noteworthy that findings from the focus group of first-episode psychosis participants revealed that perceptions of illness were not universally negative. In most cases (four out of six), participants spoke of the illness as positively life-enhancing. Three participants (two tertiary students and one university graduate) actually expressed that they were glad that their illness experience had in many ways made them a "different", "better", more "mature", and "considerate" person. One participant accounted, "I used to want to do a lot of things with no time left. After I've recovered, I've realized that that's not the way to go. I didn't have to have a second job. I didn't have to be occupied with work all the time. After I've recovered, I've learnt to manage my time much better."

As a result of the illness experience, participants have developed new values and views on life and relationships: "I've become more confident, my values have changed. I have a different value system now." "After I'd recovered, I read more and was involved in fewer activities. Simply talking to friends makes me very happy now. I've learnt to plan my life, and have a clearer grasp of things. I'm now generally smarter." Participants were better able to differentiate between "casual friends" and "closer friends" with whom they shared more intimate thoughts and feelings: "Now I know which ones I can sit down and talk to, which ones are just party friends . . . I used to just talk about my own problems and not listen to what others might have to say about theirs. Now I understand that I could offer others help just as they have helped me . . . I'm not so much different, but having grown up, become more mature, kinder and gentler, I can think more clearly now, I've grown to be more mature."

Participants have learnt to appreciate life and the value of helping others, as opposed to putting personal achievements as top priority. They have learnt to take pleasure in simple things such as exercising, reading, watching television, listening to music, going to movies, and travelling. One participant shared, "My values are different now. I used to be so preoccupied with work and study. But now I feel that I could just go home and cook after work, eat with my boyfriend, then go swimming. This kind of life is very relaxing. I'm now a contented person. I make less money, but can spend just less."

Some of them have become stronger characters and have gained a sense of being in control with better time and resource management as opposed to being overwhelmed by extending activities and responsibilities. "I used to care about the quantity of friends to a point that I'd compete with others for the longest friend list on ICQ . . . Now I look for those who have shown care for me before and those to whom I can talk. I don't like keeping so many acquaintances close by anymore." Participants have taken time to nurture existing friendships or rekindle old ones.

The findings also revealed that people with first-episode psychosis viewed psychotic illness as having a better outlook than other chronic physical illnesses: "Those other chronic [physical] conditions require long-term fights. Mental illness doesn't have to be forever. As long as you lead a normal and healthy life, you can readjust gradually. Other physical conditions can never be cured, they're lifelong."

From the experience of recovery in first-episode psychosis, there is a common theme of being better and stronger persons and being able to withstand adversity and illness, while recovery causes a desire to live each minute to the full no matter how difficult the circumstances are. Through approaching life this way, circumstances inevitably improve and problems no longer seem insurmountable. Recovery is about being loved and accepted. It is about human transformation in the deepest sense. Through coming to terms with the illness experience, people are able to change their perceptions about themselves and the world to something more positive and begin to act accordingly.

Summary

A common theme expressed by most participants in the focus group was that of becoming a better and stronger person following their illness experience. They were able to overcome the adversity of illness. From their perspective, recovery was about improving their personal outlook for the future, including having a valued role, which included:

1. Social networks, such as family or friends. The ability to sustain and resolve conflicts within relationships was crucial to recovery.
2. Employment or having meaningful vocational opportunities.
3. A personal desire to progress in life and make changes where necessary to achieve his or her goals and dreams.
4. A sense of belonging to a group or community and having a valid role to play in that group.
5. Spiritual growth and a fulfilling personal philosophy to live by.

Current services and research focus too heavily on clinical recovery, that is, symptomatic control. The current proposal that early intervention services should encourage personal growth is particularly important for young people at the critical developmental stage when they search for identity. Help should be offered not only for symptomatic management, but also in resolving personal problems, building and sustaining relationships and developing identity and status. This requires workers who understand the recovery process and are enthusiastic and able to instil hope in their clients.

Early intervention appears to have broken away from the negative approach of traditional psychiatry so far as it has adopted a far more optimistic view of recovery. However, the main focus of treatment remains symptom control and relapse prevention via medications. The need for continued medications to prevent relapse must be balanced with the individual's choice of treatment with informed risks. Any measure of coercion, either overtly or covertly, can be most damaging to individuals and can easily reinforce feelings of helplessness and powerlessness, as well as encourage avoidance in seeking help.

Recovery is a far more fundamental step forward than simply removing or suppressing symptoms. Recovery does not necessarily mean that psychotic symptoms have disappeared, but rather that the person feels more in control of their symptoms, and is able to function well and do the things he or she wants to do in life, rather than being a victim of psychosis. As seen in the findings, most participants expressed negative views about medication. The way in which medication is given can reinforce the clients' negative beliefs about themselves, that they are victims controlled by other people. An essential part of recovery is the feeling of control and not being at the mercy of others, especially people in authority or those closest to them. For example, threatening to withdraw support or active treatment from services for those refusing medication may reinforce their previous experience of rejection and powerlessness. The same may be true in families that monitor and administer medication for the client.

Stigma emerges as a major theme from the findings. No participants reported overt discrimination, but subjective, internalized stigmas about themselves were evident. Participants perceived "early psychosis" to have a more optimistic outlook than "schizophrenia". This implies that media may exert a crucial influence in the production of stereotypical images, just as it can be a powerful vehicle for changing any stigmatizing representation of schizophrenia. Thus, cooperation with the media is essential for effectively counteracting negative media coverage and addressing the lack of information on psychosis for the public.

Recovery and the hope for it could be encouraged by particular professional attitudes. The emphasis on medication to prevent relapse needs to be balanced with treatment coercion which enforces passivity and powerlessness that interfere with clients' control over recovery. Recovery can also be achieved through non-medical measures, including support from family, friends, and other parties. Instead of merely observing the clients' behaviour and trying to interpret it in terms of clinical models, more focus must be put on valuing, respecting, and understanding the person's experiences from his or her perspective.

References

Anthony, W. A. (1993). Recovery from mental illness: The guiding vision of the mental health service system in the 1990s. *Psychosocial Rehabilitation Journal, 16*(4), 11–23.

Lam, M. M., Pearson, V., Ng, R. M., Chiu, C. P., Law, C. W., & Chen, E. Y. (2010). What does recovery from psychosis mean? Perceptions of young first-episode patients. *The International Journal of Social Psychiatry*. doi: 10.1177/0020764010374418

Part VIII

Evaluation and Research

32
Database Design and Management

Kin-sheung Wong

Healthcare is one of the most information-intensive and information-demanding industries. Healthcare workers, including doctors, nurses, and other allied health workers, require large amounts of information about their clients in order to make clinical decisions and select appropriate care for clients. At the same time, healthcare planners need comprehensive service data to evaluate existing services and to implement new service strategies. The application of information technology to healthcare industries is therefore an essential element to ensure that timely and up-to-date client information is maintained and accessible when necessary.

Information Needs for Daily Operation of Early Psychosis Intervention

In Hong Kong's Early Assessment Service for Young People with Psychosis (EASY), case managers of each team handle copious phone enquires and referrals from different sources every day. They conduct first-stage assessments and arrange clinical assessments for potential clients if needed. Hence, a system is necessary to keep track of the phone enquires and referrals they handle. Case managers need to maintain regular contact with existing clients and their caregivers in order to provide appropriate psychosocial intervention and psychoeducation. Therefore, they need to keep a complete register of their clients, which includes basic demographic and essential clinical information. At the same time, different clinical and service data need to be collected via various clinical measuring scales at different intervals of the treatment programme. Moreover, as educational talks are conducted in schools and the community on a regular basis to promote public awareness of the illness, each team needs to submit various statistical reports to head office regularly so that the convener can monitor progress and effectiveness of services.

System Analysis

User requirements

A computerized system to manage the information processing of EASY is in place to meet the following needs:

1. Keep a complete and comprehensive register of clients in the service.
2. Keep a complete record of the number of phone calls received.
3. Keep a complete record of educational talks conducted.
4. Collect service-related data, such as number of relapses, admissions, and suicidal attempts.
5. Generate statistical reports on a regular basis.

Existing information infrastructure

Nowadays, most of the healthcare authorities in modern countries have already taken advantage of computerized systems to enhance efficiency and effectiveness of services. Major service providers may have their own enterprise-wide information systems, for example the Clinical Management System (CMS) in Hong Kong, to manage key healthcare information. Ideally, such information systems are multifunctional so as to support daily operations in hospitals and clinics.

System Design

System architecture

The EASY system is composed of individual databases and a master database. Each team has its own local database in the site office, which only stores that team's client information. The data from individual databases is incorporated into the master database located in the head office. A designated worker visits different site offices to collect up-to-date client information and synchronize it with the master database when he/she returns to the head office. The advantages of such an approach are:

- Each team is only able to access the information of its own clients (but not other teams' clients), enhancing privacy and confidentiality of clients' information.
- The size of individual databases is relatively small, making it easier to maintain.
- Individual system failure will not affect the integrity of the master database at head office.
- Likewise, the master database can easily be rebuilt by integrating the four individual databases in case of system failure at head office.

Table Design

A set of core data is identified and defined, and the resulting dataset is finalized and normalized into different tables in the database accordingly. The tables could be grouped into four categories as below and in Figure 32.1:

1. *Client demographic data*
   - Client table: stores basic demographic data of clients (e.g., name, sex, date of birth, address)
   - Contact table: stores clients' contact information
2. *Client clinical data*
   - Engagement table: stores the engagement works done with clients
   - Intervention table: stores the intervention done with clients
   - Clinical psychologist intervention table: stores information about intervention by clinical psychologists with clients
   - Medication table: stores the details of medications prescribed for clients
   - Admission table: stores the admission information of clients
   - Relapse table: stores the relapse information of clients
   - Suicide table: stores the suicide information of clients
   - Violence table: stores the violence records of clients
   - Works table: stores the nature of psychoeducation provided for clients
3. *Questionnaires and scales*
   - Quality of Life table: stores the data sourced from quality of life questionnaire
   - Symptoms table: stores the data collected about clients' symptoms
   - RPS table: stores the data collected for the relapse prevention programme
   - Onset table: stores the data collected on clients' onset and help-seeking

4. *Supporting tables*
   - Nurse table: stores the names of nurses
   - Doctor table: stores the names of doctors
   - Phone call table: stores the phone calls received by case managers
   - Talks table: stores the educational talk information
   - Call-by-case table: stores the number of calls from an individual case
   - Screen-by-case table: stores the number of screening section required for an individual case

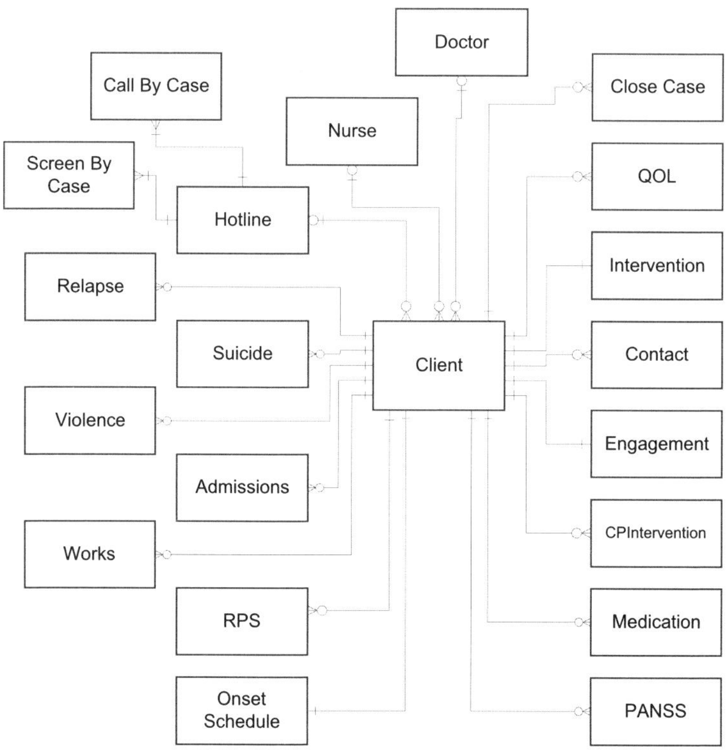

Figure 32.1

ER diagram of the EASY system

System Development

Selection of database system

In EASY, Microsoft Access is used as the backend database system for the following reasons:

1. A mature and reliable relational database management system (RDBMS) comes with the Microsoft Office package. Most of the computers used by major service providers have already installed this system.
2. Sufficient processing power to manage data is expected not to be huge.
3. It is relatively simple and easy to implement and manage when compared with other RDBMS systems.
4. Sufficient technical information and support are available on the internet via various newsgroups or Microsoft Developer Network (MSDN).

System Specification

The EASY system provides the following information processing functions:

1. Data processing – to append, edit, delete, and enquire:
   - client information
   - phone call records
   - educational talks records
2. Reports generation – to generate:
   - monthly phone call statistical reports
   - monthly educational talks reports
   - monthly case intake reports
   - monthly psychoeducation activities reports
   - client listing for team meetings
   - client contact listing for respective case managers
3. Data security:
   - adapts the nativc sccurity architecture of Microsoft Access 2000
   - users need to have an account and logon with valid password before they can open the application to access client information
   - this security measure is able to protect the confidentiality of client data and to prohibit amateur and casual users breaking into the IT system

System Implementation

The EASY system was implemented in individual site offices. Individual computers in the office are connected to the hospital network. The local database file of the team is installed on one of the computers and shares the access rights with other workstations (Figure 32.2). Since the system runs the network, case managers can open the application to access client information at any time without interrupting others' work; for example, case manager A can look for a client's address and contact phone number while case manager B is adding a new client information to the database.

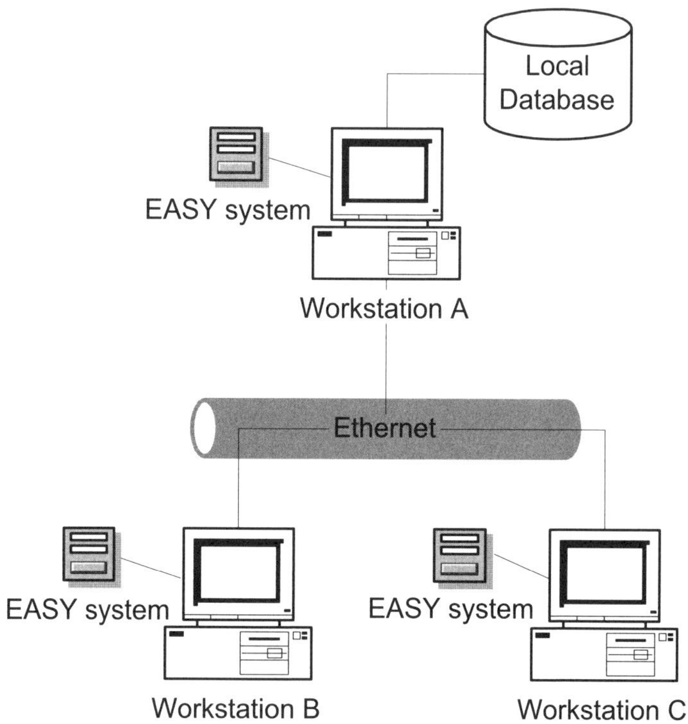

Figure 32.2

Implementation of EASY system in site office

Limitations and Challenges

Data planning

Selecting data to be stored is an extremely important step in all database applications as it not only affects the primary design of respective tables in the database, but also affects the future modification and expansion, especially in a relational database management system. In RDBMS, tables are linked together via relations, and adding new data field or new table will most likely disturb the existing relations among tables. It will add complexity to the application in retrieving data from different tables, which will then affect the stability and efficiency of the application. On the other hand, properly identified and grouped data can make data analysis or data mining easier. Therefore, careful planning of data structure can avoid a lot of data exploration and system maintenance nightmares.

User acceptance

User acceptance and cooperation is one of the most important factors that foster successful implementation of a system. User involvement throughout the entire development cycle is the key to success. Users' input in the development process better ensures that the system under development would be exactly what the users seek. Proper training could also increase user acceptance.

Missing data

Missing data is a common problem when user acceptance is low and updating client information in the system requires users' effort and cooperation. When users do not appreciate the system, they are usually reluctant to spend time entering necessary data. Missing or incorrect data definitely distorts statistical results and data representation of the service.

Summary

Early psychosis intervention service requires a computerized information system to store its client information and to support daily operations. Such a system provides basic information processing features to support the team's daily activities and generates useful statistical reports on a regular basis. Naturally, careful data planning and high user acceptance fosters the successful implementation of the system.

33

Research and Outcome Evaluation in Early Psychosis

Eric Yu-hai Chen

Research Tradition in Early Psychosis

One of the major characteristics distinguishing early psychosis from some other mental health arenas is that research forms an integral part of the early psychosis initiative.

In the last two decades, research in schizophrenia has witnessed a growing emphasis on first-episode studies. Researchers started to identify patient samples with a first onset of psychotic illness and performed various clinical, cognitive, and biological measurements. Some of these observations (particularly those focusing on biological or neurocognitive markers of the disease) were potentially affected by the patients' medication. In attempts to rule out medication effects, researchers measured these markers among first-episode patients, especially those who have never received any medication. Studies on first-episode patients revealed that, although these patients share many common characteristics with those who have suffered from the illness for a prolonged time period, the former group of patients do have some unique characteristics that interest researchers and clinicians.

Another relevant research paradigm in early psychosis is the pursuit of longitudinal high-risk studies, which often involve following up individuals with increased risk of illness onset, such as those with genetic risks (e.g., one of the parents is suffering from the disease). Researchers track patterns of onset in such high-risk groups, in an attempt to identify factors that can be observed even before the onset of the illness. Some studies are devoted to investigating the onset pattern of the illness, leading to the development of instruments that describe the evolution of symptoms over time.

Research Questions in Early Psychosis

Duration of untreated psychosis, early intervention, and outcome

While it is generally agreed that the duration of untreated psychosis (DUP) is related to treatment outcome, researchers are not just interested in the statistical relationship between the two constructs, but more importantly, in the nature of mechanisms that mediate such a relationship. If we can identify any mediating mechanisms, treatment outcomes can potentially be altered. One major question is whether the correlation between DUP and treatment outcome has a causal relationship, or whether such interrelatedness is the result of a third confounding factor that exerts effect on both DUP and treatment outcome. Some researchers have suggested premorbid personality and/or premorbid adjustment as potential confounding factor(s), which may partly explain the relationship between DUP and treatment outcomes. Clarifying the mechanism underlying the relationship between DUP and treatment outcomes will continue to be an important research question in early psychosis.

Setting aside the issue of DUP, another fundamental research question is whether intensive and specialized input during the early phase of psychosis would really improve the outcome of the illness. Randomized controlled studies, in which patients are randomly assigned to an experimental group (i.e., receiving early intervention) or a control group (i.e., receiving standard care without early intervention), with longitudinal outcome follow up, are required to answer this important question. However, this experimental design may present ethical problems, as patients assigned to the control group will have their early intervention intentionally delayed despite their diagnosis. Nevertheless, if the level of service provided is acceptable even for standard care of the given population, this kind of study may be ethically justified. A study of this kind, the Lambeth Early Onset (LEO) study, was conducted in London, and its conclusions supported the superiority of specialized teams over standard care (Craig et al., 2004).

Some researchers referred to early data that pre-dated any established finding about the effectiveness of medical treatment. Some of these studies had adopted a randomized experimental design with the assumption that medication treatment is the only effective intervention. Groups receiving other kinds of intervention (such as psychotherapy alone) were taken as control groups and one such study supported the efficacy of early medication treatment (May et al., 1981).

Besides referring to historical data sets, another approach performs an historical control study using current data. In other words, instead of a randomized design, two cohorts of patients with similar characteristics within the same population are examined, with one group pre-early intervention service development, and the other group post early intervention service. The outcome of these two groups are then compared. Studies of this kind have been conducted in Australia and Norway, supporting the effectiveness of early intervention, especially in reducing negative symptoms, improving quality of life, and shortening DUP (Johannessen et al., 2001; Larsen et al., 2001; McGorry et al., 1996). However, historical control study design has several flaws. For instance, it is vulnerable to cohort effect, namely, the apparent group differences might be due to the fact that they take place in different time periods, and some historical factors other than the early intervention itself may be at play. In other words, some social changes or general environmental factors could potentially contribute to treatment outcome and cannot be excluded.

In sum, given the ethical concerns associated with analysing and evaluating data for early psychosis, it is not always easy to investigate the outcomes of early psychosis in a stringent manner.

Primary prevention

Another popular topic in early psychosis research addresses the question whether the incidence of psychosis can be reduced if early intervention is extended to a period prior to illness onset (i.e., primary prevention of the illness). If the answer to this question is positive, psychosis will be the first mental health condition that has a preventive solution.

Nevertheless, research and solutions to primary intervention in mental health are complex. The first issue to deal with is to screen and identify individuals who will potentially develop the illness. Herein lies the relevance of the medical concept of prodrome. Retrospective scrutiny reveals the presence of certain signs and symptoms during the prodromal phase, such as functional difficulties and mood fluctuations. If individuals in the prodromal phase can be identified with the help of accurate screening techniques, researchers can investigate whether intervention strategies can reduce or even prevent the onset of illness.

In light of the significant implications associated with preventing illness onset, prodrome has become a popular research area in psychiatry. However, certain challenges arise in designing and implementing prodrome research. First, whether the prodrome can be identified accurately remains a controversial question; that is, whether certain markers or methods can be used to effectively predict the imminent onset of a psychotic illness. In fact, existing research data reveal that although some symptoms do appear before the onset of psychosis, they are far from specific. For instance, insomnia can be a prodromal symptom, but probably only a small proportion of those suffering from insomnia would eventually develop psychosis. This presents the problem of specificity; the level of specificity of the screening tool has to be taken into account when screening prodromal symptoms.

In medicine, acknowledging the fact that no screening method is absolutely specific and accurate, preventive intervention is often applied to a broader population to ensure its efficacy. This consideration leads to the concept of "number needed to treat" (NNT), namely, the number of people that an intervention should be applied to in order to prevent one person from developing the condition of interest. The NNT needs to be counterbalanced by the cost of the intervention; for example, an invasive form of intervention has to be justified by a low NNT ratio. Researchers in psychosis are constantly defining and refining the prodromal characteristics of the illness in an attempt to reduce the NNT ratio and thereby maximizing the efficacy of the intervention. The more specific rating scales for screening purposes now available are the At-Risk Mental States (Yung et al., 2005), Structured Interview for Prodromal Syndromes (SIPS; Miller et al., 2002) and Scale of Prodromal Syndromes (SOPS; Miller et al., 1999), which give an NNT ratio of about 3:1. That is, it may be possible to prevent one person from developing psychosis by applying the intervention to every three persons screened positive using these scales. In other words, two out of these three persons receiving the intervention did so "unnecessarily". Unfortunately, it is currently impossible to accurately identify which one of these three persons would actually develop psychosis at a later time.

Antipsychotic medication

The most effective intervention to manage psychosis is antipsychotic medication, which nonetheless entails the cost of side-effects even with second generation antipsychotics. Preliminary research data hint that antipsychotic medication may only delay the onset of psychosis instead of preventing it altogether. In other words, the patient may still develop psychosis upon later cessation of medications. Thus, another difficult issue is for how long medication should be prescribed in order to prevent the illness onset, and whether medication should be continued indefinitely, which induces even heavier costs.

At present, different research groups are actively seeking interventions that have fewer side-effects, such as the use of psychosocial intervention or neuroprotective agents that are not antipsychotic drugs. These possible new ways of treating psychosis remain important areas of research. In investigating the prevention of the illness, the defining criteria of prodrome must include some mild psychotic symptoms, or else the NNT ratio might be too high to justify any form of intervention. However, the inclusion of mild psychotic symptoms inevitably brings about the problem of circularity. That is, the patients under scrutiny are actually not in a prodromal phase, but are already presenting some psychotic symptoms that are transient or otherwise hidden. Thus, this kind of intervention can at most be taken as a "very early intervention" for psychosis, rather than genuine prodromal intervention. Any form of true prodromal screening and identification (e.g., without any traces of psychotic symptoms) might incur even greater costs, as the NNT would be very high. Also, such research is difficult to conduct as the progression from prodrome to the development of psychosis may take up to 10 years or more, which would demand copious research resources.

Identification of markers

Another theme of research in early psychosis is the identification of markers or predictors of outcome. There are many dimensions pertaining to outcome, including recovery, relapse, suicide, deliberate self-harm, violence, symptomatic control, quality of life, and functioning; each of these dimensions of outcome may be affected by different factors and processes. Finding markers to predict and clarify underlying mechanisms for these outcome qualities in a naturalistic sample is an important first step to uncover mechanisms that lead to poor outcome and to design intervention to prevent these adverse outcomes of the illness.

Experiential dimensions

Though recent trends in research tend to view psychotic disorders from a biological and cognitive point of view, an important perspective to be highlighted is the patients' experiential dimension. This dimension has often been delegated an insignificant role in current research, yet it is crucial in the sense that it may be indispensable in determining patient outcome, in terms of quality of life, symptomatic control, functioning, and so on. As a self-determining agent, the patients' subjective experience and decision-making should not be overlooked in the research process.

Relationship between Research and Service Delivery

Research is a multifaceted endeavour, and service development is one of the aspects closely associated with it. As contemporary healthcare adopts an evidence-based approach, sufficient local data on the specific population is needed to show the outcome when a certain kind of intervention is delivered to this population. After that, attempts are to be made to identify the predictors or markers of good and bad outcome, and then during service design, these markers should be used to identify those patients with poor outcome. If a certain marker were believed to be a mediator, it would be desirable to minimize this risk factor so as to improve overall outcome.

In clinical service, data are collected at the point of contact, and these data reveal the characteristics of the patients during a specific stage. Patients in the same illness stage are likely to be more homogenous in nature and this in turn may help identify predictors. Otherwise, noise associated with different illness stages might mask potential predictors. Therefore with a phase-specific service targeting a particular population, there is a better chance of identifying outcome predictors. In addition, phase specific cohorts may guide service delivery by testing whether intervention designs are feasible and effective. This cycle of service-generated population-specific data and data-guided service development must be re-iterated to continuously improve service outcome and quality.

References

Craig, T. K. J., Garety, P., Power, P., Rahaman, N., Colbert, S., Fornells-Ambrojo, M., Dunn, G. (2004). The Lambeth Early Onset (LEO) Team: Randomised controlled trial of the effectiveness of specialised care for early psychosis. *British Medical Journal 329*, 1067. doi: 10.1136/bmj.38246.594873.7C

Johannessen, J. O., McGlashan, T. H., Larsen, T. K., Horneland, M., Joa, I., Mardal, S., et al. (2001). Early detection strategies for untreated first-episode psychosis. [Clinical Trial, Phase I Comparative Study Multicenter Study Research Support, Non-U.S. Government Research Support, U.S. Government, P.H.S.]. *Schizophrenia Research, 51*(1), 39–46.

Larsen, T. K., McGlashan, T. H., Johannessen, J. O., Friis, S., Guldberg, C., Haahr, U., et al. (2001). Shortened duration of untreated first episode of psychosis: Changes in patient characteristics at treatment. [Research Support, Non-U.S. Government Research Support, U.S. Government, P.H.S.]. *American Journal of Psychiatry, 158*(11), 1917–1919.

May, P. R., Tuma, A. H., Dixon, W. J., Yale, C., Thiele, D. A., & Kraude, W. H. (1981). Schizophrenia: A follow-up study of the results of five forms of treatment. [Clinical Trial Randomized Controlled Trial Research Support, Non-U.S. Government Research Support, U.S. Government, Non-P.H.S. Research Support, U.S. Government, P.H.S.]. *Archives of General Psychiatry, 38*(7), 776–784.

McGorry, P. D., Edwards, J., Mihalopoulos, C., Harrigan, S. M., & Jackson, H. J. (1996). EPPIC: An evolving system of early detection and optimal management. *Schizophrenia Bulletin, 22*(2), 305–326.

Miller, T. J., McGlashan, T. H., Rosen, J. L., Somjee, L., Markovich, P. J., Stein, K., & Woods, S. W. (2002). Prospective diagnosis of the initial prodrome for schizophrenia based on the Structured Interview for Prodromal Syndromes: Preliminary evidence of interrater reliability and predictive validity. [Comparative Study Research Support, Non-U.S. Government Research Support, U.S. Government, P.H.S.]. *The American Journal of Psychiatry, 159*(5), 863–865.

Miller, T. J., McGlashan, T. H., Woods, S. W., Stein, K., Driesen, N., Corcoran, C. M., et al. (1999). Symptom assessment in schizophrenic prodromal states. [Clinical Trial Review]. *The Psychiatric Quarterly, 70*(4), 273–287.

Yung, A. R., Yuen, H. P., McGorry, P. D., Phillips, L. J., Kelly, D., Dell'Olio, M., et al. (2005) Mapping the onset of psychosis: The Comprehensive Assessment of At-Risk Mental States. [Comparative Study]. *The Australian and New Zealand Journal of Psychiatry, 39*(11–12), 964–971. doi: 10.1111/j.1440-1614.2005.01714.x

Index

Abbreviated Youth Psychosis At-Risk Questionnaire (Y-PARQ-B), 51
aberrant salience, 148
accident and emergency departments, 17, 106
acute and transient psychosis, 113, 118
adjustment reaction/disorder, 37, 97
affective psychosis, 118
affective symptoms, 93, 112, 114, 264, 285, 291, 293
age of onset, 49, 68, 70, 105
antipsychotics, 11, 132, 137, 148, 204, 263–267, 273, 305–306, 351, 370–371
  first-generation, 264, 305, 315
  recommended dose, 266–267
  second-generation/atypical, 40, 264, 306, 315
Asian Network of Early Psychosis (ANEP), 7
Asperger's syndrome, 115
assertive community treatment, 52, 54
at-risk mental state, 9, 21, 26, 33, 40–41, 48, 50–51, 93, 95–97, 103, 112, 115, 118, 123–132, 256, 263, 369–371
attunement disorder (調絃病), 56–57, 80

basic symptoms, 124, 126–127
belief modification, 168
benzodiazepines, 130, 267
bipolar affective disorder, 20, 111, 113
birth cohorts, 125–126
bizarre behaviour, 102, 117, 146–147, 248
Bonn Scale for the Assessment of Basic Symptoms (BSABS), 127
Brief Psychiatric Rating Score (BPRS), 324
bullying, 50, 165

cannabis, 115, 301
cardiovascular changes, 265
caregivers, 10–11, 22, 24, 32–33, 68–69, 71, 114, 116–117, 145, 160, 189, 191–197, 199–205, 247, 315–317, 324–327, 359
  caregivers' stress, 204–205, 257
  support worker, 250–253
care plan (*see* management plan)
caseload, 22–23, 52, 210, 305
case management, 10, 17, 21–22, 31, 52, 54, 168, 190, 210–219, 317
  accessibility, 190
  case formulation, 111, 172
  characteristics of case managers, 214–218
  development, 24
  evaluation, 213
  role of case managers, 211, 306–307, 314
  supervision model, 209–219
  training, 24, 213–214
child psychiatric team, 106

Chinese medicine, 195
client-centred services, 162, 194, 197
Clinical Management System (CMS), 360
clinical psychologists, 23, 40–41, 130, 138–139, 145, 147, 190, 219, 361
clubhouse model, 31–33, 41, 224–241
cocaine, 115
cognitive behavioural therapy (CBT), 22, 40, 53–54, 137, 145, 148, 150, 159, 161, 168–171
cognitive impairment/symptoms, 31, 40, 115, 117, 172, 230, 264
  subjective, 99, 328
cognitive remediation/training, 40–41, 137, 160, 230–233
Community Assessment of Psychic Experiences (CAPE), 51
community-based services, 11, 37–38, 49, 194, 257
Community Health Assessment Team (CHAT), 34
comorbidities, 12, 115–116, 138, 146–148, 160–161, 168, 192, 293, 301–307, 317
Comprehensive Assessment of At-Risk Mental States (CAARMS), 50–51, 53, 130–131
concealment, 142, 200–201, 203, 351–353
conceptual misalignment, 338
confidentiality, 116, 144, 242, 361, 363
consultation liaison team, 104, 106
cost-benefit analysis, 25
counselling, 31, 49–50, 52, 128, 131, 178, 209, 211, 214, 224, 231, 250
course of illness, 4, 11–12, 112, 118, 292, 342, 350
crisis management, 52, 139, 160, 209, 211, 233, 248–250
critical period, 8–9, 11, 47–48, 53–55
cultural beliefs/values, 6–7, 10, 138, 160–161, 164, 175–187, 192–193, 203, 237, 243, 248, 279
data management, 359–366
  data planning, 365
  data processing, 363
  data security, 363
  missing data, 365
  reports generation, 363
  user acceptance, 365
data system
  architecture, 360–361
  specification, 363
deinstitutionalization, 37, 323
delusional disorder, 20, 113, 118
delusions, 50–51, 102, 137, 141, 146–147, 162, 166, 168, 195, 273, 293, 313, 325, 328–329
dementia praecox, 4, 48
denial, 29, 35, 141, 179, 191, 194, 201
depot medication, 196, 276, 306
depressive symptoms, 21, 37, 47, 89, 99, 102, 108, 112, 115, 118, 124, 128, 146–147, 159, 168, 186, 192, 238, 264, 292–295, 313, 325–327, 338
destigmatization, 25, 206
detection, 49–51
  at-risk mental state, 9, 21, 42, 132
  psychosis, 8, 23, 52–53
Detection of Early Psychosis (DEEP), 127
developmental tasks, 347
diabetes, 265
diagnosis
  diagnostic criteria, 112
  diagnostic interview, 49, 111–119
  diagnostic stability, 113–114
  differential diagnosis, 117
  dual diagnosis, 303–304
  revision, 117
discrimination, 89, 132, 199, 202
dopamine D_2 occupancy, 266
drug abuse (*see* substance abuse)
drug-induced psychosis, 100, 115, 118, 302, 305

duration of untreated psychosis (DUP), 5–6, 8–9, 18–19, 25, 29, 38, 67–71, 114, 312–313, 368

Early Assessment Service for Young People with Psychosis (EASY), 17–26, 75, 93, 101, 111, 128, 137, 190, 258, 301, 359
Early Psychosis Intervention Programme (EPIP), 11, 29–35, 160, 209, 225, 235, 247
Early Psychosis Prevention and Intervention Centre (EPPIC), 304
Early Treatment of Psychosis Project (TOPP), 127
ecstasy, 115, 301
emotional changes, 97, 102, 351–352
empathic listening, 107, 116, 196, 295
employment, 41, 258, 328
  supported employment, 225, 231–233
  unemployment, 34, 88, 347, 351
empowerment, 83, 223–226, 233, 237, 245, 324, 346
endocrine disease, 118
epilepsy, 118, 327
Eppendorf Schizophrenia Inventory (ESI), 50–51, 53
explanatory model of illness, 141, 161, 163–167, 176, 200, 304
expressed emotion, 200, 253, 285, 312
extrapyramidal symptoms, 99, 264–266, 305–306, 313, 328

family experience of psychiatry illness, 68
family intervention, 247, 257
family service centres, 252
functional psychosis, 113, 115
functioning
  family, 247
  functional decline, 102, 128
  occupational/vocational, 24, 41, 89
  psychosocial, 40, 89, 335

gatekeepers, 80, 93–100
general practitioners, 30, 67, 106
genetic high-risk studies, 125–126
global assessment of functioning (GAF), 41, 130–131
global burden of disease, 47
Green Program for Recognition and Prevention of Early Psychosis (GRAPE), 54
grieving, 147
group work, 32, 237
  discussion groups, 227, 238
  group dynamics, 237, 243

hallucinations, 89, 96, 102, 108, 130, 141, 149, 168, 178, 183, 193, 293, 325, 330, 335, 350
help-seeking, 6, 9, 17, 34, 67–70, 75, 78, 81, 83, 87, 100, 141–142, 160, 163, 177, 191–192, 248, 361
  barriers, 34, 69, 75, 83
Hillside Study of Risk and Early Detection of Schizophrenia (HSREDS), 127–128
home leave, 249–250
home visit, 249
Hong Kong Early Psychosis Intervention Society (EPISO), 25, 76
hospital-based services, 37–38
hospital discharge, 294
hospitalization, 24, 313
  compulsory admission, 196
  social admission, 38
housing services (*see* residential services)

Il Bosco, 40
illness attribution (*see* explanatory model of illness)
illness experience, integration of, 343
incidence, 47
information technology, 359
insight, 102, 141, 147

International Clinical Practice Guidelines for Early Psychosis, 266
International Early Psychosis Association (IEPA), 6
intervention service
  disengagement, 192, 194–195, 305
  duration, 26
  engagement, 93, 102, 143–144, 160, 189–197
  evaluation, 12, 24, 367–372
  psychosocial, 223–224
  step-down, 26, 224
  timing, 3
Interview for the Retrospective Assessment of the Onset of Schizophrenia (IRAOS), 125

Japanese Society for Prevention and Early Intervention in Psychiatry (JSEIP), 39
Jockey Club Early Psychosis (JCEP) project, 17, 26, 76, 79–84

ketamine, 115, 301
Korean Network of Early Psychosis (K-NEP), 52–53

labelling, 96, 199
life events, 98, 292, 294, 341
lipid abnormalities, 265
long-term outcome, 5, 8, 78, 142, 304

maintenance medication, 267, 273
  duration, 285–286, 338
management plan, 10, 39, 116, 172, 209, 315
marginalization, 200, 235
media exposure to psychosis, 76
media work, 19, 25, 81
medical insurance, 55
Medication Adherence Rating Scale (MARS), 277
medication compliance, 89, 143, 273–279, 301, 305
medication discontinuation, 265, 274, 287, 326, 338
Medication Event Monitoring System (MEMS), 277
medication side-effects, 99, 118, 258–259, 274, 306, 351
mental retardation, 115
metabolic disease, 118
metaphor
  journal, 341
  spatial, 342
methamphetamine, 115
mindfulness, 149
misconceptions, 76–77, 90, 143
mode of illness development, 19, 70, 114
  acute onset, 67
  insidious onset, 69
mood symptoms (*see* affective symptoms)
multidisciplinary team, 40, 93, 139, 190

needs assessment, 140
negative symptoms, 40, 99, 114, 311–317
  attenuated, 124
  persistent, 314
  primary, 313
  secondary, 313
neuroleptics (*see* antipsychotics)
neuroticism, 146
non-affective psychosis, 113
non-government organization (NGO), 23, 75, 94, 105, 255–259, 305, 316
non-specific symptoms, 112, 124
normalization, 54, 257–258
number needed to treat (NNT), 370
nurses, 23, 38, 40–41, 101, 250, 256

obsessive-compulsive disorder, 115
occupational therapists, 32, 40, 228, 258
outcome predictors, 371
outpatient department, 106
outreach, 35, 38, 49, 93, 189–197, 190

paranoid ideas, 97
pathway to care, 5, 93, 314
peer support, 235–245
  specialists, 237, 240
perceptual changes, 102, 113
performance deterioration (*see* functioning, functional decline)
Personal and Strategic Coping Therapy for Early Psychosis (PASTE), 159–172
Personal Assistance and Crisis Evaluation (PACE) clinic, 127
personal contact, 82
personal therapy, 161, 163–167
personality changes, 103
personality disorder, 115
Peters Delusions Inventory (PDI), 50–51
phase-specific intervention, 21–23
physical exercise, 230
physical work-up, 117
Positive and Negative Syndrome Scale (PANSS), 131
positive symptoms (*see* psychotic symptoms)
premorbid functioning, 292, 313
premorbid personality, 69
prevalence, 47
Preventive through Risk Identification, Management and Education (PRIME) study, 127
Prodromal Questionnaire (PQ), 51
prodrome (*see* at-risk mental state)
psychiatrists, 17, 23, 30, 37–38, 41, 101–103, 106–108, 129, 139, 194, 201, 240, 257, 351
psychoeducation, 22, 41, 53, 141–143, 161, 224, 247–252, 263, 304, 315
psychological adjustment, 138
Psychological Intervention Programmes for Early Psychosis (PIPE), 137–150
psychopathological assessment, 101
psychosis-like experience (*see* psychotic symptoms, subclinical/subthreshold)
psychosis proneness, 126
Psychosis Recovery Inventory (PRI), 337
psychotherapy, 31, 50, 54, 159, 161, 189
psychotic symptoms
  attenuated, 99, 130
  atypical features, 118
  brief limited intermittent, 131
  drug-resistant, 138, 148–150
  personal significance, 330
  re-appraisal, 148
  residual, 99, 283
  subclinical/subthreshold, 42, 47, 124–125, 128
public awareness, 19, 25, 30, 49, 75–85, 94, 256, 317
  messages, 83–84
public education (*see* public awareness)

quality of life, 89, 185, 199, 225, 251, 264, 323, 324, 328, 346, 361, 369, 371–372

randomized controlled design, 368
rapport, 93, 102, 107, 116
reality judgment, 343
reality testing, 168
recovery, 12, 140, 144, 160, 323–331, 335–344, 345–356
  clinical recovery, 140, 346
  cognitive linguistic approach, 335–344
  consumer model, 336
  functional recovery, 140
  medical model, 336
  partial recovery, 327
  principles of recovery, 347
  psychological recovery, 346
  recovery styles, 142
  social recovery, 140, 346
  subjective experience, 274, 336–337, 345–356

Recovery in Schizophrenia Working Group, 335
recovery movement, 236, 327
referral channel, 21, 93–95, 103–107, 256
  external referral, 103–105
  internal referral, 106
  online referral, 42, 105
  self-referral, 107
  sensitivity and specificity, 95–96
rehabilitation, 223–224, 315, 325
  psychosocial, 41, 170–171
  vocational, 41, 88–89, 258
reintegration, 225, 238, 257–258
relapse, 283–287
  cost of relapse, 284
  prevention, 143–144, 273, 316
  relapse predictors, 285
  relapse rate, 24, 53, 267, 284, 301
  risk perception, 274
relational database management system (RDBMS), 363
religious beliefs, 161, 175–187
remission, 140, 273, 323, 335
renaming, 20–21, 55–58, 79–80
residential services, 224
resilience, 54
risk assessment, 295
role functioning (*see* functioning)

safety behaviour, 141
safety, staff, 196
schema
  container image, 339
  path image, 340
schizoaffective disorder, 118
school-based intervention, 49–50
school counsellors, 31, 34, 49, 93
school teachers, 49, 80, 101, 105
screening of psychosis, 21, 23, 42, 49–51
  population screening, 125–126
  telephone-based assessment, 101–109
sealing over, 125, 142, 343
secondary morbidities (*see* comorbidities)
sedation, 266
self-esteem, 132, 142, 172, 200, 209, 223, 233, 312, 328, 346–347, 351
self-harm, 98, 291–297
sijue shitiao (思覺失調), 20, 25, 108
Silver Ribbon Singapore, 30
slimming pills, 115
social anxiety, 329–330
social relationship
  interaction, 89, 97, 225
  isolation, 37, 97, 292
  network, 93
  social distance, 76
  withdrawal, 6, 112
social skills training, 170–171, 228
Social Treatment for Early Psychosis (STEP) programme, 52
social workers, 40, 80, 93, 101, 105
speech abnormality, 102
spiritualist, 193
stereotyping, 78, 199
stigma
  enacted stigma, 202
  iatrogenic stigmatization, 201
  perceived stigma/felt stigma, 200, 202, 352
  public/social stigma, 38, 77, 132, 142, 199–200
  self-stigma/internalized stigma, 132, 200–201, 204, 347
stimulants, 306, 313
strategic coping therapy, 149, 161, 168–171
Strauss and Carpenter Prognostic Scale (SCS), 89
stress management, 143
stress-vulnerability model, 54, 98, 143
substance abuse, 93, 115, 147, 301–307
  assessment, 303
  drug counselling, 307
  self-medication, 118, 302
  vulnerability hypothesis, 302
suicide, 24–25, 53, 291–297

parasuicide, 294
risk factors, 291–294
suicidal attempts, 38–39, 293, 301
suicidal ideation, 294–295
Support for the Wellness Achievement Programme (SWAP), 33
supportive therapy, 161

tardive dyskinesia, 264–265, 306
therapeutic alliance, 116, 143, 160–162, 189–190, 325
togo shitcho sho (統合失調症), 55, 80
traditional healers, 29, 176–177, 182
transition to psychosis, 128, 131
treatment
delay, 5
duration, 267
resistance, 267
response, 118, 301
triage, 106

ultra high-risk (UHR) (*see* at-risk mental state)
unengaged youth, 93

violence, 98, 200, 301
vocational training, 224, 258

weight gain, 258–259, 265, 274
workplace, 87–90, 202